The Diabetes Carbohydrate & Fat Gram Guide

Third Edition

Quick, Easy Meal Planning Using Carbohydrate & Fat Gram Counts

Lea Ann Holzmeister, RD, CDE

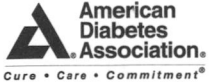

American Diabetes Association.

Cure • Care • Commitment®

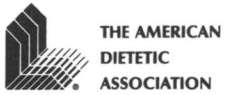

THE AMERICAN DIETETIC ASSOCIATION

Director, Book Publishing, John Fedor; *Managing Editor,* Abe Ogden; *Associate Director, Book Acquisitions,* Robert J. Anthony; *Production Manager,* Melissa Sprott; *Composition,* Circle Graphics, Inc.; *Cover Design,* Koncept, Inc.; *Printer,* Transcontinental Printing.

Printed in Canada
5 7 9 10 8 6

♾ The paper in this publication meets the requirements of the ANSI Standard Z39.48-1992 (permanence of paper).

American Diabetes Association titles may be purchased for business or promotional use or for special sales. For information, please write to Lee Romano Sequeira, Special Sales & Promotions, at the address below.

American Diabetes Association
1701 North Beauregard Street, Alexandria, Virginia 22311

The American Dietetic Association
120 South Riverside Plaza, Suite 2000, Chicago, Illinois 60606-6995

Portions of the data in the first edition were obtained from ESHA Research, Salem, OR.

Library of Congress Cataloging-in-Publication Data
Holzmeister, Lea Ann.
  The diabetes carbohydrate and fat gram guide / Lea Ann Holzmeister.— 3rd ed.
    p. cm.
  Includes bibliographical references and index.
  ISBN 13: 978-1-58040-247-7 (alk. paper)
  1. Diabetes—Diet therapy. 2. Food exchange lists. 3. Food—Carbohydrate content—Tables. 4. Food—Fat content—Tables. I. Title.

  RC662.H66 2005
  641.5'6314—dc22

                                    2005026428

The suggestions and information contained in this publication are generally consistent with the *Clinical Practice Recommendations* and other policies of the American Diabetes Association and The American Dietetic Association, but they do not represent the policy or position of the Associations or any of their boards or committees. Reasonable steps have been taken to ensure the accuracy of the information presented. However, the Associations cannot ensure the safety or efficacy of any product or service described in this publication. Individuals are advised to consult a physician or other appropriate health care professional before undertaking any diet or exercise program or taking any medication referred to in this publication. Professionals must use and apply their own professional judgment, experience, and training and should not rely solely on the information contained in this publication before prescribing any diet, exercise, or medication. The Associations—their officers, directors, employees, volunteers, and members—assume no responsibility or liability for personal or other injury, loss, or damage that may result from the suggestions or information in this publication.

Dedication

To Jeff, Erin, Adam, and Emily

Table of Contents

Preface to the Third Edition

Since the second edition of the *Diabetes Carbohydrate and Fat Gram Guide* was first published, many new food products have been introduced and fast-food restaurants have revised their menus. This third edition includes over 1500 new listings, as well as one additional nutrient category. Because of your comments and a desire by many people to monitor their intake of fat, the percent calories of fat in foods has been added for each food. In addition to fat grams, this nutrient fact will help you evaluate what percent of the total calories of a food is from fat.

America is becoming increasingly multicultural, and diabetes is taking a toll on minority populations. In addition to the ethnic foods in the second edition, three new ethnic cuisines have been added: East Indian and Pakistani, Soul, and Cajun & Creole. Many familiar ethnic foods—some of which we may not even think of as ethnic—can also be found in other sections of the book according to the type of product. For example, many prepared Mexican-, Chinese-, and Italian-American dishes can be found in the chapter "Combination Foods."

To prepare this new edition, we contacted food companies and fast-food franchises to obtain current nutrition information and product listings, scanned grocery store shelves for the newest foods and most up-to-date nutrition facts, and compiled ethnic food data from the American Diabetes Association and The American Dietetic Association's Ethnic and Regional Food Practice Series. The result is a more complete resource for anyone who is concerned about nutrition.

Acknowledgments

Thanks to Madelyn L. Wheeler, MS, RD, FADA, CDE, and Patti Bazel Geil, MS, RD, CDE, for their valuable review comments.

Introduction

Since its discovery hundreds of years ago, diabetes has been linked with what people eat. What people with diabetes are advised to eat and how they plan their meals has changed over the years, however. The latest American Diabetes Association (ADA) *Nutrition Principles and Recommendations in Diabetes* (published each January in Supplement 1 of the journal *Diabetes Care*) emphasizes attaining and maintaining the best metabolic outcomes, including:

- Blood glucose in the normal range or as close to normal as is safely possible to prevent or reduce the risk for complications of diabetes
- A lipid profile that reduces the risk for macrovascular disease
- Blood pressure levels that reduce the risk for vascular disease

The goals also recommend prevention and treatment of chronic complications of diabetes, which may require changes in eating patterns and lifestyle. People with diabetes should always consider improving health through healthy food choices and physical activity while considering personal and cultural preferences.

Many people with diabetes use some type of meal planning system to help them meet their individual nutrition goals. Just as there is no one diet that is right for everyone with diabetes, there is also no one meal planning approach that meets everyone's needs. It is important to know your own nutrition goals. A registered dietitian (RD) can help you determine your individual nutrition goals and develop a meal plan based on your food preferences, lifestyle, blood glucose and blood lipid (fat) levels, overall health, and abilities. If you're not currently seeing a dietitian, your doctor may be able to recommend one. Or visit the American Dietetic Association's web site at www.eatright.org.

Types of Meal Planning Approaches

Four types of meal-planning approaches are described in this book:
- Carbohydrate counting
- Fat gram counting
- Food exchange system
- Calorie counting

The advantages and disadvantages of each are discussed, and information about where to learn more is provided.

It is important to select a meal planning approach that you are comfortable using and that will work toward achieving your goals. You do not have to use the same approach your entire life. As your individual nutrition goals change, so may your meal planning approach. Before switching, though, it is a good idea to consult with your dietitian.

Carbohydrate Counting

Carbohydrate counting has been used for many years in Europe and is becoming increasingly popular in the United States. The three main nutrients in the foods we eat are carbohydrate, protein, and fat. The carbohydrate in foods affects your blood glucose level more than protein or fat. In carbohydrate counting, you count only carbohydrate.

To use carbohydrate counting, you must know your total carbohydrate allotment for the day. A dietitian can help you determine this. Together, you and your dietitian will make a carbohydrate counting meal plan based on your usual food intake, lifestyle, diabetes medications, and physical activity. Once you have your carbohydrate counting meal plan, you'll need to become familiar with the carbohydrate content in foods. Carbohydrate is found in many foods, such as grains, vegetables, fruits, milk, and table sugar. It is important to count all carbohydrate regardless of its source.

The two main types of carbohydrate are sugars and starches. According to ADA's nutrition recommendations, both the amount (grams) of carbohydrate as well as the type of carbohydrate in a food influence blood glucose level. However, monitoring total grams of carbohydrate and eating the same amount of carbohydrate at meals and snacks each day, remains a key strategy in achieving good blood glucose control.

Carbohydrate counting can provide some advantages over other meal planning approaches. Some people feel that focusing on only one nutrient makes this system easier. With the focus on carbohydrate, food and insulin can be matched more precisely. Matching food and insulin increases flexibility in meal and snack times. This can be particularly helpful when your appetite varies or your schedule changes. Also, insulin can be matched to carbohydrate eaten at specific times during the day. For example, some people need more insulin at breakfast for each gram of carbohydrate eaten. Thus, carbohydrate counting may be most appropriate for people who take insulin.

One disadvantage of carbohydrate counting is that when you focus only on carbohydrate, it is easy to lose sight of the overall nutritional quality of foods. For example, counting the carbohydrate in foods like bacon or sausage but ignoring their fat content may lead you to eat these fatty foods more often. Too much fat in the diet increases your risk of heart disease, cancer, and weight gain. If you pay no attention to the overall nutritional quality of foods, you may end up eating a diet that is too high in fat or protein.

To learn more about carbohydrate counting, contact your dietitian. The American Diabetes Association and The American Dietetic Association have jointly published two instructional booklets on carbohydrate counting: *Basic Carbohydrate Counting* and *Advanced Carbohydrate Counting*. You can obtain these booklets from your dietitian or by ordering them online at *http://store.diabetes.org* or *www.eatright.org*.

Fat Gram Counting

Fat gram counting has been around since the 1980s, when it was introduced as a tool to teach low-fat eating to reduce the risk of cancer. Since that time, it has also been used for heart-healthy eating for heart disease and reduced-calorie eating for weight reduction. Fat gram counting may be particularly useful for people with type 2 diabetes who are overweight. Fat provides two and a half times as many calories per gram as carbohydrate or protein.

The first step in using fat gram counting is to establish a daily calorie requirement based on your height, weight, activity level, and weight goal. Your dietitian can help you determine this. Then, based on your nutrition goals, a daily fat gram goal will be determined. In fat gram counting, you keep a record of the foods you eat and their fat content.

There are some advantages to fat gram counting. It is simple, and it allows a considerable amount of flexibility and control over your food choices. With fat gram counting, you will usually improve the overall quality of your food choices, because you will tend to select low-fat foods, such as fruits, vegetables, grains, and low-fat dairy products. Like carbohydrate counting, you are focusing on only one nutrient. This can be especially appealing when weight loss is the primary goal and other approaches have not worked.

One disadvantage of fat gram counting is that it does not take into consideration foods that may affect your blood glucose. Therefore, your blood glucose values may be inconsistent.

To learn more about fat gram counting, contact your dietitian. Your local American Heart Association may also have additional information on fat gram counting programs.

Food Exchange System

For many years, the food exchange system has been used as a meal-planning approach for people with diabetes, regardless of the type of diabetes and how it is treated. This system groups foods with similar nutritional value into lists, with the goal of helping people with diabetes eat consistent amounts of nutrients. Each food has approximately the same number of calories, carbohydrate, protein, and fat as the other foods on the same list. Any food on a list can be traded or "exchanged" for any other food on the same list.

To use the exchange system, you need an individualized meal plan that tells you how many exchanges from each list to select for meals and snacks. Your dietitian can help you design your individualized meal plan and teach you how to use this system.

The American Diabetes Association and The American Dietetic Association's *Exchange Lists for Meal Planning* booklet groups food into three broad groups: the carbohydrate group, the meat and meat substitutes group, and the fat group.

The carbohydrate group includes five lists: the starch list, the fruit list, the milk list, the other carbohydrates list, and the nonstarchy vegetable list. The meat and meat substitutes group includes four lists: the very lean list, the lean list, the medium-fat list, and the high-fat list. The fat group includes a monounsaturated fats list, a polyunsaturated fats list, and a saturated fats list. In addition to these lists, there is a free foods list, a combination foods list, and a fast foods list.

One advantage of the food exchange system is its emphasis on more than one nutrient and the importance of the overall nutritional content of foods. This system also encourages consistency in the timing and amount of your meals and snacks. People wanting to lose weight might find this approach useful for learning the caloric and fat values of foods. Food exchanges can also be used as a reference for those using carbohydrate counting. Each serving of a food in the carbohydrate group counts as 15 grams of carbohydrate.

One disadvantage of this system is the level of understanding needed to grasp the concept of "exchanging" foods. It also requires learning where a food that is not listed fits. To learn more about the food exchange system for meal planning, contact your dietitian.

Calorie Counting

Calorie counting has been used for many years as a way to achieve weight loss, weight gain, or weight maintenance. This approach is most appropriate for people who are overweight and do not take insulin. Even modest weight loss improves blood glucose levels.

To use calorie counting, you and your dietitian establish a calorie goal that will help you achieve your weight goal. Your weight goal will be based on your current weight, height, and activity level. If you desire to lose weight, your calorie goal will be set lower than your usual intake of calories. If you wish to maintain your current weight, your calorie goal will be set at a calorie level similar to your current intake of calories. You keep records of the foods you eat and their calorie content. A periodic comparison of your food records and weekly weight can give you feedback on how you are progressing toward your weight goal. These records can also help you identify problem areas. For example, you might realize after reviewing your records that you tend to overeat when away from home. Knowing this information will help you and your dietitian develop strategies for changing this behavior.

The main advantage of calorie counting is the expanded choice of foods, which gives you more flexibility in what you eat. You decide whether and how a food might fit into your meal plan. For example, say your daily calorie goal is 1,500 calories, and a food you want to eat contains 600 calories. You can eat that food as long as you plan what other foods you'll eat that day to add up to the remaining 900 calories. Your serving size, too, is based on how you want to "spend" your calories. You might decide you can work in only half a serving of pasta salad, or you might choose to have a double serving of pasta salad.

One disadvantage of calorie counting might be the amount of time involved in keeping records and calculating the calorie content of foods. Also, because this approach does not guide you toward making nutritionally balanced choices, you may end up with a high-fat diet or one low in essential vitamins and minerals. Your dietitian can provide you with basic nutrition guidelines by which to select your foods to ensure that you meet your nutrition goals as well.

Estimating Serving Sizes

The success of any meal planning approach depends on how accurately you estimate your serving sizes. Therefore, it is essential to train your eyes to do this. Equip your kitchen with measuring spoons, measuring cups, and a food scale. Use these tools to measure and weigh foods consistently for two weeks or until you have trained your eyes to recognize what a cup of pasta looks like on your plate or how much one cup of milk fills your favorite glass.

Without some practice, it is surprisingly easy to mistakenly pour yourself one cup instead of a half cup of juice. A cup of juice has twice the carbohydrate and calories of a half cup of juice. This might tip you over your calorie or carbohydrate goal. If you did this with two to three foods each day, it could spoil your efforts at weight loss and blood glucose control.

Of course, it is not practical to measure servings when you eat out in a restaurant, but training your eyes will help. Fortunately, the serving sizes of fast foods are fairly standardized among restaurants, e.g., a taco at any Taco Bell restaurant is likely to be the same size.

How Food Counts Can Work For You

The meal planning approach you select will determine what you will "count" in your diet. But using a meal planning approach to guide your food choices is only a starting point. To reach your individual goals (such as blood glucose, blood lipids, weight, general health), you need to respond every day to blood glucose changes and periodically to other indicators of your progress (such as blood lipid levels, weight gain, or weight loss).

Food Counts and Blood Glucose

Making the connection between what you eat and how it affects your blood glucose level can be a very powerful step toward achieving your blood glucose goals. Once you have recorded your food intake and blood glucose values, you can learn to analyze the data to see how individual foods and meals affect your blood glucose. You can then try adjusting food intake, physical activity, and diabetes medications.

Food Counts and Blood Lipids

Counting total fat and saturated fat in your diet while keeping tabs on your blood lipid levels (total cholesterol, HDL cholesterol, LDL cholesterol, and triglycerides) allows you to determine whether your meal plan is helping you to achieve your blood lipid goals. Suppose you have been advised to follow a diet with less than 70 grams of fat and less than 25 grams of saturated fat per day in an attempt to reduce your total cholesterol from 250 to 200 mg/dl.

By comparing your food records of fat and saturated fat intake to your blood lipid levels over time, you can determine how close you are coming to your blood lipid goals.

Using This Book of Food Counts

This book is intended to be a comprehensive listing of both generic and brand name foods that are available nationally. The nutrition information in this third edition comes from several sources, including:

- The U.S. Department of Agriculture
- The Agricultural Research Service
- The USDA National Nutrient Database for Standard Reference, Release 17
- The American Diabetes Association and The American Dietetic Association's *Exchange Lists for Meal Planning* nutrient database
- A variety of food-processing companies and fast-food franchises
- Nutrition Facts from food labels

Foods are listed alphabetically by food category and manufacturer. Nutrient information for foods from mixes (for example, puddings and cakes) reflect values after the food has been prepared according to package directions.

This book lists the calories, carbohydrate, fat, percent calories from fat, saturated fat, cholesterol, sodium, fiber, and protein of many foods. These particular nutrients were selected because they are the most commonly monitored by people with diabetes (see Table 1).

TABLE 1. American Diabetes Association Nutrient Recommendations

Calories: Most adults require 1,800 to 2,500 calories per day. However, your calorie needs are best determined by your dietitian.

Carbohydrate: Carbohydrates raise your blood glucose level. A recommended range of carbohydrate intake is 45–65% of total calories. Carbohydrate and monounsaturated fat together should provide 60–70% of your total calorie intake. Your dietitian can help you determine how much carbohydrate you need in a day.

Fat: Fat contributes to weight gain. Most people need no more than 30% of their daily calories from fat. People who are overweight should consider reducing their intake of fat. Your dietitian can help you determine what percentage of your daily calories should come from fat.

Saturated Fat: Saturated fat can raise your blood cholesterol level. Most people should get no more than 10% of their daily calories from saturated fat. Some individuals (persons with LDL cholesterol at or above 100 mg/dl) may benefit from lowering saturated fat intake to less than 7% of total calorie intake.

Cholesterol: Cholesterol, which is found in foods from animal sources, can raise your blood cholesterol level. Limit cholesterol in your diet to 300 milligrams or less daily. Some individuals (persons with LDL cholesterol at or above 100 mg/dl) may benefit from lowering dietary cholesterol to less than 200 milligrams per day.

Sodium: Sodium has been linked to high blood pressure (hypertension). People with normal blood pressure should get no more than 2,400 to 3,000 milligrams of sodium per day. People with moderately high blood pressure are advised to get 2,400 milligrams or less of sodium per day, and people with high blood pressure and kidney disease are advised to get 2,000 milligrams or less of sodium per day.

TABLE 1. American Diabetes Association Nutrient Recommendations (*Continued*)

Fiber: Daily consumption of 20–35 grams of dietary fiber from both soluble and insoluble fibers from a wide variety of food sources is recommended. Dietary fiber may be helpful in the treatment and prevention of constipation and several gastrointestinal disorders. Soluble fiber has a beneficial effect on serum lipids and provides satiety value to your diet.

Protein: Most adults, including people with diabetes, require approximately 15–20% of their calories from protein. For persons with diabetes, especially those not in optimal glucose control, the protein requirement may be greater than the Recommended Dietary Allowance, but not greater than what they usually eat.

The nutrient values you use will depend on your meal planning approach. You may need one, two, or even more of the values to figure out how a food fits in your plan. Values have been rounded to the nearest calorie, gram (g), or milligram (mg) per serving (a gram is a unit of mass and weight in the metric system; an ounce is about 30 grams). The serving sizes listed in this book are those most commonly used. Similar foods will have the same serving sizes. The serving size may be very different from the amount you serve yourself or eat. If your serving size is different, ask your dietitian to help you recalculate the numbers.

The exchange values of foods have been calculated using the "rounding off method" (Wheeler ML, Franz M, Barrier PH, Holler H, Cronmiller N, Delahanty LM: Macronutrient and energy database for the 1995 Exchange Lists for Meal Planning: A rationale for clinical practice decisions. *J Am Diet Assoc* 96:1167–1170, 1996). Table 2 shows the amount of nutrients in one serving from each list.

Some of the foods in this book have a nutrient claim, such as "reduced-fat" or "low-calorie," as part of their name. These claims have standard meanings set by the Food and Drug Administration (FDA). Some of these terms and their meanings are listed in Table 3.

TABLE 2. Nutrient Content of Exchange Lists

Groups/Lists	Carb. (g)	Prot. (g)	Fat (g)	Cal.
Carbohydrate Group				
Starch List	15	3	0–1	80
Fruit List	15	0	0	60
Milk List				
Skim/Low-Fat	12	8	0–3	90
Reduced-Fat	12	8	5	120
Whole	12	8	8	150
Other Carbohydrates List	15	varies	varies	varies
Vegetable List	5	2	0	25
Meat and Meat Substitutes Group				
Very Lean List	0	7	0–1	35
Lean List	0	7	3	55
Medium-Fat List	0	7	5	75
High-Fat List	0	7	8	100
Fat Group				
Monounsaturated Fats List	0	0	5	45
Polyunsaturated Fats List	0	0	5	45
Saturated Fats List	0	0	5	45
Free Foods List	5 or less	varies	varies	less than 20
Combination Foods List	varies	varies	varies	varies
Fast Foods List	varies	varies	varies	varies

Adapted from the American Diabetes Association and The American Dietetic Association: *Exchange Lists for Meal Planning.* Alexandria, VA, 2003, p. 5.

TABLE 3. Nutrient Claims on Food Labels

Term	Meaning
Calorie-Free	Less than 5 calories per serving
Cholesterol-Free	Less than 2 mg of cholesterol per serving and 2 g or less of saturated fat per serving
Extra Lean	Less than 5 g of fat, 2 g of saturated fat, and 95 mg of cholesterol per serving
Fat-Free	Less than 0.5 g of fat per serving
Lean	Less than 10 g of fat, 4.5 g of saturated fat, and 95 mg of cholesterol per serving
Light or Lite	33.3% fewer calories or 50% less fat per serving than comparison food
Low-Calorie	40 calories or less per serving
Low-Cholesterol	20 mg or less of cholesterol per serving and 2 g or less of saturated fat per serving
Low-Fat	3 g or less of fat per serving
Low-Saturated Fat	1 g or less of saturated fat per serving and 15% or less of calories from saturated fat
Low-Sodium	140 mg or less of sodium per serving
Reduced	25% less per serving than comparison food
Saturated Fat-Free	Less than 0.5 g of saturated fat and 0.5 g of trans fatty acids per serving
Sodium-Free	Less than 5 mg of sodium per serving
Sugar-Free	Less than 0.5 g of sugar per serving

ALCOHOL, BEER, SPIRITS, WINE

BEER

	Serving	Calories	Carb. (g)	Fat (g)	% Cal. Fat	Sat. Fat (g)	Chol. (mg)	Sod. (mg)	Fib. (g)	Prot. (g)	Servings/ Exchanges
Beer, Light	12 oz	99	5	0	0	0	0	11	0	<1	2 fat
Beer, Regular	12 oz	146	13	0	0	0	0	14	0	1	3 fat
Beer, Non-Alcoholic	12 oz	70	13	0	0	0	0	8	0	1	1 carb
Brands											
Anheuser Busch Natural Light	12 oz	95	3	0	0	0	0	9	0	<1	1 fat
Bud Light	12 oz	110	7	0	0	0	0	1	0	1	2 fat
Budweiser	12 oz	145	11	0	0	0	0	9	0	1	3 fat
Coors Light	12 oz	102	5	0	0	0	0	13	0	0	2 fat
Coors Non-Alcoholic	12 oz	65	14	0	0	0	0	7	0	0	1 carb
Coors Original	12 oz	148	11	0	0	0	0	12	0	1	3 fat
Corona Light	12 oz	105	5	0	0	0	0	NA	0	1	2 fat

ALCOHOL, BEER, SPIRITS, WINE

	Serving	Calories	Carb. (g)	Fat (g)	% Cal. Fat	Sat. Fat (g)	Chol. (mg)	Sod. (mg)	Fib. (g)	Prot. (g)	Servings/ Exchanges
Hamm's	12 oz	144	12	0	0	0	0	7	0	1	3 fat
Hamm's Golden Draft	12 oz	144	12	0	0	0	0	7	0	1	3 fat
Hamm's Special Light	12 oz	110	7	0	0	0	0	6	0	<1	2 fat
Michelob Amber Bock	12 oz	166	15	0	0	0	0	9	0	1	3 fat
Michelob Honey Lager	12 oz	175	18	0	0	0	0	9	0	2	4 fat
Michelob Lager	12 oz	155	13	0	0	0	0	9	0	1	3 fat
Michelob Light	12 oz	134	12	0	0	0	0	9	0	1	3 fat
Michelob Ultra	12 oz	95	3	0	0	0	0	9	0	<1	2 fat
Miller High Life	12 oz	143	13	0	0	0	0	7	0	1	3 fat
Miller Light	12 oz	96	3	0	0	0	0	0	0	1	2 fat
MGD	12 oz	143	13	0	0	0	0	7	0	1	3 fat
MGD Light	12 oz	110	7	0	0	0	0	0	0	<1	2 fat
Milwaukee's Best	12 oz	128	11	0	0	0	0	6	0	<1	3 fat
O'Doul's Non-Alcoholic Brew	12 oz	70	13	0	0	0	0	9	0	1	1 carb

	Serving										
O'Doul's Amber Non-Alcoholic Brew	12 oz	90	18		0	0	0	9	0	2	1 carb
Sharp's Non-Alcoholic Brew	12 oz	58	12		0	0	0	3	0	0	1 carb
COCKTAILS											
Daiquiri, Canned	4 oz	152	19		0	0	0	48	0	0	1 carb, 2 fat
Daiquiri, Prepared from Recipe	4 oz	224	8		0	0	0	8	0	0	1/2 carb, 4 fat
Martini, Prepared from Recipe	4 oz	276	2		0	0	0	4	0	0	6 fat
Pina Colada, Canned	4 oz	308	45	10	29	8	0	92	0	<1	3 carb, 1 fat
Pina Colada, Prepared from Recipe	4 oz	220	28	2	8	2	0	8	0	<1	2 carb, 1 fat
Tequila Sunrise, Canned	4 oz	136	14		0	0	0	72	0	0	1 carb, 1 fat
Whiskey Sour, Canned	4 oz	148	16		0	0	0	56	0	0	1 carb, 2 fat

ALCOHOL, BEER, SPIRITS, WINE

	Serving	Calories	Carb. (g)	Fat (g)	% Cal. Fat	Sat. Fat (g)	Chol. (mg)	Sod. (mg)	Fib. (g)	Prot. (g)	Servings/ Exchanges
LIQUEURS											
Coffee Liqueur	1 oz	117	16	0	0	0	0	3	0	0	1 carb, 1 fat
Crème de Menthe	1 oz	125	14	0	0	0	0	2	0	0	1 carb, 1 fat
Kahlua	1 oz	90	11	0	0	0	0	0	0	0	2 fat
SPIRITS											
Alcohol (Gin, Rum, Vodka, Whiskey)											
100 proof	1 oz	82	0	0	0	0	0	0	0	0	2 fat
94 proof	1 oz	76	0	0	0	0	0	0	0	0	2 fat
90 proof	1 oz	73	0	0	0	0	0	0	0	0	2 fat
86 proof	1 oz	70	0	0	0	0	0	0	0	0	2 fat
80 proof	1 oz	64	0	0	0	0	0	0	0	0	1 fat
WINE											
Wine, Champagne	4 oz	85	2	0	0	0	0	NA	0	0	2 fat
Wine, Cooking	4 oz	14	2	0	0	0	0	182	0	0	free

Food	Serving									
Wine, Dry Dessert	2 oz	90	7	0	0	0	6	0	0	2 fat
Wine, Light	4 oz	60	1	0	0	0	8	0	<1	1 fat
Wine, Non-Alcoholic	4 oz	8	1	0	0	0	8	0	<1	free
Wine, Sweet Dessert	2 oz	94	8	0	0	0	6	0	0	2 fat
Wine, Table, Red	4 oz	84	2	0	0	0	4	0	<1	2 fat
Wine, Table, Rose	4 oz	84	2	0	0	0	4	0	<1	2 fat
Wine, Table (Average all Types)	4 oz	80	1	0	0	0	4	0	0	2 fat
Wine, Table, White	4 oz	80	1	0	0	0	4	0	0	2 fat

WINE COOLERS

Brands

Bartles & Jaymes

Food	Serving									
Black Cherry	12 oz	200	32	0	0	0	5	0	0	2 carb, 1 fat
Blue Hawaiian	12 oz	179	28	0	0	0	7	0	0	2 carb, 1 fat
Classic Original	12 oz	190	29	0	0	0	0	0	0	2 carb, 1 fat
Fuzzy Navel	12 oz	230	39	0	0	0	5	0	0	2 1/2 carb, 1 fat

ALCOHOL, BEER, SPIRITS, WINE

	Serving	Calories	Carb. (g)	Fat (g)	% Cal. Fat	Sat. Fat (g)	Chol. (mg)	Sod. (mg)	Fib. (g)	Prot. (g)	Servings/ Exchanges
Margarita	12 oz	260	46	0	0	0	0	40	0	0	3 carb, 1 fat
Pina Colada	12 oz	270	48	0	0	0	0	5	0	0	3 carb, 1 fat
Strawberry Daiquiri	12 oz	220	36	0	0	0	0	5	0	0	2 1/2 carb, 1 fat

BEVERAGES, SODA, SPORTS/ENERGY DRINKS, MEAL REPLACEMENT DRINKS, COCOA, COFFEE/CREAMER, TEA

COCOA/HOT CHOCOLATE/CHOCOLATE MILK

	Serving	Calories	Carb. (g)	Fat (g)	% Cal. Fat	Sat. Fat (g)	Chol. (mg)	Sod. (mg)	Fib. (g)	Prot. (g)	Servings/ Exchanges
Hot Cocoa, Homemade	8 oz	192	27	6	28	4	20	110	3	9	1 low-fat milk, 1 carb
Hot Cocoa, Prepared from Powder	6 oz	113	24	1	8	<1	2	146	1	2	1 1/2 carb
Sugar-Free Hot Cocoa, Prepared from Powder	6 oz	56	10	<1	0	0	0	171	1	2	1/2 carb
Brands											
Carnation											
Malted Milk	3 Tbsp	90	33	2	22	1	10	80	0	5	2 carb
Hershey's											
Chocolate Raspberry Hot Cocoa	1 envelope	150	27	3	18	0.5	0	135	1	3	2 carb, 1 fat

BEVERAGES, SODA, SPORTS/ENERGY DRINKS, MEAL REPLACEMENT DRINKS, COCOA

	Serving	Calories	Carb. (g)	Fat (g)	% Cal. Fat	Sat. Fat (g)	Chol. (mg)	Sod. (mg)	Fib. (g)	Prot. (g)	Servings/ Exchanges
Fat-Free Dutch Chocolate Hot Cocoa	1 envelope	50	10	0	0	0	0	160	<1	2	1/2 carb
French Vanilla Hot Cocoa	1 envelope	140	28	2.5	16	0	0	150	0	2	2 carb, 1 fat
Nestle											
Butterfinger Hot Cocoa	1 envelope	120	23	3	23	2	0	160	<1	<1	1 1/2 carb, 1 fat
Fat-Free Hot Cocoa	2 Tbsp	25	5	0	0	0	0	120	<1	1	free
Hot Cocoa with Mini Marshmallows	1 envelope	80	15	3	34	2	0	160	<1	<1	1 carb, 1 fat
Nesquik Chocolate	2 Tbsp	90	19	1	11	<1	0	30	<1	1	1 carb
Nesquik with Marshmallows Hot Cocoa	1 envelope	130	23	3	21	2.5	0	180	1	2	1 1/2 carb, 1 fat
Nesquik No-Sugar-Added Chocolate	2 Tbsp	40	7	1	25	<1	0	85	1	1	1/2 carb

	Serving										Exchanges
Milk Chocolate Hot Cocoa	1 envelope	80	15	2.5	28	1.5	0	180	<1	<1	1 carb, 1 fat
Rich Chocolate Hot Cocoa	1 envelope	80	15	3	34	2	0	170	<1	<1	1 carb, 1 fat
Ovaltine											
Malted Milk Drink, Chocolate Malt	4 Tbsp	80	18	0	0	0	0	115	<1	1	1 carb
Malted Milk Drink, Rich Chocolate	4 Tbsp	80	19	0	0	0	0	140	0	<1	1 carb
Swiss Miss											
Milk Chocolate Hot Cocoa, All Varieties	1 envelope	120	23	2.5	19	0.5	0	150	<1	1	1 1/2 carb, 1 fat
No-Sugar-Added Hot Cocoa	1 envelope	60	10	1	15	0	0	170	1	2	1/2 carb
COFFEE											
Coffee, Brewed	8 oz	9	0	2	100	0	0	2	0	0	free
Coffee, Instant	8 oz	8	<1	0	0	0	0	8	0	0	free

BEVERAGES, SODA, SPORTS/ENERGY DRINKS, MEAL REPLACEMENT DRINKS, COCOA

	Serving	Calories	Carb. (g)	Fat (g)	% Cal. Fat	Sat. Fat (g)	Chol. (mg)	Sod. (mg)	Fib. (g)	Prot. (g)	Servings/ Exchanges
Brands											
Folgers											
Café Latte, All Varieties	2 scoops	100	14	5	45	2	5	80–110	0	2	1 carb, 1 fat
Cappuccino Mix, All Varieties	3 tsp	80–90	15–16	2.5	25	0.5	0	85–95	0	1	1 carb, 1 fat
General Foods											
Cappuccino Café Mocha	1 envelope	100	18	3	27	0.5	0	45	0	<1	1 carb, 1 fat
Cappuccino Coolers	1 Tbsp	60	15	0	0	0	0	0	0	0	1 carb
Chai Latte	2 Tbsp	110	20	4	33	1	0	95–110	0	0	1 carb, 1 fat
International Coffees, All Varieties	1 1/3 Tbsp	50–70	10–12	1.5–3	38	0.5	0	30–55	0	0–1	1 carb, 1/2 fat
International Coffees, Sugar-Free, Fat-Free, All Varieties	1 1/3 Tbsp	25	5	0	0	0	0	35–65	0	0	free

Hills Brothers

Cappuccino	3 Tbsp	120	19	3.5–4.5	30	0	0	1–125	0–1	2	1 carb, 1 fat

Nescafe

Frothe Coffee House Drink	3 Tbsp	90	14	3	30	0.5	0	170	0	1	1 carb, 1 fat
Iced Java Coffee Syrup	2 Tbsp	0	20	0	0	0	0	0	0	0	1 carb

Starbucks

Caramel Frappuccino Coffee Drink	9.5 oz bottle	200	37	3.5	16	2	15	110	0	7	2 1/2 carb, 1 fat
Coffee Frappuccino Coffee Drink	9.5 oz bottle	200	37	3.5	16	2	15	110	0	7	2 1/2 carb, 1 fat
Doubleshot Coffee Drink	6.5 oz can	140	18	6	39	3.5	20	70	0	4	1 carb, 1 fat
Mocha Frappuccino Coffee Drink	9.5 oz bottle	190	35	3.5	17	2.5	15	105	2	7	2 1/2 carb, 1 fat
Mocha Lite Frappuccino Coffee Drink	9.5 oz bottle	110	14	3.5	29	2.5	15	105	0	7	1 carb, 1 fat

BEVERAGES, SODA, SPORTS/ENERGY DRINKS, MEAL REPLACEMENT DRINKS, COCOA

	Serving	Calories	Carb. (g)	Fat (g)	% Cal. Fat	Sat. Fat (g)	Chol. (mg)	Sod. (mg)	Fib. (g)	Prot. (g)	Servings/ Exchanges
Vanilla Frappuccino Coffee Drink	9.5 oz bottle	200	37	3.5	16	2	15	110	0	7	2 1/2 carb, 1 fat
COFFEE CREAMER											
Brands											
Creamora											
Dulce De Leche	4 tsp	60	9	2.5	42	2.5	0	25	0	0	1/2 carb, 1 fat
Lite & Creamy	1 tsp	10	1	0	0	0	0	5	0	0	free
No Carb Original	1 tsp	15	0	1.5	67	1.5	0	0	0	0	free
Nutty for Hazelnut	4 tsp	25	<1	2.5	100	2.5	0	0	0	0	1 fat
Ooh-La-La Vanilla	4 tsp	25	<1	2.5	100	2.5	0	0	0	0	1 fat
Original	1 tsp	10	<1	1	100	1	0	10	0	0	free
Nestle Coffee-Mate (Powder)											
Fat Free	1 tsp	10	2	0	0	0	0	0	0	0	free
French Vanilla	4 tsp	60	9	3	42	2	0	15	0	0	1/2 carb, 1 fat

Hazelnut	4 tsp	60	9	3	42	2.5	0	15	0	1/2 carb, 1 fat
Original	1 tsp	10	1	0.5	50	0.5	0	0	0	free
Vanilla Caramel	4 tsp	60	9	3	42	2.5	0	15	0	1/2 carb, 1 fat
Nestle Coffee-Mate (Liquid)										
Café Mocha	1 Tbsp	40	5	2	50	0	0	5	0	1 fat
French Vanilla	1 Tbsp	40	5	2	50	0	0	5	0	1 fat
Hazelnut, Carb Select, Fat-Free	1 Tbsp	15	2	0	0	0	0	0	0	free
Irish Crème, Fat-Free	1 Tbsp	25	5	0	0	0	0	0	0	free
Original	1 Tbsp	20	2	1	50	0	0	0	0	free
Vanilla Caramel	1 Tbsp	40	5	2	50	0.5	0	10	0	1 fat
OTHER DRINKS AND MIXES										
Fruit Punch Drink, Canned	8 oz	117	30	0	0	0	0	94	0	2 carb
Fruit Punch Drink, Prepared from Frozen Concentrate	8 oz	114	29	0	0	0	0	10	0	2 carb

BEVERAGES, SODA, SPORTS/ENERGY DRINKS, MEAL REPLACEMENT DRINKS, COCOA

	Serving	Calories	Carb. (g)	Fat (g)	% Cal. Fat	Sat. Fat (g)	Chol. (mg)	Sod. (mg)	Fib. (g)	Prot. (g)	Servings/ Exchanges
Fruit Punch Juice Drink, Prepared from Frozen Concentrate	8 oz	124	30	0	0	0	0	12	0	0	2 carb
Fruit Punch-Flavor Drink, Prepared from Powder	8 oz	97	25	0	0	0	0	8	0	0	1 1/2 carb
Lemonade, Pink, Prepared from Frozen Concentrate	8 oz	99	26	0	0	0	0	7	0	0	2 carb
Lemonade, White, Prepared from Frozen Concentrate	8 oz	131	34	0	0	0	0	7	0	0	2 carb
Lemonade, Prepared from Powder	8 oz	103	26	0	0	0	0	11	0	0	2 carb
Lemonade-Flavored Drink, Prepared from Powder	8 oz	112	29	0	0	0	0	19	0	0	2 carb

Brands								
Country Time								
Lemonade, Prepared from Powder	8 oz	60	16	0	0	0	25	0	1 carb
Raspberry Lemonade	8 oz	80	19	0	0	0	0	0	1 carb
Sugar-free Lemonade	8 oz	5	0	0	0	0	0	0	free
Crystal Light								
Crystal Light Bottles	8 oz	5	0	0	0	0	10	0	free
Crystal Light Fruit Flavored Drinks or Lemonades, and Teas	8 oz	5	0	0	0	0	0–5	0	free
Kool-Aid								
Drink Mix from Powder, All Varieties	8 oz	60–70	16–17	0	0	0	0–5	0	1 carb
Snapple								
Lemonade, All Varieties	8 oz	110–130	28–33	0	0	0	50	0	2 carb

BEVERAGES, SODA, SPORTS/ENERGY DRINKS, MEAL REPLACEMENT DRINKS, COCOA

	Serving	Calories	Carb. (g)	Fat (g)	% Cal. Fat	Sat. Fat (g)	Chol. (mg)	Sod. (mg)	Fib. (g)	Prot. (g)	Servings/ Exchanges
Juice Drinks, All Varieties	8 oz	90–120	25–30	0	0	0	0	10–40	0	0	2 carb
Tang											
Orange Drink Mix, Prepared from Powder	8 oz	95	24	0	0	0	0	0	0	0	1 1/2 carb
Sugar-Free Orange Drink Mix, Prepared from Powder	8 oz	5	0	0	0	0	0	0	0	0	free
SODA DRINKS											
Cola Drinks											
Small Drink	16 oz	207	53	0	0	0	0	20	0	0	2 1/2 carb
Medium Drink	22 oz	284	73	0	0	0	0	27	0	0	5 carb
Large Drink	32 oz	413	106	0	0	0	0	39	0	0	7 carb
Extra Large Drink	44 oz	568	146	0	0	0	0	54	0	0	10 carb
Club Soda	12 oz	0	0	0	0	0	0	75	0	0	free

Cream Soda	12 oz	189	49	0	45	0	3 carb
Diet Cola with Aspartame	12 oz	4	<1	0	21	0	free
Ginger Ale	12 oz	124	32	0	26	0	3 carb
Grape Soda	12 oz	160	42	0	56	0	3 carb
Lemon-Lime Soda	12 oz	147	38	0	40	0	2 1/2 carb
Orange Soda	12 oz	179	46	0	45	0	3 carb
Root Beer	12 oz	152	39	0	48	0	2 1/2 carb
Tonic Water	12 oz	124	32	0	15	0	2 carb

Brands

7-Up

7-Up	12 oz	140	39	0	75	0	2 1/2 carb
7-Up, Cherry	12 oz	140	39	0	38	0	2 1/2 carb
7-Up, Upside Down (Caffeinated)	12 oz	170	46	0	70	0	3 carb

A&W

A&W Root Beer	12 oz	170	46	0	45	0	3 carb

BEVERAGES, SODA, SPORTS/ENERGY DRINKS, MEAL REPLACEMENT DRINKS, COCOA

	Serving	Calories	Carb. (g)	Fat (g)	% Cal. Fat	Sat. Fat (g)	Chol. (mg)	Sod. (mg)	Fib. (g)	Prot. (g)	Servings/ Exchanges
A&W Cream Soda	12 oz	165	41	0	0	0	0	NA	0	0	3 carb
Barq's Root Beer	12 oz	160	45	0	0	0	0	70	0	0	3 carb
Canada Dry Ginger Ale, All Flavors	12 oz	135	33	0	0	0	0	NA	0	0	2 carb
Coca-Cola											
Cherry Coke	12 oz	150	42	0	0	0	0	40	0	0	3 carb
Cocoa-Cola Classic	12 oz	140	39	0	0	0	0	50	0	0	2 1/2 carb
Diet Coke	12 oz	0	0	0	0	0	0	40	0	0	free
Diet Coke with Lime	12 oz	0	0	0	0	0	0	40	0	0	free
Vanilla Coke	12 oz	150	42	0	0	0	0	40	0	0	3 carb
Diet Rite	12 oz	0	0	0	0	0	0	0	0	0	free
Dr. Pepper	12 oz	150	40	0	0	0	0	55	0	0	2 1/2 carb
Fanta											
Fanta Grape	12 oz	176	44	0	0	0	0	14	0	0	3 carb

Fanta Orange	12 oz	177	45	0	0	0	14	0	3 carb
Fresca	12 oz	3	<1	0	0	0	2	0	free
Hansen's Soda, Average	12 oz	168	42	0	0	0	0	0	3 carb
All Flavors									

Mountain Dew

Mountain Dew	12 oz	170	46	0	0	0	70	0	3 carb
Mountain Dew Code Red	12 oz	170	47	0	0	0	105	0	3 carb
Mr. Pibb	12 oz	146	36	0	0	0	11	0	2 carb
MUG Root Beer	12 oz	160	43	0	0	0	65	0	3 carb
New York Seltzer Soda,	8 oz	80	21	0	0	0	15	0	1 1/2 carb
All Varieties									

Pepsi

Diet Pepsi	12 oz	0	0	0	0	0	35	0	free
Pepsi	12 oz	150	41	0	0	0	35	0	3 carb
Pepsi Twist	12 oz	150	42	0	0	0	55	0	3 carb
Pepsi Vanilla	12 oz	160	43	0	0	0	40	0	3 carb

BEVERAGES, SODA, SPORTS/ENERGY DRINKS, MEAL REPLACEMENT DRINKS, COCOA

	Serving	Calories	Carb. (g)	Fat (g)	% Cal. Fat	Sat. Fat (g)	Chol. (mg)	Sod. (mg)	Fib. (g)	Prot. (g)	Servings/ Exchanges
Wild Cherry Pepsi	12 oz	160	43	0	0	0	0	35	0	0	3 carb
Slice Orange	12 oz	190	50	0	0	0	0	55	0	0	3 carb
Sprite											
Berryclear Sprite ReMix	12 oz	140	38	0	0	0	0	65	0	0	2 1/2 carb
Diet Sprite	12 oz	0	0	0	0	0	0	35	0	0	free
Sprite	12 oz	140	38	0	0	0	0	70	0	0	2 1/2 carb
Tropical Sprite Re Mix	12 oz	150	40	0	0	0	0	55	0	0	2 1/2 carb
Sunkist Orange	12 oz	190	52	0	0	0	0	45	0	0	3 carb
Squirt	12 oz	140	39	0	0	0	0	50	0	0	2 1/2 carb
TAB	12 oz	0	0	0	0	0	0	40	0	0	free

SPORTS/ENERGY DRINKS AND MEAL REPLACEMENT

Brands

	Serving	Calories	Carb. (g)	Fat (g)	% Cal. Fat	Sat. Fat (g)	Chol. (mg)	Sod. (mg)	Fib. (g)	Prot. (g)	Servings/ Exchanges
Accelerade	1 scoop (makes 12 oz)	140	26	1	6	0	0	190	0	7	2 carb

Food	Serving	Cal	Carb (g)	Fat (g)	% Cal Fat	Sat Fat (g)	Chol (mg)	Sodium (mg)	Fiber (g)	Prot (g)	Exchanges/Choices
All Sport Body Quencher	8 oz	70	20	0	0	0	0	55	0		1 carb
AMP Energy Drink	8.4 oz	120	32	0	0	0	0	75	0		2 carb
Aquafina Essentials	8 oz	40	11	0	0	0	0	15	0		1/2 carb
Baxter Healthcare Pulse Heart Health Water	16.9 oz	38	9	0	0	0	0	0	6	0	1/2 carb
Baxter Healthcare Pulse Men's Health Formula	6.9 oz	38	0	0	0	0	0	0	0	0	1/2 carb
Baxter Healthcare Pulse Women's Health Water	6.9 oz	19	4	0	0	0	0	0	0	0	1/2 carb
Boost	8 oz	240	41	4	15	0.5	5	130	0	10	3 carb
Boost Breeze	8 oz	160	31	0	0	0	0	50	0	8	2 carb
Boost with Fiber	8 oz	240	42	4	15	0.5	5	170	3	10	3 carb
Boost Plus	8 oz	360	45	14	35	1.5	10	170	<1	14	3 carb, 1 med-fat meat, 2 fat
Carnation Instant Breakfast Powder Mix, All Varieties	1 pkt	130	27	0-1	0	0	<5	80-160	0-1	5	2 carb

BEVERAGES, SODA, SPORTS/ENERGY DRINKS, MEAL REPLACEMENT DRINKS, COCOA

	Serving	Calories	Carb. (g)	Fat (g)	% Cal. Fat	Sat. Fat (g)	Chol. (mg)	Sod. (mg)	Fib. (g)	Prot. (g)	Servings/ Exchanges
Carnation Instant Breakfast Ready-to-Drink	9.8 oz can	200–220	31–38	3	14	0–1	0–5	170–230	0–1	12	2 carb, 1 med-fat meat
Carnation Instant Breakfast Carb Conscious Powder, All Varieties	1 pkt	70	12	0–1	0	0	<5	70–75	<1	4 to 5	1 carb
Choice dm	8 oz	220	24	10	41	1.5	0	200	3	9	1 1/2 carb, 1 med-fat meat, 1 fat
Cott Emerge	8.5 oz	100	25	0	0	0	0	25	0	0	1 1/2 carb
CytoSport Cytomax	1 pkt (makes 8 oz)	160	30	0	0	0	0	140	0	0	2 carb
CytoSport Cytomax Lite	1 pkt (makes 8 oz)	80	16	0	0	0	0	65	0	0	1 carb
Gatorade, All Varieties	8 oz	50	14	0	0	0	0	110	0	0	1 carb
Gatorade Propel Fitness Water	8 oz	10	3	0	0	0	0	35	0	0	free

Glaceau Vitamin Water, All Varieties	8 oz	50	13	0	0	0	0	0	0	1 carb
Gookinaid E.R.G.	1 Tbsp	38	10	0	0	0	0	64	0	1/2 carb
GU20 Hydration Drink	1 pkg (24 oz)	150	39	0	0	0	0	360	0	2 1/2 carb
Hansen's Original Formula Energy	8.2 oz	110	32	0	0	0	0	25	0	2 carb
Hansen's Power Functional Beverage	8.2 oz	110	32	0	0	0	0	25	0	2 carb
Hydrolyte	1 Tbsp (makes 8 oz)	38	10	0	0	0	0	64	0	1/2 carb
Impact Water Plus	8 oz	0	0	0	0	0	0	0	0	free
Kasha GoLean Shakes Ready-to-Drink (Vanilla)	10.8 oz can	220	36	2.5	0	10	0	330	7	2 1/2 carb, 1 lean meat
KMX Energy Drink, All Varieties	8.4 oz	120	31	0	0	0	0	75	0	2 carb
Powerade (All Varieties)	8 oz	70	19	0	0	0	0	55	0	1 carb

BEVERAGES, SODA, SPORTS/ENERGY DRINKS, MEAL REPLACEMENT DRINKS, COCOA

	Serving	Calories	Carb. (g)	Fat (g)	% Cal. Fat	Sat. Fat (g)	Chol. (mg)	Sod. (mg)	Fib. (g)	Prot. (g)	Servings/ Exchanges
Powerade Light	8 oz	25	7	0	0	0	0	55	0	0	1/2 carb
Red Bull Energy Drink	8.3 oz	112	28	0	0	0	0	215	0	<1	2 carb
Reebok Flavored Fitness Water (All Varieties)	23.6 oz	30	1	0	0	0	0	0	0	0	
Reebok Natural Fitness Water	23.6 oz	0	0	0	0	0	0	0	0	0	free
Rockstar Energy Drink	8 oz	110	29	0	0	0	0	35	0	0	2 carb
RW Knudsen											
Recharge Plus Energy Drink	8 oz	80	18	0	0	0	0	25	0	1	1 carb
Recharge Sports Beverage (All Varieties)	8 oz	80	18	0	0	0	0	25	0	<1	1 carb
Simply Nutritious Ginkgo Alert	8 oz	120	29	0	0	0	0	20	0	0	2 carb

Simply Nutritious Ginseng Boost	8 oz	120	29	0	0	0	0	20	0	0	2 carb
Simply Nutritious VitaJuice	8 oz	120	29	0	0	0	0	35	0	2	2 carb

Ross Products

Enlive	8.1 oz	300	65	0	0	0	<5	65	0	10	4 carb
Ensure	8 oz	250	40	6	22	<1	<5	200	0	9	2 1/2 carb, 1 fat
Ensure Fiber	8 oz	250	42	6	22	<1	<5	200	3	9	2 1/2 carb, 1 fat
Ensure High Calcium	8 oz	225	31	6	24	<1	<5	290	0	12	2 carb, 1 med-fat meat
Ensure Light	8 oz	200	33	3	14	<1	<5	200	0	10	2 carb, 1 fat
Ensure Plus	8 oz	360	50	11	28	1	<5	240	0	13	3 carb, 2 fat
Glucerna Shake	8 oz	220	29	9	37	1	<5	210	3	10	2 carb, 2 fat
Glucerna Weight Loss Shake	11 oz	290	39	11	34	1	<5	NA	4	13	2 1/2 carb, 1 med-fat meat, 1 fat

Slim Fast

Powder Shakes	1 scoop	100	20	1	9	0.5	5	110	2	5	1 carb

BEVERAGES, SODA, SPORTS/ENERGY DRINKS, MEAL REPLACEMENT DRINKS, COCOA

	Serving	Calories	Carb. (g)	Fat (g)	% Cal. Fat	Sat. Fat (g)	Chol. (mg)	Sod. (mg)	Fib. (g)	Prot. (g)	Servings/ Exchanges
Powder Shakes with Soy Protein	1 scoop	170	25	2	11	1	0	270	5	15	1 1/2 carb, 1 lean meat
Ready-to-Drink, All Varieties	10.8 oz can	210–220	35–42	2.5–3	11	0.5–1	5	220	5	10	3 carb
Ready-to-Drink with Soy Protein	11.3 oz can	220	46	1	4	0	<5	180	5	7	3 carb
Ultra Powder Shakes, All Varieties	1 scoop	120	23–25	0–1.5	8	0–0.5	0–5	100–130	4–5	5	1 1/2 carb
Snapple Elements											
Enhanced Water (Berry or Lemon)	8 oz	40	10	0	0	0	0	10	0	0	1/2 carb
Enhanced Water (Lime or Orange)	8 oz	40	10	0	0	0	0	80	0	0	1/2 carb
Juice Drinks (Fire, Meteor, Rain, Sun)	8 oz	120	29	0	0	0	0	10	0	0	2 carb

Snapple-A-Day Meal Replacement, Strawberry Banana	11.3 oz can	210	43	0	0	0	150	5	7	3 carb
Snapple-A-Day Meal Replacement, Blueberry or Mango Lime	11.3 oz can	90	16	0	0	0	150	7	7	1 carb
Vitamin Supreme	8 oz	150	44	0	0	0	10	0	0	3 carb
SoBe										
Adrenaline Rush Energy Drink	8 oz	140	35	0	0	0	60	0	0	2 carb
Cranberry Grapefruit Elixir	8 oz	100	28	0	0	0	10	0	0	2 carb
Energy	8 oz	120	32	0	0	0	15	0	0	2 carb
Liz Blizz	8 oz	130	33	0	0	0	55	0	0	2 carb
Lizard Fuel	8 oz	130	33	0	0	0	20	0	0	2 carb
Lizard Lightning	8 oz	130	0	0	0	0	20	0	0	2 carb

BEVERAGES, SODA, SPORTS/ENERGY DRINKS, MEAL REPLACEMENT DRINKS, COCOA

	Serving	Calories	Carb. (g)	Fat (g)	% Cal. Fat	Sat. Fat (g)	Chol. (mg)	Sod. (mg)	Fib. (g)	Prot. (g)	Servings/ Exchanges
Twinlab Ultra Fuel	4 scoops (makes 16 oz)	400	99	0	0	0	0	60	0	0	6 1/2 carb
US Energy Drink	8 oz	110	29	0	0	0	0	15	0	0	2 carb
TEA											
Tea, Brewed	8 oz	2	<1	0	0	0	0	7	0	0	free
Tea, Camomile, Brewed	8 oz	2	<1	0	0	0	0	2	0	0	free
Tea, Instant	8 oz	2	<1	0	0	0	0	7	0	0	free
Brands											
Arizona Brand											
Arnold Palmer Lite Iced Tea	8 oz	50	14	0	0	0	0	25	0	0	1 carb
Diet Green Tea with Ginseng	8 oz	0	<1	0	0	0	0	20	0	0	free
Green Tea with Ginseng & Honey	8 oz	70	18	0	0	0	0	20	0	0	1 carb

Iced Tea	8 oz	90	25	0	0	0	20	0	1 1/2 carb
Iced Tea with Ginseng Extract	8 oz	60	15	0	0	0	20	0	1 carb
Iced Tea & Fruit Punch	8 oz	100	25	0	0	0	26	0	1 1/2 carb
Country Time									
Lemonade Iced Tea	8 oz	90	22	0	0	0	10	0	1 1/2 carb
Crystal Light									
Crystal Light Iced Tea Mixes, All Varieties	8 oz	5	0	0	0	0	0	0	free
Lipton									
Blackberry Flavored Tea Bags	1	0	<1	0	0	0	0	0	free
Calorie Free Iced Tea Mix	1 tsp	0	0	0	0	0	5	0	free
Carb Options Flavored Iced Tea Mix	1/8 tub	0	0	0	0	0	0	0	free
Diet Iced Tea Mix, All Varieties	1 Tbsp	5	1	0	0	0	0	0	free

BEVERAGES, SODA, SPORTS/ENERGY DRINKS, MEAL REPLACEMENT DRINKS, COCOA

	Serving	Calories	Carb. (g)	Fat (g)	% Cal. Fat	Sat. Fat (g)	Chol. (mg)	Sod. (mg)	Fib. (g)	Prot. (g)	Servings/ Exchanges
Instant Unsweetened Tea	2 tsp	0	0	0	0	0	0	0	0	0	free
Regular Tea Bags	1	0	0	0	0	0	0	0	0	0	free
Sugar Sweetened Tea Mix	1 1/3 Tbsp	70–80	18–19	0	0	0	0	0	0	0	1 carb
Nestea											
Sugar Sweetened Iced Tea Mix	1 1/3 Tbsp	60	15	0	0	0	0	0	0	0	1 carb
Unsweetened Iced Tea Mix	2 tsp	0	0	0	0	0	0	0	0	0	free
Snapple											
Fruit Flavored Sweetened Tea, All Varieties	8 oz	100–110	25–28	0	0	0	0	10	0	0	2 carb
Just Plain Tea Unsweetened	8 oz	0	0	0	0	0	0	10	0	0	free

BREAD, BAGELS, ROLLS, TORTILLAS, BISCUITS, PANCAKES, WAFFLES, STUFFING, CROUTONS

	Serving	Calories	Carb. (g)	Fat (g)	% Cal. Fat	Sat. Fat (g)	Chol. (mg)	Sod. (mg)	Fib. (g)	Prot. (g)	Servings/ Exchanges
Bagel	1/2	98	19	<1	0	0	0	190	<1	4	1 strch
Bagel, Cinnamon Raisin	1	195	39	1	5	<1	0	229	2	7	2 1/2 strch
Biscuit	2 1/2-inch piece	127	17	6	43	<1	0	368	<1	2	1 strch, 1 fat
Bread, Buckwheat	1 slice	71	13	1	13	<1	<1	100	<1	2	1 strch
Bread, Butter Croissant	1	231	26	12	47	7	43	424	2	5	2 strch, 2 fat
Bread, Cheese	1 slice	71	12	1	13	<1	2	144	<1	2	1 strch
Bread, Corn	2-oz piece	152	25	4	24	<1	23	375	1	4	1 strch, 1 fat
Bread, Cracked Wheat	1 slice	65	12	1	14	<1	0	135	1	2	1 strch
Bread, French	1 slice	69	13	<1	0	<1	0	152	<1	2	1 strch
Bread, Indian Fry	5 inch	296	48	9	27	2	0	626	2	6	3 strch, 2 fat
Bread, Italian	1 slice	81	15	1	11	<1	0	175	<1	3	1 strch

BREAD, BAGELS, ROLLS, TORTILLAS, BISCUITS, PANCAKES, WAFFLES, STUFFING, CROUTONS

	Serving	Calories	Carb. (g)	Fat (g)	% Cal. Fat	Sat. Fat (g)	Chol. (mg)	Sod. (mg)	Fib. (g)	Prot. (g)	Servings/ Exchanges
Bread, Mixed-Grain	1 slice	65	12	<1	0	<1	0	127	2	3	1 strch
Bread, Oat Bran	1 slice	71	12	1	13	<1	0	122	1	3	1 strch
Bread, Oatmeal	1 slice	72	13	1	13	<1	0	162	1	2	1 strch
Bread, Pita	1/2, 6-inch piece	83	17	<1	0	<1	0	161	<1	3	1 strch
Bread, Pita, Whole-Wheat	1	170	35	2	11	<1	0	239	5	6	2 strch
Bread, Potato	1 slice	69	13	<1	0	<1	<1	143	<1	2	1 strch
Bread, Pumpernickel	1 slice	80	15	1	11	<1	0	215	2	3	1 strch
Bread, Raisin	1 slice	71	14	1	13	<1	0	101	1	2	1 strch
Bread, Rye	1 slice	83	16	1	11	<1	0	211	2	3	1 strch
Bread, Sourdough	1 slice	69	13	<1	0	<1	0	152	<1	2	1 strch
Bread, Sweet Potato	1 slice	72	13	2	25	<1	14	228	<1	2	1 strch
Bread, Triticale	1 slice	63	12	<1	0	<1	0	136	2	2	1 strch
Bread, Vienna	1 slice	69	13	<1	0	<1	0	152	<1	2	1 strch

Bread, Wheat Bran	1 slice	89	17	1	10	<1	0	175	1	3	1 strch
Bread, White	1 slice	67	12	<1	0	<1	0	134	<1	2	1 strch
Bread, White, Reduced-Calorie	2 slices	96	20	1	9	<1	0	208	4	4	1 strch
Bread, Whole-Wheat	1 slice	70	13	1	13	<1	0	149	2	3	1 strch
Bread Sticks, Crisp	2, 4-inch pieces	82	14	2	22	<1	0	131	<1	2	1 strch
Bread Stuffing	1/3 cup	117	14	6	46	1	0	359	2	2	1 strch, 1 fat
Bread Stuffing, Homemade	1/3 cup	129	17	6	42	1	0	353	2	3	1 strch, 1 fat
Bun, Hamburger	1/2	61	11	1	15	<1	0	120	<1	2	1 strch
Bun, Hot Dog	1/2	61	11	1	15	<1	0	120	<1	2	1 strch
Crepe/French Pancake	1	239	22	13	49	4	163	274	<1	9	1 1/2 strch, 3 fat
Croutons	1 cup	122	22	2	15	<1	0	209	<1	4	1 strch, 1 fat
Dinner Roll/Bun, French	1	105	19	2	17	<1	0	231	1	3	1 strch
Dinner Roll/Bun, Wheat	1	98	16	2	18	<1	0	122	1	3	1 strch
Dumpling, Plain	medium	42	7	1	21	<1	1	105	<1	1	1/2 strch

BREAD, BAGELS, ROLLS, TORTILLAS, BISCUITS, PANCAKES, WAFFLES, STUFFING, CROUTONS

	Serving	Calories	Carb. (g)	Fat (g)	% Cal. Fat	Sat. Fat (g)	Chol. (mg)	Sod. (mg)	Fib. (g)	Prot. (g)	Servings/ Exchanges
Egg Bread/Challah	1 slice	115	19	2	16	<1	20	197	<1	4	1 strch
English Muffin	1/2	67	13	<1	0	<1	0	132	<1	2	1 strch
French Toast, Frozen	1 slice	126	19	4	29	1	48	292	<1	4	1 strch, 1 fat
French Toast, Homemade with 2% Milk	1 slice	149	16	7	42	2	75	311	<1	5	1 strch, 1 fat
Pancakes, From Mix	2	166	22	6	33	2	54	384	1	6	1 strch, 1 fat
Popover, Homemade with Whole Milk	1	90	11	3	30	1	47	81	<1	4	1 strch, 1 fat
Pretzel, Soft	2 oz	190	38	2	9	<1	2	772	<1	5	2 1/2 strch
Roll, Plain	1	85	14	2	21	<1	0	148	<1	2	1 strch
Roll, Submarine/Hoagie	1, 5-oz piece	392	75	4	9	<1	0	783	4	12	5 strch
Roll, Whole-Wheat	1	75	15	1	12	<1	0	167	2	3	1 strch
Scone	1, 1 1/2-oz piece	150	19	7	42	2	51	246	<1	4	1 strch, 1 fat

Food	Serving									
Scone, Whole-Wheat	1	145	13	7	43	2	50	174	3	5	1 strch, 1 fat
Taco Shells	2	122	15	6	44	<1	0	95	2	2	1 strch, 1 fat
Tortilla, Corn	1, 6-inch piece	56	12	<1	0	<1	0	40	1	1	1 strch
Tortilla, Flour	1, 7-inch piece	114	20	3	24	<1	0	167	1	3	1 strch
Tortilla, Flour	1, 10 1/2-inch piece	185	32	4	19	1	0	272	2	5	2 strch, 1 fat
Tortilla, Whole-Wheat	1	73	20	<1	0	<1	0	171	2	3	1 strch
Waffles, Blueberry	1, 4-inch piece	97	16	3	28	<1	18	272	<1	3	1 strch, 1 fat
Waffles, from Mix	1, 4 1/2-inch piece	145	7	7	43	1	35	256	<1	4	1 strch, 1 fat
Waffles, Homemade	1	218	25	11	45	2	52	383	1	6	1 1/2 strch, 2 fat
Waffles, Low-Fat	1, 4 1/2-inch piece	80	17	<1	0	<1	0	270	<1	3	1 strch

BREAD, BAGELS, ROLLS, TORTILLAS, BISCUITS, PANCAKES, WAFFLES, STUFFING, CROUTONS

	Serving	Calories	Carb. (g)	Fat (g)	% Cal. Fat	Sat. Fat (g)	Chol. (mg)	Sod. (mg)	Fib. (g)	Prot. (g)	Servings/ Exchanges
Brands											
Aunt Jemima											
Pancake/Waffle Mix, Buckwheat	1/4 cup	120	22	1	8	0	0	560	4	5	1 1/2 strch
Pancake/Waffle Mix, Buttermilk	1/3 cup	190	31	2	9	<1	10	480	2	6	2 strch
Pancake/Waffle Mix, Original	1/3 cup	150	28	<1	0	0	0	620	1	4	2 strch
Pancake/Waffle Mix, Whole Wheat	1/4 cup	130	28	<1	0	0	0	560	3	6	2 strch
Ballard											
Extra Light Oven-Ready Biscuit Dough	1	50	10	<1	0	<1	0	165	<1	1	1/2 strch

Extra Light Oven-Ready Biscuit Dough, Buttermilk	1	50	13	<1	0	<1	0	165	<1	1	1/2 strch
Betty Crocker											
Bisquick, Original	1/3 cup	160	25	6	34	1	NA	490	NA	3	1 1/2 strch, 1 fat
Bisquick, Reduced-Fat	1/3 cup	140	27	3	19	<1	NA	500	<1	3	2 strch, 1 fat
Health Valley											
Fat-Free Scones, Cinnamon Raisin	1	180	43	0	0	0	0	190	5	4	3 strch
Fat-Free Scones, Cranberry Orange	1	180	43	0	0	0	0	190	5	4	3 strch
Fat-Free Scones, Blueberry	1	180	43	0	0	0	0	190	5	4	3 strch
Jiffy											
Corn Bread Mix, Honey	1/4 cup	160	28	4	23	2	NA	320	1	2	2 strch
Corn Bread Mix, Fat-Free	1/4 cup	120	27	0	0	0	0	410	1	2	2 strch

BREAD, BAGELS, ROLLS, TORTILLAS, BISCUITS, PANCAKES, WAFFLES, STUFFING, CROUTONS

	Serving	Calories	Carb. (g)	Fat (g)	% Cal. Fat	Sat. Fat (g)	Chol. (mg)	Sod. (mg)	Fib. (g)	Prot. (g)	Servings/ Exchanges
Kellogg's Eggo											
French Toast Sticks	2 slices	220	36	6	23	2	20	550	1	5	2 1/2 strch, 1 fat
Waffles, Apple Cinnamon	2	190	30	6	28	2	15	370	1	4	2 strch, 1 fat
Waffles, Blueberry	2	190	30	6	28	2	20	370	1	4	2 strch, 1 fat
Waffles, Buttermilk	2	190	28	7	33	2	20	420	2	5	2 strch, 1 fat
Waffles, Chocolate Chip	2	200	32	7	32	2	15	380	1	4	2 strch, 1 fat
Waffles, Cinnamon Toast	3	270	46	8	27	2	20	480	1	5	3 strch, 2 fat
Waffles, Homestyle	2	190	29	7	33	2	20	440	2	5	2 strch, 1 fat
Waffles, Low Carb	2	190	15	11	53	2	0	350	7	15	1 strch, 2 fat
Waffles, Low-Fat Homestyle	2	160	31	3	17	<1	15	300	1	5	2 strch, 1 fat
Waffles, Low-Fat Nutri-Grain	2	140	28	3	19	<1	0	430	3	5	2 strch, 1 fat
Waffles, Minis Homestyle	12	260	38	9	31	2	25	600	2	7	2 1/2 strch, 2 fat

Waffles, Nutri-Grain	2	170	28	5	26	1	0	420	3	5	2 strch, 1 fat
Waffles, Special K	3	190	37	1	5	0	0	400	1	8	2 1/2 strch
Waffles, Strawberry	2	190	32	6	28	2	15	400	1	4	2 strch, 1 fat
Waffles, Toaster Swirlz Strawberry Minis	4	110	19	3	23	<1	5	210	<1	2	1 strch, 1 fat

Marshall's

Biscuits, Buttermilk	2	170	19	9	48	2	NA	380	0	2	1 strch, 2 fat
Biscuits, Homestyle	1	120	16	5	38	1	NA	270	0	2	1 strch, 1 fat

Mission

Flour Tortilla, 96% Fat Free Whole Wheat	1	140	26	3	14	<1	0	380	2	4	2 strch, 1 fat
Flour Tortilla, Low Carb Fajita Size	1	80	12	2	23	0	0	220	7	3	1 strch

Old El Paso

Taco Shells, Corn	3	150	20	7	42	2	0	135	1	2	1 strch, 1 fat

BREAD, BAGELS, ROLLS, TORTILLAS, BISCUITS, PANCAKES, WAFFLES, STUFFING, CROUTONS

	Serving	Calories	Carb. (g)	Fat (g)	% Cal. Fat	Sat. Fat (g)	Chol. (mg)	Sod. (mg)	Fib. (g)	Prot. (g)	Servings/Exchanges
Ortega											
Taco Shells, Corn	2	120	19	5	38	<1	0	190	2	2	1 strch, 1 fat
Tostada Shells	2	140	19	6	39	1	0	180	1	2	1 strch, 1 fat
Pepperidge Farm											
Bagel, Cinnamon Raisin	1	270	57	1	3	0	0	450	3	8	4 strch
Bagel, Everything	1	270	55	2	7	<1	0	550	3	9	3 1/2 strch
Bagel, Multi-Grain	1	270	55	2	7	0	0	470	5	9	3 1/2 strch
Bread, 100% Whole Wheat Thin Slice	1 slice	70	11	1	13	0	0	95	2	3	1 strch
Bread, Carb Style 100% Whole Wheat	1 slice	60	8	2	30	0	0	170	3	5	1/2 strch
Bread, Carb Style 7-Grain	1 slice	60	8	2	30	0	0	150	3	5	1/2 strch
Bread, Cinnamon Swirl	1 slice	90	14	3	30	<1	0	115	2	3	1 strch, 1 fat
Bread, Family Pumpernickel	1 slice	80	15	1	11	<1	0	230	2	3	1 strch

Food	Serving										
Bread, Farmhouse Buttertopped White	1 slice	110	21	2	16	0	<1	240	<1	3	1 1/2 strch
Bread, Farmhouse Golden Potato	1 slice	110	22	1	8	<1	0	220	1	3	1 1/2 strch
Bread, Farmhouse Honey Wheatberry	1 slice	110	20	2	16	0	0	200	2	4	1 strch
Bread, Farmhouse Soft Oatmeal	1 slice	110	21	1	8	0	0	200	1	4	1 1/2 strch
Bread, Farmhouse Sweet Buttermilk	1 slice	110	22	1	8	0	0	210	1	4	1 1/2 strch
Bread, Jewish Rye Party Bread	1 slice	130	25	1	7	0	0	440	3	4	1 1/2 strch
Bread, Light Style 7-Grain	1 slice	140	28	1	6	0	0	260	3	6	2 strch
Bread, Oatmeal	1 slice	60	11	1	15	0	0	160	1	2	1 strch
Bread, Original White Thin Sliced	1 slice	70	13	2	26	0	0	135	1	2	1 strch

BREAD, BAGELS, ROLLS, TORTILLAS, BISCUITS, PANCAKES, WAFFLES, STUFFING, CROUTONS

	Serving	Calories	Carb. (g)	Fat (g)	% Cal. Fat	Sat. Fat (g)	Chol. (mg)	Sod. (mg)	Fib. (g)	Prot. (g)	Servings/ Exchanges
Bread, Raisin Cinnamon Swirl	1 slice	80	14	2	23	0	0	105	1	3	1 strch
Bread, Seedless Rye	1 slice	80	15	1	11	<1	0	210	1	3	1 strch
Buns, Sandwich with Sesame Seeds	1	130	22	3	21	1	0	220	1	5	1 1/2 strch, 1 fat
English Muffin, 100% Whole Wheat	1	130	26	<1	0	0	0	210	3	6	2 strch
Mini Bagel, Blueberry Swirl	1	120	24	<1	0	0	0	190	<1	4	1 1/2 strch
Mini Bagel, Brown Sugar Cinnamon	1	120	24	<1	0	0	0	150	2	4	1 1/2 strch
Mini Bagel, Plain	1	110	22	<1	0	0	0	200	1	4	1 1/2 strch
Rolls, Carb Style Hamburger	1	110	17	1	8	0	<5	190	3	7	1 strch

Food											
Rolls, French, Hot & Crusty Seven Grain	1	80	19	2	23	0	0	270	2	4	1 strch
Rolls, French, Hot & Crusty	1	100	20	1	9	0	0	220	1	4	1 strch
Rolls, Hamburger	1	120	21	3	23	1	0	220	1	5	1 1/2 strch, 1 fat
Rolls, Hot & Crusty Club	1	130	24	2	14	0	0	250	1	4	1 1/2 strch
Rolls, Hot & Crusty Sourdough	1	100	19	1	9	0	0	240	1	4	1 strch
Rolls, Parker House Dinner	1	80	14	2	23	0	0	95	<1	3	1 strch
Rolls, Soft Hoagie with Sesame Seeds	1	200	33	5	23	2	0	320	2	7	2 strch, 1 fat
Pillsbury											
Biscuits (Frozen), Butter Tastin'	1	180	21	9	45	3	NA	570	1	4	1 1/2 strch, 2 fat
Biscuits (Frozen), Southern Style	1	180	21	9	45	3	NA	570	1	4	1 1/2 strch, 2 fat

BREAD, BAGELS, ROLLS, TORTILLAS, BISCUITS, PANCAKES, WAFFLES, STUFFING, CROUTONS

	Serving	Calories	Carb. (g)	Fat (g)	% Cal. Fat	Sat. Fat (g)	Chol. (mg)	Sod. (mg)	Fib. (g)	Prot. (g)	Servings/ Exchanges
Biscuits, Buttermilk	3	150	29	2	12	0	NA	540	<1	4	2 strch
Biscuits, Country	3	150	29	2	12	0	NA	540	<1	4	2 strch
Bread, Crusty French Loaf	1 slice	150	27	2	12	<1	na	370	<1	5	2 strch
Breadsticks, Garlic	2	180	25	7	35	1	NA	580	<1	4	1 1/2 strch, 1 fat
Breadsticks, Parmesan	2	180	24	7	35	1	NA	570	<1	5	1 1/2 strch, 1 fat
Cornbread Twists	1	130	17	6	42	2	NA	340	0	3	1 strch, 1 fat
Crescent Rolls, Original	1	110	11	6	49	2	NA	220	0	2	1 strch, 1 fat
Crescent Rolls, Reduced-Fat	1	100	12	5	45	1	NA	230	0	2	1 strch, 1 fat
Dinner Rolls, Traditional	1	110	18	2	16	0	NA	270	<1	4	1 strch
Pizza Crust	1/5 can	150	27	2	12	0	NA	410	<1	4	2 strch
Pillsbury Grands!											
Biscuits, Buttermilk	1	190	24	9	43	2	NA	600	<1	4	1 1/2 strch, 2 fat
Biscuits, Butter Tastin'	1	190	23	9	43	2	NA	600	<1	4	1 1/2 strch, 2 fat
Biscuits, Flaky	1	200	25	9	41	2	NA	580	<1	4	1 1/2 strch, 2 fat

Biscuits, Reduced-Fat Buttermilk	1	170	26	6	32	1	NA	590	<1	4	2 strch, 1 fat

Pillsbury Hungry Jack

Biscuits, Buttermilk	1	100	14	4	36	1	NA	360	0	2	1 strch, 1 fat
Biscuits, Cinnamon & Sugar	1	110	17	4	33	1	NA	280	1	2	1 strch, 1 fat

Progresso

Bread Crumbs, Italian-Style	1/4 cup	110	20	2	16	0	0	430	1	4	1 strch
Bread Crumbs, Parmesan	1/4 cup	100	17	2	18	0	0	870	1	4	1 strch
Bread Crumbs, Plain	1/4 cup	110	19	2	16	0	0	210	1	4	1 strch

Rhodes

Biscuits, AnyTime! Blueberry with Frosting	1	240	37	11	41	1	NA	440	1	3	2 1/2 strch, 2 fat
Biscuits, AnyTime! Buttermilk	1	200	25	10	45	2	NA	490	1	3	1 1/2 strch, 2 fat

BREAD, BAGELS, ROLLS, TORTILLAS, BISCUITS, PANCAKES, WAFFLES, STUFFING, CROUTONS

	Serving	Calories	Carb. (g)	Fat (g)	% Cal. Fat	Sat. Fat (g)	Chol. (mg)	Sod. (mg)	Fib. (g)	Prot. (g)	Servings/ Exchanges
Shake 'N Bake											
Coating Mix, Classic Italian	1/8 pkt	35	7	<1	0	0	0	280	0	1	1/2 strch
Coating Mix, Original Chicken	1/8 pkt	40	7	1	23	0	0	220	0	<1	1/2 strch
Coating Mix, Original Pork	1/8 pkt	45	8	<1	0	0	0	230	0	1	1/2 strch
Stove Top											
Stuffing Mix for Pork	1/2 cup	170	21	9	48	2	0	540	<1	4	1 strch, 2 fat
Stuffing Mix for Turkey	1/2 cup	170	21	9	48	2	0	530	<1	4	1 strch, 2 fat
Stuffing Mix, Chicken Flavor	1/2 cup	170	20	9	48	2	0	520	<1	4	1 strch, 2 fat
Stuffing Mix, Corn Bread	1/2 cup	170	21	8	48	2	0	580	1	3	1 1/2 strch, 2 fat
Stuffing Mix, Low-Sodium Chicken	1/2 cup	180	21	9	45	2	0	340	<1	4	1 1/2 strch, 2 fat
Stuffing Mix, Savory Herbs	1/2 cup	170	20	9	48	2	0	530	1	4	1 strch, 2 fat

BREAKFAST CEREAL, READY-TO-EAT CEREAL, HOT CEREAL

	Serving	Calories	Carb. (g)	Fat (g)	% Cal. Fat	Sat. Fat (g)	Chol. (mg)	Sod. (mg)	Fib. (g)	Prot. (g)	Servings/ Exchanges
Bulgur	1/2 cup	76	17	<1	0	0	0	5	4	3	1 strch
Corn Grits, White or Yellow, Cooked	1/2 cup	73	16	<1	0	<1	0	0	<1	2	1 strch
Cream of Rice, Cooked	1/2 cup	64	14	<1	0	<1	0	1	<1	1	1 strch
Cream of Rye, Cooked	1/2 cup	54	12	<1	0	<1	0	175	2	1	1 strch
Cream of Wheat, Cooked	1/2 cup	66	14	<1	0	<1	0	71	<1	2	1 strch
Farina, Cooked	1/2 cup	59	12	<1	0	<1	0	0	2	2	1 strch
Granola, Homemade	1/2 cup	285	32	15	47	3	0	15	6	9	2 strch, 3 fat
Honey Bran Cereal	1 cup	60	14	<1	0	<1	0	101	2	2	1 strch
Kasha or Buckwheat Groats, Cooked	1/2 cup	91	20	<1	0	<1	0	4	2	3	1 strch
Millet, Cooked	1/4 cup	72	14	<1	0	<1	0	1	<1	2	1 strch
Multi-Grain Cereal, Cooked	1/2 cup	100	20	1	9	<1	0	380	2	3	1 strch

BREAKFAST CEREAL, READY-TO-EAT CEREAL, HOT CEREAL

	Serving	Calories	Carb. (g)	Fat (g)	% Cal. Fat	Sat. Fat (g)	Chol. (mg)	Sod. (mg)	Fib. (g)	Prot. (g)	Servings/ Exchanges
Oatmeal Cereal, Cooked	1/2 cup	73	13	1	12	<1	0	1	2	3	1 strch
Wheatena, Cooked	1/2 cup	68	15	<1	0	<1	0	3	3	2	1 strch
Brands											
General Mills											
Basic 4	1 cup	200	42	3	25	0	0	320	3	4	3 strch
Boo Berry	1 cup	120	26	1	8	0	0	190	0	1	2 strch
Cheerios	1 cup	110	22	2	16	0	0	210	3	3	1 1/2 strch
Cheerios, Apple Cinnamon	3/4 cup	120	25	2	13	0	0	120	1	2	1 1/2 strch
Cheerios, Berry Burst Strawberry	1 cup	110	24	2	14	0	0	180	2	3	1 1/2 strch
Cheerios, Berry Burst Strawberry Banana	1 cup	110	24	2	14	0	0	180	3	3	1 1/2 strch
Cheerios Berry Burst Triple Berry	1 cup	110	24	2	14	0	0	180	2	3	1 1/2 strch

Cheerios, Frosted	1 cup	120	26	1	8	0	0	210	1	2	2 strch
Cheerios, Honey Nut	1 cup	120	24	2	13	0	0	210	2	3	1 1/2 strch
Cheerios Plus, Multi-Grain	1 cup	110	24	1	9	0	0	200	3	3	1 1/2 strch
Chex, Corn	1 cup	110	25	<1	0	0	0	280	1	2	2 strch
Chex, Frosted	3/4 cup	110	26	<1	5	0	0	180	0	1	2 strch
Chex, Honey Nut	3/4 cup	120	26	1	4	0	0	220	0	2	2 strch
Chex, Multi-Bran	1 cup	190	46	2	8	0	0	360	7	4	3 strch
Chex, Rice	1 1/4 cup	120	26	0	4	0	0	270	<1	2	2 strch
Chex, Wheat	1 cup	180	40	1	6	0	0	420	5	5	2 1/2 strch
Cinnamon Toast Crunch	3/4 cup	130	24	4	23	<1	0	210	1	1	1 1/2 strch
Cinnamon Toast Crunch, Reduced-Sugar	3/4 cup	120	24	3	21	0	0	190	2	1	1 1/2 strch, 1 fat
Cocoa Puffs	1 cup	120	26	2	13	0	0	160	1	1	2 strch
Cocoa Puffs, Reduced-Sugar	1 cup	120	25	2	13	0	0	220	1	1	1 1/2 strch
Cookie Crisp	1 cup	120	26	1	8	0	0	170	1	1	2 strch

BREAKFAST CEREAL, READY-TO-EAT CEREAL, HOT CEREAL

	Serving	Calories	Carb. (g)	Fat (g)	% Cal. Fat	Sat. Fat (g)	Chol. (mg)	Sod. (mg)	Fib. (g)	Prot. (g)	Servings/ Exchanges
Count Chocula	1 cup	120	26	1	8	0	0	170	1	1	2 strch
Country Corn Flakes	1 cup	110	26	<1	5	0	0	270	1	2	2 strch
Fiber One	1/2 cup	60	24	1	17	0	0	105	14	2	1 1/2 strch
Fiber One, Honey Clusters	1 1/4 cup	170	47	1	6	0	0	170	14	3	3 strch
Frankenberry	1 cup	120	27	1	4	0	0	190	0	1	2 strch
French Toast Crunch	3/4 cup	120	26	2	8	0	0	150	1	1	2 strch
Golden Grahams	3/4 cup	120	25	1	8	0	0	270	1	1	1 1/2 strch
Honey Nut Clusters	3/4 cup	210	47	3	12	0	0	280	3	4	3 strch
Kaboom	1 1/4 cup	120	25	1	8	0	0	190	1	1	1 1/2 strch
Kix	1 1/3 cup	120	26	1	8	0	0	220	1	2	1 1/2 strch
Kix, Berry Berry	3/4 cup	120	26	2	13	0	0	160	1	1	2 strch
Lucky Charms	1 cup	120	25	1	8	0	0	200	1	2	1 1/2 strch
Lucky Charms, Chocolate	1 cup	120	26	1	8	0	0	160	1	1	2 strch
Nature Valley Low-Fat Fruit Granola	2/3 cup	210	44	3	13	0	0	210	3	4	3 strch, 1 fat

Oatmeal Crisp, Almond	1 cup	220	42	5	18	<1	0	250	4	5	3 strch, 1 fat
Oatmeal Crisp, Apple Cinnamon	1 cup	210	45	2	10	<1	0	270	4	5	3 strch
Oatmeal Crisp, Raisin	1 cup	210	44	2	10	<1	0	220	3	5	3 strch
Oatmeal Crisp, Triple Berry	1 cup	210	45	3	10	<1	0	260	5	5	3 strch, 1 fat
Peanut Butter Toast Crunch	3/4 cup	130	23	4	23	<1	0	210	1	2	1 1/2 strch, 1 fat
Raisin Nut Bran	1 1/4 cup	200	44	3	10	<1	0	270	5	4	3 strch
Reese's Peanut Butter Puffs	3/4 cup	130	24	4	23	<1	0	200	1	2	1 1/2 strch, 1 fat
Shrek	1 cup	120	27	<1	4	0	0	160	0	1	2 strch
Team Cheerios	1 cup	110	25	1	9	0	0	200	2	2	1 1/2 strch
Total Brown Sugar & Oat	3/4 cup	110	25	<1	9	0	0	200	1	2	1 1/2 strch
Total Corn Flakes	1 1/3 cup	110	26	<1	5	0	0	210	1	2	2 strch
Total Protein	3/4 cup	120	11	4	25	0	0	270	3	13	1 strch, 1 med-fat meat
Total Raisin Bran	1 cup	170	42	1	6	0	0	240	5	3	3 strch
Total Whole-Grain	3/4 cup	100	24	1	10	0	0	190	3	2	2 strch

BREAKFAST CEREAL, READY-TO-EAT CEREAL, HOT CEREAL

	Serving	Calories	Carb. (g)	Fat (g)	% Cal. Fat	Sat. Fat (g)	Chol. (mg)	Sod. (mg)	Fib. (g)	Prot. (g)	Servings/ Exchanges
Trix	1 cup	120	26	2	17	0	0	190	1	1	2 strch
Trix, Reduced-Sugar	1 cup	120	26	2	13	0	0	180	1	1	2 strch
Wheaties	1 cup	110	24	1	9	0	0	220	3	3	1 1/2 strch
Health Valley											
Amazing Apple! with Cinnamon Hot Cereal	1 pkg	210	41	2	10	0	0	230	4	9	3 strch
Apple Cinnamon Soy O's	1 cup	180	31	2	11	0	0	230	3	11	2 strch
Bananas Gone Nuts! Crunches & Flakes Cereal	3/4 cup	200	41	2	13	0	0	30	4	5	3 strch
Blueberry Bliss Crunches & Flakes	3/4 cup	200	41	3	13	0	0	100	4	5	3 strch, 1 fat
Cranberry Crunch	3/4 cup	200	41	3	13	0	0	30	4	5	3 strch, 1 fat
Empower Cereal	1 cup	200	42	3	13	0	0	170	6	6	3 strch, 1 fat

Heart Wise	1 cup	200	36	3	13	0	0	120	5	11	2 1/2 strch, 1 fat
Low-Fat Date Almond Flavor Granola	2/3 cup	180	43	1	6	0	0	90	6	5	3 strch
Low-Fat Tropical Fruit Granola	2/3 cup	180	43	1	6	0	0	90	6	5	3 strch
Maple Madness! with Raisins Hot Cereal	1 pkg	240	47	2	8	0	0	290	4	9	3 strch
Organic Amaranth Flakes	3/4 cup	100	24	0	0	0	0	90	4	3	1 1/2 strch
Organic Blue Corn Flakes	3/4 cup	100	24	0	0	0	0	10	3	3	1 1/2 strch
Organic Golden Flax Cereal	3/4 cup	190	38	3	16	0	0	80	6	6	2 1/2 strch, 1 fat
Slender Cereal	1 cup	180	35	2	8	0	0	130	4	10	2 strch
Terrific 10 Grain! Hot Cereal	1 pkg	220	41	3	11	0	0	210	5	12	3 strch, 1 fat

Kashi

GoLean	1 cup	140	30	1	7	0	0	85	10	13	2 strch
GoLean Crunch	1 cup	190	36	3	13	0	0	95	8	9	2 1/2 strch, 1 fat

BREAKFAST CEREAL, READY-TO-EAT CEREAL, HOT CEREAL

	Serving	Calories	Carb. (g)	Fat (g)	% Cal. Fat	Sat. Fat (g)	Chol. (mg)	Sod. (mg)	Fib. (g)	Prot. (g)	Servings/ Exchanges
Good Friends	1 cup	170	43	2	12	0	0	130	12	5	3 strch
Good Friends Cinna-Raisin Crunch	1 cup	170	41	2	9	0	0	105	8	4	3 strch
Heart to Heart	3/4 cup	110	25	2	14	0	0	90	5	4	1 1/2 strch
Heart to Heart Apple Cinnamon Hot Cereal	1 pkt	160	33	2	13	0	0	130	5	4	2 strch
Heart to Heart Golden Brown Maple Hot Cereal	1 pkt	160	33	2	13	0	0	95	5	4	2 strch
Heart to Heart Oatmeal Raisin Spice Hot Cereal	1 pkt	150	33	2	13	0	0	100	4	3	2 strch
Honey Puffed Kashi	1 cup	120	25	1	8	0	0	6	2	3	1 1/2 strch
Kashi Medley	3/4 cup	120	26	1	8	0	0	75	3	3	2 strch
Kashi Pilaf	1/2 cup	170	30	3	15	0	0	15	6	6	2 strch, 1 fat
Organic Promise Autumn Wheat	1 cup	190	45	1	5	0	0	0	6	5	3 strch

Organic Promise Cranberry Sunshine	1 cup	110	26	1	9	0	0	100		2	2 strch
Organic Promise Strawberry Fields	1 cup	120	28	0	0	0	0	200		1	2 strch
Puffed Kashi	1 cup	70	15	<1	7	0	0	0		1	1 strch
Seven in the Morning	1/2 cup	210	47	2	7	0	0	260		7	3 strch
Kellogg's											
All-Bran	1/2 cup	80	23	1	13	0	0	80	10	4	1 1/2 strch
All-Bran with Extra Fiber	1/2 cup	50	20	1	20	0	0	120	13	3	1 strch
Apple Jacks	1 cup	130	30	<1	0	0	0	150	1	1	2 strch
Cinnamon Krunchers	3/4 cup	130	23	4	23	<1	0	150	<1	1	1 1/2 strch, 1 fat
Cocoa Krispies	3/4 cup	120	27	1	8	<1	0	190	1	1	2 strch
Complete Oat Bran Flakes	3/4 cup	110	23	1	9	0	0	210	4	3	1 1/2 strch
Complete Wheat Bran Flakes	3/4 cup	90	23	<1	0	0	0	210	5	3	1 1/2 strch
Corn Flakes	1 cup	100	24	0	0	0	0	200	1	2	1 1/2 strch

BREAKFAST CEREAL, READY-TO-EAT CEREAL, HOT CEREAL

	Serving	Calories	Carb. (g)	Fat (g)	% Cal. Fat	Sat. Fat (g)	Chol. (mg)	Sod. (mg)	Fib. (g)	Prot. (g)	Servings/ Exchanges
Corn Pops	1 cup	120	28	0	0	0	0	120	0	1	2 strch
Cracklin' Oat Bran	3/4 cup	200	35	7	30	3	0	150	6	4	2 strch, 2 fat
Crispix	1 cup	110	25	0	0	0	0	210	<1	2	2 strch
Crunchy Blends Low-Fat Granola	2/3 cup	220	48	3	14	1	0	150	3	5	3 strch, 1 fat
Froot Loops	1 cup	120	28	1	8	<1	0	150	1	1	2 strch
Froot Loops, 1/3 Less Sugar	1 1/4 cup	120	28	1	8	<1	0	180	1	2	2 strch
Froot Loops, Marshmallow Alien Berry	1 cup	130	29	1	8	<1	0	115	<1	1	2 strch
Frosted Flakes	3/4 cup	120	28	0	0	0	0	150	1	1	2 strch
Frosted Flakes, 1/3 Less Sugar	1 cup	120	28	0	0	0	0	180	<1	1	2 strch
Fruit Harvest, Banana Berry	3/4 cup	120	25	2	15	2	0	140	1	2	1 1/2 strch

Food	Serving	Cal.							Exchange
Fruit Harvest, Peach Strawberry	3/4 cup	110	26	0	0	0	170	1	2	2 strch
Fruit Harvest, Strawberry Blueberry	3/4 cup	110	25	0	0	0	140	1	2	1 1/2 strch
Honey Smacks	3/4 cup	100	24	<1	0	0	50	1	2	2 strch
Mini Swirlz-Cinnamon Bun	1 cup	120	25	2	17	0	115	1	2	1 1/2 strch
Mini-Wheats, Apple Cinnamon	3/4 cup	180	44	1	6	0	20	5	4	3 strch
Mini-Wheats, Blueberry	3/4 cup	180	43	1	6	0	20	5	4	3 strch
Mini-Wheats, Frosted Original	5 biscuits	180	41	1	6	0	5	5	5	3 strch
Mini-Wheats, Frosted Bite Size	24 biscuits	200	48	1	5	0	5	6	6	3 strch
Mini-Wheats, Frosted Maple & Brown Sugar	24 biscuits	190	44	1	5	0	0	5	4	3 strch

BREAKFAST CEREAL, READY-TO-EAT CEREAL, HOT CEREAL

	Serving	Calories	Carb. (g)	Fat (g)	% Cal. Fat	Sat. Fat (g)	Chol. (mg)	Sod. (mg)	Fib. (g)	Prot. (g)	Servings/ Exchanges
Mini-Wheats, Frosted Vanilla Crème Bite Size	24 biscuits	180	43	1	6	0	0	0	5	4	3 strch
Product 19	1 cup	100	25	0	0	0	0	210	1	2	1 1/2 strch
Raisin Bran	1 cup	190	45	2	9	0	0	350	7	5	3 strch
Raisin Bran Crunch	1 cup	190	45	1	5	0	0	210	4	3	3 strch
Rice Krispies	1 1/4 cup	120	29	0	0	0	0	320	0	2	2 strch
Rice Krispies, Razzle Dazzle	3/4 cup	110	25	0	0	0	0	170	0	1	1 1/2 strch
Rice Krispies Treats	3/4 cup	120	26	2	15	0	0	190	0	1	2 strch
Scooby-Doo! Berry Bones	1 cup	130	28	1	8	0	0	230	<1	1	2 strch
Smart Start, Healthy Heart	1 1/4 cup	230	49	2	9	0	0	140	5	6	3 strch
Smart Start, Soy Protein	1 cup	200	40	2	8	0	0	260	4	10	2 1/2 strch

Special K	1 cup	110	23	0	0	0	220	1	6	1 1/2 strch
Special K Low-Carb Lifestyle	3/4 cup	100	14	3	30	<1	110	5	10	1 strch, 1 med-fat meat
Special K Red Berries	1 cup	110	25	0	0	0	220	1	3	1 1/2 strch
Special K Vanilla Almond	1 cup	110	25	2	16	0	160	1	2	1 1/2 strch
SpongeBob SquarePants	1 cup	120	26	1	8	0	120	<1	2	2 strch

Malt-O-Meal

Berry Colossal Crunch	3/4 cup	120	26	2	13	0	210	1	1	2 strch
Cocoa Roos	3/4 cup	120	27	1	8	0	190	0	1	2 strch
Corn Bursts	1 cup	120	29	0	0	0	120	0	1	2 strch
Crispy Rice	1 1/4 cup	130	26	0	0	0	320	0	2	2 strch
Frosted Flakes	3/4 cup	120	28	0	0	0	200	1	1	2 strch
Frosted Mini Spooners	1 cup	190	45	1	5	0	0	6	5	3 strch
Golden Puffs	3/4 cup	100	25	0	0	0	40	<1	2	2 strch
Hot Wheat Cereal, Chocolate	3 Tbsp dry	120	27	<1	0	0	0	1	4	2 strch

BREAKFAST CEREAL, READY-TO-EAT CEREAL, HOT CEREAL

	Serving	Calories	Carb. (g)	Fat (g)	% Cal. Fat	Sat. Fat (g)	Chol. (mg)	Sod. (mg)	Fib. (g)	Prot. (g)	Servings/ Exchanges
Hot Wheat Cereal, Maple & Brown Sugar	3 Tbsp dry	120	28	0	0	0	0	0	1	3	2 strch
Hot Wheat Cereal, Quick Original	3 Tbsp dry	120	26	<1	0	0	0	0	1	5	2 strch
Puffed Rice	1 cup	60	13	0	0	0	0	0	0	1	1 strch
Puffed Wheat	1 cup	50	11	0	0	0	0	0	1	2	1 strch
Toasty O's	1 cup	110	22	2	14	0	0	280	3	4	1 1/2 strch
Toasty O's, Apple & Cinnamon	3/4 cup	120	25	2	13	0	0	160	1	2	1 1/2 strch
Toasty O's, Honey & Nut	1 cup	110	24	1	8	0	0	270	2	3	1 1/2 strch
Tootie Fruities	1 cup	120	28	1	8	0	0	150	1	1	2 strch
Post											
100% Bran	1/3 cup	80	22	1	13	0	0	125	9	4	1 1/2 strch
Alpha-Bits	1 cup	130	27	2	14	0	0	210	1	3	2 strch

Alpha-Bits, Marshmallow	1 cup	120	25	1	8	0	0	160	0	2	1 1/2 strch
Banana Nut Crunch	1 cup	240	44	6	23	<1	0	200	5	5	3 strch, 1 fat
Blueberry Morning	1 1/4 cup	230	43	4	16	0	0	240	2	4	3 strch, 1 fat
Bran Flakes	3/4 cup	100	24	<1	0	0	0	220	5	3	1 1/2 strch
Cocoa Pebbles	3/4 cup	120	25	2	15	1	0	180	0	1	1 1/2 strch
Fruity Pebbles	3/4 cup	110	24	1	9	<1	0	160	0	<1	1 1/2 strch
Fruity Pebbles, 1/2 the Sugar	3/4 cup	110	22	2	9	1	0	230	0	1	1 1/2 strch
Golden Crisp	3/4 cup	110	25	0	0	0	0	40	<1	2	1 1/2 strch
Grape Nuts	1/2 cup	200	47	1	5	0	0	310	6	7	3 strch
Grape Nuts Flakes	3/4 cup	110	24	1	9	0	0	120	3	3	1 1/2 strch
Great Grains, Crunchy Pecan	1/2 cup	220	38	6	27	1	0	180	4	5	2 1/2 strch, 1 fat
Great Grains, Raisin/Date/Pecan	1/2 cup	210	40	4	19	0	0	130	4	4	2 1/2 strch, 1 fat
Honey Bunches of Oats	3/4 cup	120	25	2	15	0	0	170	2	2	1 1/2 strch, 1 fat

BREAKFAST CEREAL, READY-TO-EAT CEREAL, HOT CEREAL

	Serving	Calories	Carb. (g)	Fat (g)	% Cal. Fat	Sat. Fat (g)	Chol. (mg)	Sod. (mg)	Fib. (g)	Prot. (g)	Servings/ Exchanges
Honey Bunches of Oats & Almonds	3/4 cup	130	25	3	21	0	0	170	2	3	1 1/2 strch, 1 fat
Honeycombs	1 1/3 cup	110	26	<1	0	0	0	220	<1	2	2 strch
Marshmallow Mania Pebbles	3/4 cup	110	25	<1	0	0	0	60	<1	1	1 1/2 strch
Raisin Bran	1 cup	190	47	1	5	0	0	300	8	4	3 strch
Shredded Wheat	2 biscuits	160	37	1	6	0	0	0	6	5	2 1/2 strch
Shredded Wheat 'n Bran	1 1/4 cup	200	48	2	8	0	0	0	8	7	3 strch
Shredded Wheat, Frosted	1 cup	180	43	1	6	0	0	0	5	4	3 strch
Shredded Wheat, Honey Nut	1 cup	200	43	2	8	0	0	70	4	5	3 strch
Quaker											
100% Natural Low-Fat Granola with Raisins	2/3 cup	210	45	3	12	1	0	140	3	4	3 strch, 1 fat

Food	Serving										Exchanges
100% Natural Granola, Oats, Honey & Raisin	1/2 cup	210	37	6	26	2	0	25	3	5	2 1/2 strch, 1 fat
100% Natural Granola, Regular	1/2 cup	210	35	7	30	2	0	25	3	5	2 strch, 1 fat
Apple Zaps	1 cup	120	27	1	8	0	0	135	1	1	2 strch
Cap'n Crunch	3/4 cup	110	23	2	16	0	0	200	1	1	1 1/2 strch
Cap'n Crunch Swirled Berries	1 cup	100	22	2	18	0	0	180	1	1	1 1/2 strch
Cap'n Crunch Peanut Butter	3/4 cup	110	21	3	25	<1	0	200	1	2	1 1/2 strch, 1 fat
Cap'n Crunch Crunchberries	3/4 cup	110	22	2	14	0	0	180	1	1	1 1/2 strch
Cinnamon Crunch	1 cup	120	25	2	15	0	0	230	1	2	1 1/2 strch
Cocoa Blasts	1 cup	130	29	1	8	<1	0	140	1	1	2 strch
Essentials Oat Bran	1 1/4 cup	210	43	3	12	<1	0	210	6	7	3 strch, 1 fat
Essentials, Oatmeal Squares	1 cup	210	44	3	12	<1	0	250	5	6	3 strch, 1 fat

BREAKFAST CEREAL, READY-TO-EAT CEREAL, HOT CEREAL

	Serving	Calories	Carb. (g)	Fat (g)	% Cal. Fat	Sat. Fat (g)	Chol. (mg)	Sod. (mg)	Fib. (g)	Prot. (g)	Servings/ Exchanges
Frosted Flakers	3/4 cup	120	28	0	0	0	0	200	0	1	2 strch
Frosted Oats	1 cup	110	23	2	16	0	0	230	1	2	1 1/2 strch
Frosted Shredded Wheat	1 cup	200	45	1	5	0	0	0	4	5	3 strch
Fruitangy Oh's	1 cup	120	27	1	8	0	0	150	1	2	2 strch
Honey Grahams	3/4 cup	110	23	2	16	0	0	230	1	2	1 1/2 strch
Honey Nut Oats	3/4 cup	110	24	1	9	0	0	220	1	2	1 1/2 strch
Hot Oat Bran	1/2 cup	150	25	3	17	<1	0	0	6	7	1 1/2 strch, 1 fat
Instant Hot Oatmeal	1 pkt	100	19	2	18	0	0	80	3	4	1 1/2 strch, 1 fat
Instant Hot Oatmeal, Apple & Cinnamon	1 pkt	130	27	2	12	<1	0	170	3	3	2 strch
Instant Hot Oatmeal, Apple & Cinnamon, Lower Sugar	1 pkt	110	22	2	14	<1	0	170	3	3	1 1/2 strch
Instant Hot Oatmeal, Apple Crisp	1 pkt	150	31	2	21	<1	0	220	3	3	2 strch

Instant Hot Oatmeal, Breakfast Blast	1 pkt	150	26	2	13	<1	0	250	2	3	2 strch
Instant Hot Oatmeal, Cinnamon Roll	1 pkt	160	32	3	16	<1	0	240	3	4	2 strch, 1 fat
Instant Hot Oatmeal, Cinnamon Spice	1 pkt	170	35	2	12	<1	0	250	3	4	2 1/2 strch
Instant Hot Oatmeal, Dinosaur Eggs	1 pkt	200	38	4	18	2	0	250	3	4	2 1/2 strch, 1 fat
Instant Hot Oatmeal, Maple/Brown Sugar	1 pkt	160	33	2	13	0	0	190	3	4	2 strch
Instant Hot Oatmeal, Maple/Brown Sugar, Lower Sugar	1 pkt	120	24	2	17	<1	0	270	3	4	2 strch
Instant Hot Oatmeal, Peaches & Cream	1 pkt	140	27	3	19	<1	0	190	2	3	2 strch

BREAKFAST CEREAL, READY-TO-EAT CEREAL, HOT CEREAL

	Serving	Calories	Carb. (g)	Fat (g)	% Cal. Fat	Sat. Fat (g)	Chol. (mg)	Sod. (mg)	Fib. (g)	Prot. (g)	Servings/ Exchanges
Instant Hot Oatmeal, Raisin/Date/Walnut	1 pkt	140	27	3	18	<1	0	240	2	3	2 strch
Instant Hot Oatmeal, Strawberries & Cream	1 pkt	140	27	3	18	<1	0	190	2	3	2 strch
Instant Hot Oatmeal Express, Baked Apple	1 cup	200	42	3	13	<1	0	320	4	4	2 strch, 1 fat
Instant Hot Oatmeal Express, Cinnamon Roll	1 cup	210	41	4	14	<1	0	250	3	4	3 strch, 1 fat
Instant Hot Oatmeal Express, Golden Brown Sugar	1 cup	200	42	3	13	<1	0	290	3	5	3 strch, 1 fat
Kretschmer Honey Crunch Wheat Germ	1 2/3 Tbsp	50	8	1	20	0	0	0	1	4	1/2 strch
Kretschmer Wheat Bran	1/4 cup	30	10	1	33	0	0	0	7	3	1/2 strch

Food	Serving										Exchanges
Kretschmer Wheat Germ	2 Tbsp	50	6	1	20	0	0	0	2	4	1/2 strch
Life	3/4 cup	120	25	2	15	0	0	150	2	3	1 1/2 strch
Life, Cinnamon	3/4 cup	120	25	2	15	0	0	160	2	3	1 1/2 strch
Life, Honey Graham	3/4 cup	120	25	2	13	0	0	160	2	3	1 1/2 strch
Multi-Grain Hot Cereal	1/2 cup	130	29	1	8	0	0	0	5	5	2 strch
Nutrition for Women Apple Cinnamon	1 pkt	170	35	2	12	<1	0	310	3	5	2 strch
Nutrition for Women Golden Brown Sugar	1 pkt	160	32	3	16	<1	0	330	3	6	2 strch, 1 fat
Nutrition for Women Vanilla Cinnamon	1 pkt	160	32	2	13	<1	0	290	3	5	2 strch
Oat Bran	1 1/4 cup	210	43	3	13	<1	0	210	6	7	3 strch
Oh's, Honey Graham	3/4 cup	110	23	2	18	<1	0	160	1	1	1 1/2 strch
Old-Fashioned Hot Oats	1/2 cup	150	27	3	18	<1	0	0	4	5	2 strch, 1 fat
Popeye Puffed Rice	1 cup	50	12	0	0	0	0	0	0	1	1 strch
Popeye Puffed Wheat	1 1/4 cup	50	11	0	0	0	0	0	1	2	1 strch

BREAKFAST CEREAL, READY-TO-EAT CEREAL, HOT CEREAL

	Serving	Calories	Carb. (g)	Fat (g)	% Cal. Fat	Sat. Fat (g)	Chol. (mg)	Sod. (mg)	Fib. (g)	Prot. (g)	Servings/ Exchanges
Quick Hot Oats	1/2 cup	150	27	3	18	<1	0	0	4	5	2 strch, 1 fat
Rice Crisps	1 cup	110	26	0	0	NA	0	290	0	2	2 strch
Shredded Wheat	3 biscuits	220	50	2	8	<1	0	0	7	7	3 strch
Sweet Puffs	1 cup	130	30	1	8	0	0	80	2	2	2 strch
Toasted Oatmeal, Honey Nut	1 cup	190	40	3	14	NA	0	180	3	4	2 1/2 strch, 1 fat
Toasted Oatmeal, Original	1 cup	190	40	2	9	NA	0	220	4	5	2 1/2 strch
Toasted Oatmeal Squares, Cinnamon	1 cup	230	47	3	12	NA	0	270	5	8	3 strch, 1 fat
Toasted Oatmeal Squares, Regular	1 cup	220	43	3	12	NA	0	260	4	7	3 strch, 1 fat
Toasted Oats	1 cup	110	23	2	16	NA	0	280	2	3	1 1/2 strch
Unprocessed Bran	1/3 cup	35	11	0	0	0	0	0	8	3	1 strch

CAKE, PIE, COOKIES, BROWNIES

	Serving	Calories	Carb. (g)	Fat (g)	% Cal. Fat	Sat. Fat (g)	Chol. (mg)	Sod. (mg)	Fib. (g)	Prot. (g)	Servings/ Exchanges
Angel Food Cake	1 piece	129	29	<1	0	<1	0	255	<1	3	2 carb
Apple Brown Betty	3/4 cup	264	46	8	27	4	17	295	4	4	3 carb, 2 fat
Apple Turnover	1	289	36	15	47	4	0	- 262	1	3	2 1/2 carb, 3 fat
Brownie	1 small	115	18	5	39	1	15	88	<1	1	1 carb, 1 fat
Brownie with Nuts	2-inch square	140	20	7	45	1	9	83	<1	1	1 carb, 1 fat
Cake, Chocolate with Chocolate Icing	1 piece	234	35	11	42	3	29	214	2	3	2 carb, 2 fat
Cake, Frosted	2-inch square	175	29	6	31	2	18	194	NA	2	2 carb, 1 fat
Cake, German Chocolate with Icing	1 slice	404	55	21	47	5	53	369	2	4	3 1/2 carb, 4 fat
Cake, Pound with Butter	1 piece	110	14	6	49	3	63	113	<1	2	1 carb, 1 fat
Cake, Unfrosted	2-inch square	97	16	3	28	<1	18	168	NA	2	1 carb, 1 fat

CAKE, PIE, COOKIES, BROWNIES

	Serving	Calories	Carb. (g)	Fat (g)	% Cal. Fat	Sat. Fat (g)	Chol. (mg)	Sod. (mg)	Fib. (g)	Prot. (g)	Servings/ Exchanges
Cake, White with White Icing	1 piece	266	45	10	34	4	6	166	<1	2	3 carb, 2 fat
Cake, Yellow with Chocolate Icing	1 piece	243	36	11	42	3	35	216	1	2	2 1/2 carb, 2 fat
Cake/Wafer Ice Cream Cone	1	17	3	<1	0	<1	0	6	<1	<1	free
Cheesecake	1/12 cake	257	20	18	63	9	44	166	<1	4	1 carb, 4 fat
Chocolate Chips, Semisweet	1/4 cup	201	27	13	58	8	0	5	3	2	2 carb, 3 fat
Cobbler, Apple	3 × 3-inch piece	199	35	6	27	1	1	304	2	2	2 carb, 1 fat
Cobbler, Cherry	3 × 3-inch piece	198	34	6	27	1	1	311	1	2	2 carb, 1 fat
Cobbler, Peach	3 × 3-inch piece	204	37	6	26	1	1	308	2	2	2 1/2 carb, 1 fat

Coconut Macaroons	1 2-inch	97	17	3	28	3	0	59	<1	<1	1 carb, 1 fat
Coffee Cake, Cinnamon with Crumb Topping	1 piece	263	29	15	51	3	20	221	1	4	2 carb, 3 fat
Cookies	1 3-inch	142	19	7	44	2	10	103	<1	2	1 carb, 1 fat
Cookies, Chocolate Chip	1	78	9	5	58	1	5	55	<1	<1	1/2 carb, 1 fat
Cookies, Fat-Free	2	68	16	<1	0	0	0	51	2	2	1 carb
Cookies, Fortune	2	61	13	<1	0	<1	2	44	<1	<1	1 carb
Cookies, Lady Fingers	4	161	26	4	22	1	161	65	<1	5	2 carb, 1 fat
Cookies, Oatmeal	1	81	12	3	33	<1	0	69	<1	1	1 carb, 1 fat
Cookies, Peanut Butter	1	73	8	4	49	<1	4	64	<1	1	1/2 carb, 1 fat
Cookies, Sandwich with Creme Filling	2	94	14	4	38	<1	NA	120	NA	1	1 carb, 1 fat
Cookies, Shortbread	4	161	21	8	44	2	6	146	<1	2	1 1/2 carb, 2 fat
Cookies, Snickerdoodle	1	81	12	4	44	2	9	68	<1	<1	1 carb, 1 fat
Cookies, Soft Raisin	1	60	10	2	30	<1	<1	51	<1	<1	1/2 carb
Cookies, Sugar	1	72	10	3	38	2	8	54	<1	<1	1/2 carb, 1 fat

CAKE, PIE, COOKIES, BROWNIES

	Serving	Calories	Carb. (g)	Fat (g)	% Cal. Fat	Sat. Fat (g)	Chol. (mg)	Sod. (mg)	Fib. (g)	Prot. (g)	Servings/ Exchanges
Crepe, Chocolate-Filled	1	119	15	5	38	2	58	148	<1	4	1 carb, 1 fat
Crepe, Fruit-Filled	1	131	21	4	27	1	63	124	<1	4	1 1/2 carb, 1 fat
Crisp, Apple, Homemade	1/2 cup	230	46	5	20	1	0	257	2	3	3 carb, 1 fat
Crisp, Cherry	3 × 3-inch piece	146	24	6	37	<1	0	74	1	2	1 1/2 carb, 1 fat
Crisp, Peach	3 × 3-inch piece	155	27	5	29	<1	0	70	2	2	2 carb, 1 fat
Cupcake, Chocolate with Chocolate Icing	1	154	23	7	41	2	19	140	1	2	1 1/2 carb, 1 fat
Cupcake, Frosted	1 small	172	28	6	31	NA	NA	161	NA	2	2 carb, 1 fat
Custard, Homemade	1/2 cup	148	15	7	42	3	123	109	0	7	1 carb, 1 fat
Gingersnaps	3	87	16	2	21	<1	0	137	<1	1	1 carb
Marshmallows	4 large	90	23	<1	0	0	0	13	<1	<1	1 1/2 carb
Pie, Fruit, 2-Crust	1/6	290	43	13	40	2	0	300	NA	2	3 carb, 3 fat
Pie, Pumpkin or Custard	1/8	168	19	4	21	1	21	209	NA	4	1 carb, 2 fat

CAKE/PIE/CHEESECAKE

Brands

Betty Crocker

Brownie Mix, Carb Monitor, Walnut Brownie	1/16 recipe	160	20	11	63	2	25	90	4	2	1 carb, 2 fat
Brownie Mix, Chocolate Fudge	1/20 recipe	170	24	7	35	2	20	105	0	2	1 1/2 carb, 1 fat
Cake Mix, Chocolate Fudge	1/12 recipe	270	35	13	44	3	55	350	1	3	2 carb, 3 fat
Cake Mix, French Vanilla	1/12 recipe	240	35	10	38	3	55	280	0	1	2 carb, 2 fat

Claim Jumper

Chocolate Motherlode 6-Layer Cake	1 slice	460	63	22	43	6	40	320	1	5	4 carb, 4 fat

Comstock

Pie Filling, Cherry Light	1/3 cup	60	15	0	0	0	0	15	1	0	1 carb

CAKE, PIE, COOKIES, BROWNIES

	Serving	Calories	Carb. (g)	Fat (g)	% Cal. Fat	Sat. Fat (g)	Chol. (mg)	Sod. (mg)	Fib. (g)	Prot. (g)	Servings/ Exchanges
Pie Filling, More Fruit, Apple	1/3 cup	80	20	0	0	0	0	40	1	0	1 carb
Pie Filling, More Fruit, Blueberry	1/3 cup	80	21	0	0	0	0	45	1	0	1 carb
Pie Filling, More Fruit, Cherry	1/3 cup	90	23	0	0	0	0	70	0	0	1 1/2 carb
Pie Filling, More Fruit, Peach	1/3 cup	80	19	0	0	0	0	15	1	1	1 carb
Pie Filling, Red Ruby Cherry	1/3 cup	90	23	0	0	0	0	25	1	0	1 1/2 carb
Pie Filling, Strawberry	1/3 cup	100	23	0	0	0	0	25	1	0	1 carb
Delizza											
Belgian Mini Cream Puffs	6	291	15	24	74	14	NA	77	1	4	1 carb, 5 fat

Edwards

Caramel Dulce de Leche Cheesecake (singles)	1 slice	290	26	19	59	8	60	230	0	4	2 carb, 4 fat
Chocolate Butter Pecan Pie	1 piece	560	63	32	52	14	90	270	2	55	4 carb, 6 fat
Chocolate Marble Cheesecake (singles)	1 slice	290	23	20	62	8	70	220	0	4	1 1/2 carb, 4 fat
Chocolate Sundae Pie	1 piece	450	47	28	56	14	10	310	1	5	3 carb, 6 fat
Georgia Pecan Pie	1 piece	470	60	20	38	4	30	580	0	3	4 carb, 4 fat
Key Lime Pie	1 piece	440	57	22	43	14	40	330	2	7	4 carb, 4 fat
Lemon Meringue Pie	1 piece	350	62	8	20	3	45	250	0	8	4 carb, 2 fat
Mocha Mudslide Pie	1 piece	430	51	24	49	12	15	330	2	5	3 1/2 carb, 5 fat
Original Cheesecake (singles)	1 slice	290	23	21	66	9	70	220	0	4	1 1/2 carb, 4 fat
Pecan Cheesecake	1 slice	530	59	27	45	8	75	540	0	5	4 carb, 5 fat
Pumpkin Cheesecake	1 slice	520	51	32	56	15	75	460	2	8	3 1/2 carb, 6 fat

CAKE, PIE, COOKIES, BROWNIES

	Serving	Calories	Carb. (g)	Fat (g)	% Cal. Fat	Sat. Fat (g)	Chol. (mg)	Sod. (mg)	Fib. (g)	Prot. (g)	Servings/ Exchanges
Strawberry Marble Cheesecake (singles)	1 slice	280	25	18	61	7	60	220	0	4	1 1/2 carb, 4 fat
Sweet Potato Pie	1 piece	420	61	18	38	6	35	270	2	4	4 carb, 4 fat
Turtle Pie	1 piece	520	60	29	50	14	15	390	1	5	4 carb, 6 fat
Entenmann's											
Cake, Fudge Chocolate	1 slice	280	42	12	39	4	15	250	2	3	3 carb, 2 fat
Cake, Louisiana Crunch	1 slice	340	49	15	41	4	55	310	<1	3	3 carb, 3 fat
Coffee Cake, Cheese-Filled Crumb	1 slice	210	26	10	43	3	35	200	<1	4	2 carb, 2 fat
Hostess											
Ding Dongs	2	370	46	19	46	12	15	250	2	3	3 carb, 4 fat
Ho Hos	2	250	34	12	31	8	20	150	1	2	2 carb, 2 fat
Twinkies	1	150	26	5	30	2	20	200	0	1	2 carb, 1 fat

Libby's

	Serving										
Pie Filling, Apple	1/3 cup	80	20	0	0	0	0	10	0	0	1 carb
Pie Filling, Blueberry	1/3 cup	80	19	0	0	0	0	0	1	0	1 carb
Pie Filling, Cherry	1/3 cup	90	22	0	0	0	0	0	0	0	1 1/2 carb

Marie Callender's

	Serving										
Apple Crumb Cobbler	4 oz	320	41	17	47	3	0	170	3	2	3 carb, 3 fat
Banana Cream Pie	1 piece	300	32	18	53	8	45	200	2	3	2 carb, 4 fat
Berry Cobbler	4 oz	370	42	22	54	3	0	180	5	2	3 carb, 4 fat
Cherry Crumb Cobbler	4 oz	330	43	18	48	4	0	190	3	2	3 carb, 4 fat
Cherry Crunch Pie	1 piece	340	52	15	38	3	0	240	3	2	3 1/2 carb, 3 fat
Chocolate Satin Pie	1 piece	440	40	31	64	14	70	240	2	4	2 1/2 carb, 6 fat
Coconut Cream Pie	1 piece	320	34	20	56	10	40	180	2	3	2 carb, 4 fat
Dutch Apple Pie	1 piece	320	45	16	44	2	0	180	4	2	3 carb, 3 fat
Key Lime Pie	1 piece	390	53	17	38	9	20	180	0	6	3 1/2 carb, 3 fat
Lattice Apple Pie	1 piece	330	42	18	48	2	0	160	2	2	3 carb, 4 fat
Lemon Meringue Pie	1 piece	290	48	10	31	2	45	160	1	3	3 carb, 2 fat

CAKE, PIE, COOKIES, BROWNIES

	Serving	Calories	Carb. (g)	Fat (g)	% Cal. Fat	Sat. Fat (g)	Chol. (mg)	Sod. (mg)	Fib. (g)	Prot. (g)	Servings/ Exchanges
Peach Cobbler	4 oz	350	37	22	57	3	0	150	4	2	2 1/2 carb, 4 fat
Pecan Pie	1 piece	410	52	22	46	2	40	250	3	4	3 1/2 carb, 4 fat
Pumpkin Pie	1 piece	350	46	14	37	2	35	240	3	6	3 carb, 3 fat
Razzleberry Pie	1 piece	360	43	21	53	3	0	180	5	2	3 carb, 4 fat
Wild Blueberry Pie	1 piece	350	39	20	51	3	0	120	2	2	2 1/2 carb, 4 fat
Mrs. Smith's											
Apple Caramel Fliplt Cake	1 slice	480	90	13	25	2	5	510	2	3	6 carb, 3 fat
Blackberry Cobbler	1 piece	260	43	10	35	2	0	250	2	2	3 carb, 2 fat
Boston Cream Pie	1 piece	210	31	9	38	2	25	160	0	2	2 carb, 2 fat
Caramel Caribou Cream Pie	1 piece	460	50	27	52	15	35	350	1	5	3 carb, 5 fat
Carrot Cake	1 slice	300	37	16	50	3	30	360	1	3	2 1/2 carb, 3 fat
Chocolate Caramel Fliplt Cake	1 slice	580	84	25	38	7	70	450	1	5	5 1/2 carb, 5 fat

Deep Dish Blueberry Crumb Pie	1 piece	320	49	13	38	2	0	320	2	3	3 carb, 3 fat
Deep Dish Caramel Apple Pie	1 piece	290	41	13	41	2	0	320	3	2	3 carb, 3 fat
Homemade Pumpkin Pie	1 piece	290	42	12	38	3	40	370	2	4	3 carb, 2 fat
Pumpkin Streusel Pie	1 piece	370	52	16	41	3	30	400	2	5	3 1/2 carb, 3 fat
Strawberry Delight Fliplt Cake	1 slice	380	73	9	21	1	5	400	1	3	5 carb, 2 fat
Pepperidge Farm											
Apple Turnover	1	290	36	15	45	4	0	230	2	4	2 1/2 carb, 3 fat
Cherry Turnover	1	280	34	15	46	4	0	250	1	4	2 carb, 3 fat
Chocolate Fudge 3-Layer Cake	1 slice	250	31	11	40	3	30	160	1	3	2 carb, 2 fat
Coconut 3-Layer Cake	1 slice	250	35	11	40	3	25	115	0	2	2 carb, 2 fat
Pillsbury											
Frosting, Chocolate Fudge	2 Tbsp	140	21	6	36	2	0	110	<1	0	1 1/2 carb, 1 fat

CAKE, PIE, COOKIES, BROWNIES

	Serving	Calories	Carb. (g)	Fat (g)	% Cal. Fat	Sat. Fat (g)	Chol. (mg)	Sod. (mg)	Fib. (g)	Prot. (g)	Servings/ Exchanges
Frosting, Vanilla	2 Tbsp	150	23	6	36	2	0	70	0	0	1 1/2 carb, 1 fat
Rich's											
New York Style Chocolate Iced Éclair	1	210	24	11	48	9	40	80	0	2	1 1/2 carb, 2 fat
Sara Lee											
All Butter Pound Cake	1 slice	300	37	16	47	9	105	160	0	4	2 1/2 carb, 3 fat
Apple Pie	1 piece	340	46	16	41	3	0	310	1	3	3 carb, 3 fat
Blueberry Pie	1 piece	360	53	15	39	3	0	260	2	3	3 1/2 carb, 3 fat
Caramel Applenut Deep Dish Pie	1 piece	370	45	18	43	4	15	170	2	9	3 carb, 4 fat
Cherry Pie	1 piece	320	44	14	41	2	0	260	0	4	3 carb, 3 fat
Chocolate-Dipped Original Cheesecake Bites	5	480	40	33	63	24	75	290	2	6	2 1/2 carb, 7 fat
Coconut Layer Cake	1 slice	260	33	14	46	10	15	210	1	2	2 carb, 3 fat

Crumb Coffee Cake	1 slice	190	30	8	37	1	20	150	0	2	2 carb, 2 fat
Double Chocolate Layer Cake	1 slice	260	33	13	42	9	10	230	2	3	2 carb, 3 fat
Dutch Apple Pie	1 piece	350	53	15	37	3	0	320	2	3	3 1/2 carb, 3 fat
French Cheesecake	1 slice	410	41	25	56	16	25	330	1	6	3 carb, 5 fat
Fruits of the Forest Deep Dish Pie	1 piece	340	41	17	47	6	15	190	0	5	3 carb, 3 fat
Mince Pie	1 piece	370	55	15	38	2	0	400	2	3	3 1/2 carb, 3 fat
New York Style Cheesecake	1 slice	500	50	30	54	16	90	520	0	8	3 carb, 6 fat
Orchard Apple Deep Dish Pie	1 piece	400	43	24	55	8	15	440	3	3	3 carb, 5 fat
Original Cream Cheesecake	1 slice	340	38	18	47	9	60	320	1	7	2 1/2 carb, 4 fat
Peach Pie	1 piece	330	50	13	36	3	0	250	2	3	3 carb, 3 fat
Pumpkin Pie	1 piece	260	37	11	28	2	30	460	2	4	2 1/2 carb, 2 fat

CAKE, PIE, COOKIES, BROWNIES

	Serving	Calories	Carb. (g)	Fat (g)	% Cal. Fat	Sat. Fat (g)	Chol. (mg)	Sod. (mg)	Fib. (g)	Prot. (g)	Servings/ Exchanges
Raspberry Pie	1 piece	360	50	16	39	3	0	250	3	4	3 carb, 3 fat
Southern Pecan Pie	1 piece	520	70	24	42	4	45	480	3	5	4 1/2 carb, 5 fat
Southern Sweet Potato Pie	1 piece	280	45	10	32	3	35	420	2	4	3 carb, 2 fat
Vanilla Layer Cake	1 slice	260	32	14	46	10	15	210	0	2	2 carb, 3 fat
Weight Watchers Smart Ones											
Chocolate Chip Cookie Dough Sundae	1	190	35	4	21	2	5	120	1	3	2 carb, 1 fat
Chocolate Éclair	1	150	25	4	23	1	30	170	1	2	1 1/2 carb, 1 fat
Double Fudge Brownie Parfait	1	190	39	2	12	2	10	170	2	6	2 1/2 carb
New York Style Cheesecake	1	150	21	5	30	2	15	140	1	6	1 1/2 carb, 1 fat

COOKIES/BROWNIES

Brands

Archway

Apple-Filled Oatmeal	1	100	16	3	27	<1	0	105	1	1	1 carb, 1 fat
Apricot-Filled	1	100	16	3	27	2	5	80	0	1	1 carb, 1 fat
Coconut Macaroon	1	100	12	6	54	5	0	40	1	1	1 carb, 1 fat
Date-Filled Oatmeal	1	100	17	3	27	<1	0	160	1	1	1 carb, 1 fat
Dutch Cocoa	1	100	16	3	27	1	0	85	1	1	1 carb, 1 fat
Frosted Lemon	1	100	16	4	36	1	0	100	0	<1	1 carb, 1 fat
Ginger Snap	5	150	23	5	30	1	0	120	0	1	1 1/2 carb, 1 fat
Gourmet Oatmeal Pecan	1	130	16	6	42	2	0	105	<1	2	1 carb, 1 fat
Iced Molasses	1	114	20	3	24	1	0	130	0	1	1 carb, 1 fat
Iced Oatmeal	4	120	20	4	30	2	0	150	1	1	1 carb, 1 fat
Oatmeal	1	110	17	3	25	2	0	85	1	2	1 carb, 1 fat
Oatmeal Raisin	1	110	17	4	33	1	0	100	<1	1	1 carb, 1 fat
Pecan Ice Box	1	120	15	6	45	2	0	75	0	1	1 carb, 1 fat

CAKE, PIE, COOKIES, BROWNIES

	Serving	Calories	Carb. (g)	Fat (g)	% Cal. Fat	Sat. Fat (g)	Chol. (mg)	Sod. (mg)	Fib. (g)	Prot. (g)	Servings/ Exchanges
Reduced-Fat Ginger Snap	5	140	25	3	19	1	0	140	0	1	1 1/2 carb, 1 fat
Rocky Road	1	130	18	6	42	2	10	70	<1	2	1 carb, 1 fat
Soft Sugar Drop	1	90	15	3	30	1	0	80	0	1	1 carb, 1 fat
Sugar-Free Chocolate Chip	1	110	16	5	41	1	0	65	0	1	1 carb, 1 fat
Sugar-Free Oatmeal	1	110	16	5	41	1	0	75	<1	1	1 carb, 1 fat
Sugar-Free Peanut Butter	1	100	12	5	45	2	0	85	1	2	1 carb, 1 fat
Sugar-Free Rocky Road	1	100	12	5	45	2	0	85	1	2	1 carb, 1 fat
Estee											
Chocolate Chip	4	150	21	7	42	2	0	30	0	2	1 1/2 carb, 1 fat
Coconut	4	140	19	6	38	2	0	25	0	2	1 carb, 1 fat
Fudge	4	150	19	7	42	1	0	45	0	2	1 carb, 1 fat
Lemon	4	140	19	6	39	0	0	25	0	2	1 carb, 1 fat
Oatmeal Raisin	4	130	19	5	35	1	0	25	1	2	1 carb, 1 fat
Shortbread	4	130	22	4	28	1	0	150	0	2	1 1/2 carb, 1 fat

Vanilla Sandwich	3	160	35	5	28	1	0	35	0	2	2 carb, 1 fat
Sugar-Free Vanilla Crème Wafers	5	155	21	8	46	2	0	10	0	1	1 1/2 carb, 2 fat

Famous Amos

Chocolate Chip	4	130	18	6	42	2	0	90	0	2	1 carb, 1 fat
Chocolate Chip & Pecans	4	140	17	7	45	2	0	90	<1	2	1 carb, 1 fat

Fifty50

Butter	4	160	20	8	45	5	25	65	<1	2	1 carb, 2 fat
Chocolate Chip	4	170	17	10	53	3	0	50	<1	2	1 carb, 2 fat
Fudge Brownie	4	160	19	8	45	1	0	20	<1	2	1 carb, 2 fat
Hearty Oatmeal	4	140	20	6	39	1	0	55	<1	2	1 carb, 1 fat
Peanut Butter	4	160	19	7	39	1	0	25	<1	3	1 carb, 1 fat
Sugar-Free Vanilla Crème Wafers	6	150	20	9	54	2	0	35	<1	1	1 carb, 2 fat

Ghirardelli

Dark Chocolate Chip Almond	1	200	24	11	50	4	10	170	0	3	1 1/2 carb, 2 fat

CAKE, PIE, COOKIES, BROWNIES

	Serving	Calories	Carb. (g)	Fat (g)	% Cal. Fat	Sat. Fat (g)	Chol. (mg)	Sod. (mg)	Fib. (g)	Prot. (g)	Servings/ Exchanges
Milk Chocolate Chip	1	200	26	10	45	3	5	170	0	2	2 carb, 2 fat
Girl Scout											
All Abouts	2	150	20	7	42	3	0	90	<1	2	1 carb, 1 fat
Aloha Chips	3	160	19	9	51	2	0	120	<1	2	1 carb, 2 fat
Do-Si-Dos Peanut Butter Sandwiches	3	180	23	8	40	2	0	150	1	3	1 1/2 carb, 2 fat
Ole-Ole	5	140	20	7	45	2	0	100	0	1	1 carb, 1 fat
Samoas Caramel deLites	2	140	19	7	45	6	0	85	1	1	1 carb, 1 fat
Tagalongs Peanut Butter Patties	2	150	16	8	48	5	0	115	1	2	1 carb, 2 fat
Thin Mints	4	160	20	9	51	6	0	140	1	1	1 carb, 2 fat
Trefoils Shortbread	4	130	18	6	42	1	0	135	<1	1	1 carb, 1 fat
Health Valley											
Fat-Free Apple Spice	3	100	24	0	0	0	0	50	3	2	1 1/2 carb

Fat-Free Old-Fashioned Healthy Chip	3	100	24	0		0	0	40	4	3	1 1/2 carb
Fat-Free Raisin Oatmeal	3	100	24	0		0	0	50	3	2	1 1/2 carb
Keebler											
Chips Deluxe	1	80	9	4	45	1	0	60	0	1	1/2 carb, 1 fat
Chips Deluxe Chocolate Lovers	1	90	11	5	50	2	5	80	0	1	1 carb, 1 fat
Chips Deluxe Coconut	1	80	10	5	56	2	0	45	<1	1	1 carb, 1 fat
Chips Deluxe Crunchy Walnut	1	90	9	6	60	1	0	60	<1	1	1/2 carb, 1 fat
Chips Deluxe Soft 'n Chewy	1	80	11	3	34	1	0	60	0	1	1 carb, 1 fat
Chips Deluxe with Peanut Butter Cups	1	80	9	5	56	2	0	45	0	1	1/2 carb, 1 fat
E.L. Fudge Fudge Sandwich	2	120	17	5	38	1	0	115	<1	1	1 carb, 1 fat

CAKE, PIE, COOKIES, BROWNIES

	Serving	Calories	Carb. (g)	Fat (g)	% Cal. Fat	Sat. Fat (g)	Chol. (mg)	Sod. (mg)	Fib. (g)	Prot. (g)	Servings/ Exchanges
E.L. Fudge Butter Sandwich	2	120	17	6	45	1	0	70	<1	1	1 carb, 1 fat
Ernie's Animal Crackers	1 box	250	41	9	32	1	0	290	1	4	3 carb, 2 fat
Fudge Shoppe Deluxe Grahams	3	140	19	7	45	4	0	105	<1	1	1 carb, 1 fat
Fudge Shoppe Fudge Sticks	3	150	19	8	48	4	0	55	0	1	1 carb, 2 fat
Fudge Shoppe Fudge Strips	3	160	21	8	45	4	0	140	<1	1	1 1/2 carb, 2 fat
Fudge Shoppe Grasshopper	4	150	19	7	42	4	0	85	<1	2	1 carb, 1 fat
Golden Vanilla Wafers	8	150	20	7	42	2	120	120	<1	1	1 carb, 1 fat
Mini Chips Deluxe	4	150	19	8	48	3	0	90	<1	2	1 carb, 2 fat
Mini E.L. Fudge Fudge Sandwich	7	130	21	6	42	2	0	75	0	1	1 1/2 carb, 1 fat

Mini Rainbow Chips Deluxe	4	150	19	8	48	2	<5	100	<1	2	1 carb, 2 fat
Mini Sandies Pecan Shortbread	4	160	17	10	56	2	<5	100	<1	2	1 carb, 2 fat
Rainbow Vanilla Wafers	8	130	20	5	35	1	0	125	0	1	1 carb, 1 fat
Sandies Almond Shortbread	1	80	9	5	56	1	5	50	0	1	1/2 carb, 1 fat
Sandies Pecan Shortbread	1	80	9	5	56	1	0	75	<1	<1	1/2 carb, 1 fat
Sandies Reduced-Fat Pecan Shortbread	1	80	11	3	34	<1	0	60	0	<1	1 carb, 1 fat
Sesame Street Animal Crackers	7	130	21	4	28	1	0	140	<1	2	1 1/2 carb, 1 fat
Soft Batch Chocolate Chip	1	80	10	4	45	1	0	70	<1	<1	1/2 carb, 1 fat
Vienna Fingers Crème Filled	2	140	21	6	39	2	0	105	0	2	1 1/2 carb, 1 fat
Vienna Fingers Fudge Thins	4	160	22	7	39	3	0	140	<1	1	1 1/2 carb, 1 fat

CAKE, PIE, COOKIES, BROWNIES

	Serving	Calories	Carb. (g)	Fat (g)	% Cal. Fat	Sat. Fat (g)	Chol. (mg)	Sod. (mg)	Fib. (g)	Prot. (g)	Servings/ Exchanges
La Choy											
Fortune Cookies	4	112	<1	<1	0	<1	0	11	26	2	2 carb
Mother's											
Almond Shortbread	3	180	19	11	55	4	0	115	1	2	1 carb, 2 fat
Animal Parade	9	135	20	6	40	4	0	75	0	1	1 carb, 1 fat
Checkerboard Wafers	8	150	20	8	48	2	0	40	1	1	1 carb, 2 fat
Circus Animals	6	140	20	6	39	7	0	55	1	1	1 carb, 1 fat
Cocadas Coconut	5	150	20	7	42	3	5	140	2	2	1 carb, 1 fat
Coffee Cremes	2	180	26	7	35	4	0	100	1	2	2 carb, 1 fat
Cookie Parade	4	140	18	7	45	4	0	95	2	1	1 carb, 1 fat
Double Fudge Sandwich	2	180	24	9	45	5	0	110	2	2	1 1/2 carb, 2 fat
English Tea Sandwich	2	180	26	7	35	4	0	100	1	2	2 carb, 1 fat
Gaucho Peanut Butter	2	190	22	10	47	3	0	200	2	3	1 1/2 carb, 2 fat
Iced Oatmeal	2	130	22	4	28	2	0	160	1	1	1 1/2 carb, 1 fat

Oatmeal Butterscotch	2	120	19	5	38	2	0	140	1	2	1 carb, 1 fat
Oatmeal Raisin	5	150	20	7	42	2	5	125	2	2	1 carb, 1 fat
Old Fashioned Chocolate Chip	2	160	20	8	45	3	10	105	0	2	1 carb, 2 fat
Old Fashioned Iced Oatmeal	2	130	22	4	28	2	0	160	1	2	1 1/2 carb, 1 fat
Old Fashioned Macaroons	2	150	18	8	48	4	0	80	2	1	1 carb, 2 fat
Old Fashioned Oatmeal	2	110	17	5	41	2	0	150	1	1	1 carb, 1 fat
Old Fashioned Sugar	2	140	19	6	39	2	0	75	1	1	1 carb, 1 fat
Old Fashioned Walnut Fudge	2	130	16	7	48	3	0	90	1	1	1 carb, 1 fat
Peanut Butter	2	150	15	9	54	3	0	115	0	3	1 carb, 2 fat
Rainbow Wafers	8	150	20	8	48	2	0	40	1	1	1 carb, 2 fat
Striped Shortbread	3	170	22	8	42	5	0	75	1	2	1 1/2 carb, 2 fat
Sugared Lemon	2	150	18	8	48	2	0	70	0	2	1 carb, 2 fat
Taffy Sandwich	2	180	25	8	40	2	0	160	2	2	1 1/2 carb, 2 fat
Vanilla Crème	2	180	26	7	35	4	0	100	1	2	2 carb, 1 fat

CAKE, PIE, COOKIES, BROWNIES

	Serving	Calories	Carb. (g)	Fat (g)	% Cal. Fat	Sat. Fat (g)	Chol. (mg)	Sod. (mg)	Fib. (g)	Prot. (g)	Servings/ Exchanges
Mrs. Fields											
Milk Chocolate Chip	1	280	38	13	42	8	15	180	<1	3	2 1/2 carb, 3 fat
Semi-Sweet Chocolate	1	280	32	13	42	8	15	200	1	2	2 carb, 3 fat
Murray Sugar Free											
Chocolate Chip	3	150	20	8	48	3	<5	130	<1	2	1 carb, 2 fat
Chocolate Sandwich	3	120	18	7	53	2	0	110	<1	2	1 carb, 1 fat
Cremes Sandwich	3	120	19	6	45	2	0	55	2	1	1 carb, 1 fat
Lemon Sandwich	3	120	19	6	45	2	0	55	1	1	1 carb, 1 fat
Oatmeal	3	140	20	7	45	2	0	170	<1	2	1 carb, 1 fat
Peanut Butter	3	150	18	7	42	1	<5	160	1	3	1 carb, 1 fat
Shortbread	8	140	22	6	39	1	0	140	1	2	1 1/2 carb, 1 fat
Vanilla Wafers	9	120	23	4	30	1	0	85	<1	2	1 1/2 carb, 1 fat
Nabisco											
Barnum's Animals	10	140	23	4	26	<1	0	150	<1	2	1 1/2 carb, 1 fat

Biscos Sugar Wafers	8	140	21	6	39	1	0	40	0	<1	1 1/2 carb, 1 fat
Café Cremes Cappuccino Sandwich	2	160	22	8	45	1	0	130	0	2	1 1/2 carb, 2 fat
Café Cremes Vanilla Sandwich	2	160	22	7	40	1	0	130	0	2	1 1/2 carb, 1 fat
Café Cremes Vanilla Fudge Sandwich	2	200	27	10	45	2	0	140	1	2	2 carb, 2 fat
Chips Ahoy! Candy Blasts	1	80	9	4	45	2	0	60	0	<1	1/2 carb, 1 fat
Chips Ahoy! Chewy	3	170	24	8	42	2	0	125	<1	1	1 1/2 carb, 2 fat
Chips Ahoy! Chunky	1	80	10	4	45	1	0	35	0	1	1/2 carb, 1 fat
Chips Ahoy! Peanut Butter	1	80	9	4	45	2	0	60	0	<1	1/2 carb, 1 fat
Chips Ahoy! Real Chocolate Chip	3	160	21	8	45	2	0	105	1	2	1 1/2 carb, 2 fat
Chips Ahoy! Reduced-Fat Real Chocolate Chip	3	140	22	5	32	1	0	150	<1	2	1 1/2 carb, 1 fat
Lorna Doone Shortbread	4	140	19	7	45	1	0	130	<1	2	1 carb, 1 fat

CAKE, PIE, COOKIES, BROWNIES

	Serving	Calories	Carb. (g)	Fat (g)	% Cal. Fat	Sat. Fat (g)	Chol. (mg)	Sod. (mg)	Fib. (g)	Prot. (g)	Servings/ Exchanges
Mallomars	2	120	17	4	38	2	0	35	<1	1	1 carb, 1 fat
Mini Chips Ahoy! Real Chocolate Chip	5	150	20	7	42	2	0	95	<1	2	1 carb, 1 fat
Mini Oreo Bite Size!	9	140	21	6	39	1	0	150	1	1	1 1/2 carb, 1 fat
Newtons Apple	2	90	21	0	0	0	0	65	0	1	1 1/2 carb
Newtons Fat-Free Fig	2	90	22	0	0	0	0	115	1	1	1 1/2 carb
Newtons Fig	2	110	22	2	16	0	0	115	1	1	1 1/2 carb
Newtons Peach Apricot Cobblers	1	70	17	0	0	0	0	55	0	1	1 carb
Newtons Raspberry	2	90	21	0	0	0	0	100	<1	1	1 1/2 carb
Newtons Strawberry	2	90	21	0	0	0	0	95	0	1	1 1/2 carb
Nilla Wafers Original	8	140	21	6	39	1	0	115	0	1	1 1/2 carb, 1 fat
Nilla Wafers Reduced-Fat	8	120	24	2	15	0	0	105	0	1	1 1/2 carb
Nutter Butter	2	130	18	5	35	1	0	110	1	2	1 carb, 1 fat

Nutter Butter Bites	10	150	20	6	36	1	0	125	1	3	1 carb, 1 fat
Nutter Butter Peanut Butter Crème Patties	5	160	17	9	51	1	0	80	1	4	1 carb, 2 fat
Old Fashioned Ginger Snaps	4	120	22	2	8	<1	0	230	0	1	1 1/2 carb
Oreo Chocolate Crème	2	150	20	7	42	2	0	130	<1	1	1 carb, 1 fat
Oreo Double Stuf	2	140	19	7	45	1	0	150	0	1	1 carb, 1 fat
Oreo Fudge Mint Covered	1	90	12	4	40	1	0	70	<1	1	1 carb, 1 fat
Oreo Original Chocolate Sandwich	3	160	23	7	39	2	0	220	1	2	1 1/2 carb, 1 fat
Oreo Reduced-Fat Chocolate Sandwich	3	130	25	3	21	1	0	190	1	1	1 1/2 carb, 1 fat
Pecanz	1	90	9	5	50	1	<5	50	0	1	1/2 carb, 1 fat
Pinwheels	1	130	21	5	35	2	0	35	<1	1	1 1/2 carb, 1 fat
Ritz Bits Sandwiches	12	150	22	6	36	1	0	140	<1	1	1 1/2 carb, 1 fat
S'mores											

CAKE, PIE, COOKIES, BROWNIES

	Serving	Calories	Carb. (g)	Fat (g)	% Cal. Fat	Sat. Fat (g)	Chol. (mg)	Sod. (mg)	Fib. (g)	Prot. (g)	Servings/Exchanges
Teddy Grahams, All Varieties	24	130	23	4	28	1	0	150	<1	2	1 1/2 carb, 1 fat
Teddy Grahams Bearwiches, Honey	2	130	19	5	35	1	0	90	0	1	1 carb, 1 fat
Nabisco SnackWell's											
Chocolate Chip Bite Size	13	130	22	4	28	1	0	160	1	2	1 1/2 carb, 1 fat
Chocolate Sandwich	2	110	20	3	25	<1	0	210	<1	1	1 carb, 1 fat
Coconut Crème	2	110	19	4	33	1	0	80	1	1	1 carb, 1 fat
Crème Sandwich	2	110	20	3	25	<1	0	130	0	2	1 carb, 1 fat
Devil's Food Cookie Cakes	1	50	12	0	0	0	0	30	0	1	1 carb
Lemon Crème Sandwich	3	130	23	6	42	1	0	150	0	1	1 1/2 carb, 1 fat
Mint Crème	2	110	19	3	25	1	0	70	<1	1	1 carb, 1 fat
Sugar-Free Chocolate Sandwich	3	130	23	6	42	2	0	170	1	2	1 1/2 carb, 1 fat

Sugar-Free Shortbread	3	130	21	5	35	1	5	150	<1	2 1 1/2 carb, 1 fat
Pepperidge Farm										
Apricot Raspberry Verona	3	140	22	6	39	2	5	110	0	2 1 1/2 carb, 1 fat
Bordeaux	3	130	19	5	35	2	0	95	<1	2 1 carb, 1 fat
Brussels	3	150	20	7	42	3	0	80	1	2 1 carb, 1 fat
Butter Chessman	3	120	18	4	38	3	0	80	0	2 1 carb, 1 fat
Chocolate Chunk Tahoe	1	140	15	8	51	3	10	90	0	2 1 carb, 2 fat
Chocolate Hazelnut Crème Filled Pirouettes	2	130	19	6	42	4	0	60	<1	1 1 carb, 1 fat
Dessert Bliss Chocolate Almond	3	170	22	8	42	2	<5	75	1	2 1 1/2 carb, 2 fat
Dessert Bliss Cookies & Crème	3	170	22	8	42	2	0	60	<1	1 1 1/2 carb, 2 fat
Geneva	3	160	19	9	51	3	0	95	1	2 1 carb, 2 fat
Lemon Nut Crunch	3	170	18	9	47	2	0	60	2	2 1 carb, 2 fat
Milano	3	180	20	10	50	3	0	80	0	2 1 carb, 2 fat

CAKE, PIE, COOKIES, BROWNIES

	Serving	Calories	Carb. (g)	Fat (g)	% Cal. Fat	Sat. Fat (g)	Chol. (mg)	Sod. (mg)	Fib. (g)	Prot. (g)	Servings/ Exchanges
Raspberry Chantilly	2	120	23	3	23	1	0	115	<1	1	1 1/2 carb, 1 fat
Salzburg Chocolate Mocha	2	150	21	6	36	2	0	65	1	2	1 1/2 carb, 1 fat
Shortbread	2	140	16	7	45	2	0	105	<1	2	1 carb, 1 fat
Soft Baked Chocolate Chunk Nantucket	1	150	20	8	48	3	0	95	0	2	1 carb, 2 fat
Soft Baked Chocolate Chunk Sausalito	1	160	19	8	45	3	10	85	0	2	1 carb, 2 fat
Spritzer	5	140	21	7	45	<1	<5	60	0	1	1 1/2 carb, 1 fat
Sugar	3	140	20	6	39	1	0	90	0	2	1 carb, 1 fat
Weight Watchers											
50% Less Fat Chocolate Sandwich	3	140	23	4	26	1	0	160	1	2	1 1/2 carb, 1 fat

Chocolate Chip	2	140	22	5	32	2	0	90	1	2	1 1/2 carb, 1 fat
Fat-Free Raspberry Fruit Filled	1	70	16	0	0	0	0	45	0	1	1 carb
Oatmeal Raisin	2	120	22	2	15	0	0	90	1	2	1 1/2 carb
Vanilla Sandwich	3	140	25	3	19	1		80	1	1	1 1/2 carb, 1 fat

CANDY, SWEETS

	Serving	Calories	Carb. (g)	Fat (g)	% Cal. Fat	Sat. Fat (g)	Chol. (mg)	Sod. (mg)	Fib. (g)	Prot. (g)	Servings/ Exchanges
Almond Roca	1 oz	124	19	5	36	3	3	51	<1	2	1 carb, 1 fat
Almonds, Chocolate-Coated	1/4 cup	234	16	18	69	3	<1	24	4	5	1 carb, 4 fat
Almonds, Sugar-Coated	7	129	20	5	35	<1	0	6	1	2	1 carb, 1 fat
Butterscotch	5 pieces	119	29	1	8	<1	3	13	0	<1	2 carb
Candy Corn	26 pieces	140	36	0	0	0	0	80	0	0	2 1/2 carb
Caramel Apple	1 medium	255	56	4	14	3	3	111	4	2	1 fruit, 4 carb, 1 fat
Caramels	3	116	23	3	23	2	2	74	<1	1	1 1/2 carb, 1 fat
Chewing Gum	1 piece	10	3	0	0	0	0	<1	0	0	free
Chewing Gum, Sugar-Free	1 piece	11	4	<1	0	0	0	<1	0	0	free
Cherries, Chocolate-Covered	2	110	18	4	33	3	0	15	2	<1	1 carb, 1 fat
Divinity, Homemade	1 oz	98	25	3	28	<1	0	13	0	<1	1 1/2 carb, 1 fat

Food	Serving	Cal.	Carb.								Exchanges/Choices
Fruit Leather	0.5 oz	49	12	<1	0	<1	0	9	<1	<1	1 carb
Fudge, Chocolate, Homemade	1 oz	108	23	3	25	1	4	18	4	4	1 1/2 carb, 1 fat
Fudge, Chocolate Marshmallow, Homemade	1 oz	118	20	5	38	3	7	29	0	<1	1 carb, 1 fat
Fudge, Chocolate with Nuts, Homemade	1 oz	124	20	6	44	3	6	27	<1	<1	1 carb, 1 fat
Fudge, Vanilla, Homemade	1 oz	105	23	2	17	<1	5	19	0	<1	1 1/2 carb
Fudge, Vanilla with Nuts, Homemade	1 oz	118	21	4	31	1	4	17	<1	<1	1 1/2 carb, 1 fat
Gumdrops	10 small	139	36	0	0	0	0	16	0	0	2 1/2 carb
Gummy Bears	10 small	85	22	0	0	0	0	15	0	0	1 1/2 carb
Hard Candy, All Flavors	1 oz	106	28	0	0	0	0	11	0	0	2 carb
Jellybeans	10	40	10	<1	0	0	0	3	0	0	1/2 carb
Lollipops	1	22	6	0	0	0	0	2	0	0	1/2 carb

CANDY, SWEETS

	Serving	Calories	Carb. (g)	Fat (g)	% Cal. Fat	Sat. Fat (g)	Chol. (mg)	Sod. (mg)	Fib. (g)	Prot. (g)	Servings/ Exchanges
Milk Chocolate Bar with Almonds	1.5 oz	216	22	14	58	7	8	30	3	4	1 1/2 carb, 3 fat
Milk Chocolate Bar with Peanuts	1.5 oz	235	16	18	69	5	4	17	2	7	1 carb, 4 fat
Mint Patty, Chocolate-Covered	1 small	28	5	<1	0	<1	0	<1	<1	<1	1/2 carb
Peanut Brittle, Homemade	1 oz	129	20	5	35	1	4	128	<1	2	1 carb, 1 fat
Peanuts, Milk Chocolate-Covered	1/4 cup	193	18	13	60	5	3	15	2	5	1 carb, 3 fat
Peanuts, Yogurt-Covered	1/4 cup	194	16	13	60	3	1	15	2	4	1 carb, 3 fat
Penuche Brown Sugar Fudge with Nuts, Homemade	1 oz	112	22	3	24	<1	2	28	<1	<1	1 1/2 carb

Praline, Homemade	1 oz	129	18	7	49	<1	0	18	<1	<1	1 carb, 1 fat
Raisins, Milk Chocolate-Covered	1/4 cup	185	33	7	34	4	1	17	2	2	2 carb, 1 fat
Raisins, Yogurt-Covered	1/4 cup	190	34	6	28	4	4	21	2	2	2 carb, 1 fat
Taffy, Homemade	1 oz	107	26	<1	0	<1	3	25	0	0	2 carb
Toffee, Homemade	1 oz	154	18	9	53	6	30	53	0	0	1 carb, 2 fat
Truffles, Homemade	1 oz	138	13	10	65	5	15	20	<1	2	1 carb, 2 fat
Brands											
BreathSavers											
Breath Mints	4 mints	60	16	0	0	0	0	0	0	0	1 carb
Cadbury's											
Caramello Bar	1.6-oz bar	220	29	10	41	6	10	60	<1	3	2 carb, 2 fat
Concorde											
Bit-O-Honey Chews	6	186	39	4	19	NA	<1	124	NA	1	2 1/2 carb, 1 fat
Hershey's											
5th Avenue Bar	2-oz bar	290	35	14	43	4	0	125	2	5	2 carb, 3 fat

CANDY, SWEETS

	Serving	Calories	Carb. (g)	Fat (g)	% Cal. Fat	Sat. Fat (g)	Chol. (mg)	Sod. (mg)	Fib. (g)	Prot. (g)	Servings/ Exchanges
Almond Joy	1.6-oz bar	220	27	12	49	8	0	65	2	2	2 carb, 2 fat
Chocolate Candy, Sugar-Free	5 pieces	170	25	13	71	8	5	5	2	1	1 1/2 carb, 3 fat
Chocolate Kisses	9	230	24	13	51	8	10	35	1	3	1 1/2 carb, 3 fat
Cookies & Cream Bar	1.5-oz bar	230	26	12	47	6	5	95	0	4	2 carb, 2 fat
Good & Plenty Licorice	1.8 oz	170	43	0	0	0	0	120	0	<1	3 carb
Heath Toffee Bar	1.4-oz bar	210	24	12	52	5	10	125	<1	1	1 1/2 carb, 2 fat
Jolly Rancher Hard Candy, Sugar-Free	4 pieces	35	13	0	0	0	0	0	0	0	1 carb
Kit Kat Bar	1.5-oz bar	220	27	11	45	7	<5	25	<1	3	2 carb, 2 fat
Krackel Bar	1.5-oz bar	210	28	10	43	6	<5	50	<1	2	2 carb, 2 fat
Milk Chocolate Bar	1.5-oz bar	230	25	13	51	9	10	40	1	3	1 1/2 carb, 3 fat
Milk Chocolate Bar, Symphony	1.5-oz bar	230	24	13	51	8	10	40	<1	4	1 1/2 carb, 3 fat
Milk Duds	13	170	28	6	29	3	0	85	0	1	2 carb, 1 fat

Mr. Goodbar	1.75-oz bar	270	27	16	53	7	5	20	2	1 1/2 carb, 3 fat
Reese's Peanut Butter Cups	2 cups	230	23	13	51	5	<5	130	1	1 1/2 carb, 3 fat
Reese's Peanut Butter Cups, Sugar-Free	5 pieces	170	23	12	65	5	<5	115	2	1 1/2 carb, 2 fat
Reese's Pieces	1.5 oz	220	26	11	45	7	0	80	5	2 carb, 2 fat
Reese's sticks	1.5-oz bar	230	23	13	51	5	<5	115	4	1 1/2 carb, 3 fat
Rolo Caramel	1.7 oz	210	31	9	39	7	5	85	2	2 carb, 2 fat
Skor Bar	1.4 oz	210	24	12	51	7	15	120	1	1 1/2 carb, 2 fat
Special Dark Sweet Chocolate Bar	1.5 oz	220	25	12	49	7	<5	0	2	1 1/2 carb, 3 fat
Tootsie Rolls	6 bite-size	160	33	3	17	4	0	40	<1	2 carb
Twizzlers, Strawberry	4 pieces	160	36	1	6	0	0	130	1	2 1/2 carb
Whatchamacallit Bar	1.6 oz	230	29	11	43	8	<5	125	3	2 carb, 2 fat
Whoppers Chocolate Malted Milk Balls	0.75 oz	100	16	4	36	3	0	70	<1	1 carb, 1 fat

CANDY, SWEETS

	Serving	Calories	Carb. (g)	Fat (g)	% Cal. Fat	Sat. Fat (g)	Chol. (mg)	Sod. (mg)	Fib. (g)	Prot. (g)	Servings/ Exchanges
York Peppermint Pattie	1 pattie	160	32	3	16	2	0	10	<1	<1	2 carb, 1 fat
Kraft											
Butter Mints	7 mints	60	14	0		0	0	25	0	0	1 carb
Caramels	5	160	30	4	23	1	<5	130	0	2	2 carb, 1 fat
Fudgies	5	180	32	5	25	3	0	90	0	1	2 carb, 1 fat
M&M Mars											
3 Musketeers Bar	2.13-oz bar	260	46	8	28	5	5	110	1	2	3 carb, 2 fat
M&M's, Chocolate	1.7 oz	240	34	10	38	6	5	30	1	2	2 carb, 2 fat
M&M's, Peanut	1.74 oz	250	30	13	47	5	5	25	2	5	2 carb, 3 fat
Milky Way Bar	2.05-oz bar	270	41	10	33	5	5	95	1	2	3 carb, 2 fat
Snickers Bar	2.07-oz bar	280	35	14	45	5	5	140	1	4	3 carb, 3 fat
Starburst Fruit Chews	2.07-oz bar	240	48	5	19	1	0	0	0	0	3 carb, 1 fat
Twix Caramel Cookie Bar	2-oz bar	280	37	14	45	5	5	115	1	3	2 1/2 carb, 3 fat

Nestlé

100 Grand Bar	1.5-oz bar	200	30	8	36	5	10	75	1	2	2 carb, 2 fat
Baby Ruth Bar	2.1-oz bar	270	36	13	43	7	0	130	2	4	2 1/2 carb, 3 fat
Buncha Crunch Bar	1.4-oz bar	200	26	10	45	6	10	60	<1	2	2 carb, 2 fat
Butterfinger Bar	2.1-oz bar	270	42	11	37	5	0	130	1	3	3 carb, 2 fat
Butterfinger BB's	1.7-oz bag	230	33	9	35	6	0	95	1	2	2 carb, 2 fat
Chunky Bar	1.4-oz bar	210	24	11	47	6	5	20	1	3	1 1/2 carb, 2 fat
Crunch Bar	1.4-oz bar	230	29	12	47	7	10	65	<1	2	2 carb, 2 fat
Demet's Turtles	1	83	10	5	54	2	<5	16	<1	1	1/2 carb, 1 fat
Goobers Chocolate-Covered Peanuts	1.38-oz bag	210	20	13	56	5	5	15	1	4	1 carb, 3 fat
Milk Chocolate Bar	1.5-oz bar	220	26	13	53	8	10	25	<1	2	1 carb, 2 fat
Mocha Crunch	1.3-oz bar	200	21	12	54	7	10	65	0	2	1 1/2 carb, 2 fat
Oh Henry! Bar	0.9-oz bar	120	16	5	38	3	<5	60	0	2	1 carb, 1 fat
Pearson Nips, Caramel	2	60	11	2	30	1	0	40	0	0	1 carb
Pearson Nips, Chocolate	2	60	11	2	30	1	0	40	0	0	1 carb

CANDY, SWEETS

	Serving	Calories	Carb. (g)	Fat (g)	% Cal. Fat	Sat. Fat (g)	Chol. (mg)	Sod. (mg)	Fib. (g)	Prot. (g)	Servings/ Exchanges
Pearson Nips, Chocolate Parfait	2	60	10	2	30	1	0	30	0	0	1 carb
Pearson Nips, Coffee	2	50	10	2	36	2	0	40	0	0	1 carb
Pearson Nips, Peanut Butter Parfait	2	60	10	2	30	2	0	45	0	<1	1 carb
Pecan Turtles, Sugar-Free	3 pieces	160	19	11	63	6	<5	110	1	2	1 carb, 2 fat
Raisinets	1.58-oz box	190	31	8	38	5	<5	15	1	2	2 carb, 2 fat
Sno Caps	2.3-oz box	300	48	13	39	8	0	0	3	2	3 carb, 3 fat
Treasures with Butterfinger	3 pieces	180	24	9	45	5	5	40	<1	2	1 1/2 carb, 2 fat
Treasures, Caramel	3 pieces	180	22	9	45	6	5	55	<1	1	1 1/2 carb, 2 fat
Treasures, Peanut Butter	4 pieces	250	23	17	61	7	5	90	1	4	1 1/2 carb, 3 fat
Turtles Caramel Chocolate	2	160	20	9	51	3	<5	30	<1	2	1 carb, 2 fat
White Crunch	1.4 oz	220	23	13	53	8	10	70	0	3	1 1/2 carb, 3 fat

Peter Paul

Almond Joy Bar	1.76-oz bar	240	29	13	49	8	0	70	2	2	2 carb, 3 fat
Mounds Bar	1.9-oz bar	250	31	13	47	11	0	80	3	2	2 carb, 2 fat

Planters

Peanut Bar	1.6-oz bar	230	22	14	55	2	0	70	2	6	1 1/2 carb, 3 fat

Russell Stover

Mint Patties, Sugar-Free	3 pieces	180	27	11	55	8	0	27	1	2	2 carb, 2 fat
Peanut Butter Cups, Sugar-Free	4 pieces	180	17	13	67	6	0	135	2	4	1 carb, 3 fat
Pecan Delights, Sugar-Free	2 pieces	150	17	11	67	6	0	30	3	2	1 carb, 2 fat

Sweet' Low

Fruits 'n Crème	3-4 pieces	35	13	1	26	0	0	85	0	0	1 carb

Y & S

Nibs Cherry	2.25 oz	220	49	2	8	0	0	135	0	2	3 carb

CHEESE, COTTAGE CHEESE, CREAM CHEESE

	Serving	Calories	Carb. (g)	Fat (g)	% Cal. Fat	Sat. Fat (g)	Chol. (mg)	Sod. (mg)	Fib. (g)	Prot. (g)	Servings/ Exchanges
American Processed	1 oz	106	<1	9	76	6	27	406	0	6	1 high-fat meat
Cheddar	1 oz	114	<1	9	71	6	<1	176	0	7	1 high-fat meat
Cheddar/Colby, Low-Fat	1 oz	49	<1	2	37	2	6	174	0	7	1 lean meat
Cheese, Fat-Free	1 oz	37	3	0	0	0	0	384	0	6	1 very lean meat
Colby & Monterey Jack	1 oz	111	0	9	73	6	30	192	0	7	1 high-fat meat
Cottage Cheese, 2%, Reduced-Fat	1/4 cup	50	2	1	18	<1	5	227	0	8	1 very lean meat
Cottage Cheese, 4.5%	1/4 cup	54	1	2	33	2	8	213	0	7	1 lean meat
Cottage Cheese, Dry	1/4 cup	31	<1	<1	0	<1	2	5	0	6	1 very lean meat
Cottage Cheese, Nonfat	1/4 cup	35	3	0	0	0	5	210	0	7	1 very lean meat
Feta	1 oz	74	1	6	73	4	25	313	0	4	1 med-fat meat
Goat Cheese, Semi-Soft	1 oz	103	<1	9	79	6	22	146	0	6	1 high-fat meat
Monterey Jack	1 oz	106	0	9	76	5	27	152	0	7	1 high-fat meat
Mozzarella, Light	1 oz	65	0	3	42	2	15	180	0	8	1 lean meat

Mozzarella, Part-Skim	1 oz	72	<1	5	63	3	16	132	0	7	1 med-fat meat
Parmesan, Grated	2 Tbsp	46	<1	3	59	2	8	186	0	4	1 lean meat
Ricotta, Part-Skim	1/4 cup	86	3	5	52	3	19	78	0	7	1 med-fat meat
String Cheese Stick	1	72	<1	5	63	3	16	132	0	7	1 med-fat meat
Swiss	1 oz	107	1	8	67	5	26	74	0	8	1 high-fat meat
Yogurt Cheese	1 oz	22	3	<1	0	<1	<1	22	0	2	free
Brands											
Alpine Lace											
Cheddar Cheese, Reduced-Fat	1 oz	90	0	7	67	5	20	200	0	7	1 high-fat meat
CO-JACK Semisoft Cheese, Reduced-Fat	1 oz	90	1	7	70	7	20	135	0	6	1 high-fat meat
Feta Cheese, Reduced-Fat	1 oz	50	1	3	50	2	10	370	0	6	1 lean meat
Hot Pepper American, Reduced-Fat, Reduced-Sodium	1 oz	90	1	6	67	5	20	300	0	6	1 med-fat meat

CHEESE, COTTAGE CHEESE, CREAM CHEESE

	Serving	Calories	Carb. (g)	Fat (g)	% Cal. Fat	Sat. Fat (g)	Chol. (mg)	Sod. (mg)	Fib. (g)	Prot. (g)	Servings/ Exchanges
Mozzarella, Low Moisture, Reduced-Fat	1 oz	70	1	5	64	3	20	250	0	6	1 med-fat meat
Muenster, Reduced-Sodium	1 oz	110	1	9	74	5	25	85	0	7	1 high-fat meat
Provolone, Reduced-Fat, Reduced-Sodium	1 oz	90	1	6	67	4	15	480	0	7	1 med-fat meat
Swiss, Reduced-Fat	1.25 oz	110	0	7	55	5	25	75	0	10	1 high-fat meat
Yellow American, Reduced-Fat, Reduced-Sodium	1 oz	90	1	6	67	5	20	300	0	6	1 med-fat meat
White American, Reduced-Fat, Reduced-Sodium	1 oz	90	1	6	67	5	20	300	0	6	1 med-fat meat

Athenos

Blue Cheese	3 Tbsp	110	2	9	73	6	30	400	<1	7	1 high-fat meat
Gorgonzola	3 Tbsp	110	2	9	73	6	30	400	<1	7	1 high-fat meat
Traditional Feta	1/4 cup	90	2	7	67	4	20	380	<1	5	1 medium fat meat

Breakstone

Cottage Cheese, 1/2% Dry Curd	1/4 cup	45	3	0	0	0	<5	90	0	7	1 very lean meat
Cottage Cheese, Fat-Free	1/2 cup	80	6	0	0	0	5	440	0	13	2 very lean meat
Cottage Cheese, 2% Low-Fat, Small Curd	1/2 cup	90	4	3	30	2	15	390	0	13	2 lean meat
Cottage Cheese, 4% Milkfat, Large Curd	1/2 cup	120	5	5	38	3	25	400	0	13	2 lean meat
Cottage Cheese, 4% Milkfat, Small Curd	1/2 cup	120	5	5	38	3	25	400	0	13	2 lean meat
Cream Cheese, Temp-Tee Whipped	2 Tbsp	80	<1	8	90	5	25	70	0	2	2 fat

CHEESE, COTTAGE CHEESE, CREAM CHEESE

	Serving	Calories	Carb. (g)	Fat (g)	% Cal. Fat	Sat. Fat (g)	Chol. (mg)	Sod. (mg)	Fib. (g)	Prot. (g)	Servings/ Exchanges
Ricotta	1/4 cup	110	3	8	65	5	25	90	0	7	1 high-fat meat
Di Giorno											
100% Romano, Grated	2 tsp	20	0	2	90	1	5	75	0	2	free
100% Romano, Shredded	2 Tbsp	20	0	2	90	1	5	70	0	2	free
100% Parmesan, Shredded	2 Tbsp	20	0	2	90	1	5	75	0	2	free
Knudsen											
Cottage Cheese, 2% Lowfat	1/2 cup	100	5	3	27	2	15	430	0	14	2 very lean meat
Cottage Cheese, Free	1/2 cup	80	7	0	0	0	5	430	0	13	2 very lean meat
Creamed Cottage Cheese, 4%, Small Curd	1/2 cup	120	5	5	38	3	25	430	0	13	2 lean meat
Kraft											
Baby Swiss	1 oz	110	0	9	74	6	25	110	0	7	1 high-fat meat

	Serving	Calories	Carb (g)	Fat (g)	% Fat	Sat. Fat (g)	Chol (mg)	Sodium (mg)	Fiber (g)	Prot (g)	Exchanges
Cheddar	1 oz	120	0	10	75	6	30	180	0	6	1 high-fat meat
Cheddar Cheese Sticks, Mild Cheddar	1 stick	120	0	10	75	6	30	180	0	6	1 high-fat meat
Cheddar, Fat-Free, Shredded	1/4 cup	40	1	0	0	0	<5	270	0	9	1 very lean meat
Cheddar, Natural 2% Reduced-Fat	1 oz	90	<1	6	56	4	20	240	0	7	1 med-fat meat
Cheddar, Shredded	1/4 cup	110	1	9	74	6	25	180	0	6	1 high-fat meat
Cheddar, 2% Reduced-Fat Mild, Shredded	1/4 cup	80	<1	6	63	4	20	230	0	7	1 med-fat meat
Cheddar, Natural 2% Reduced-Fat Sharp	1 oz	90	<1	6	60	4	20	240	0	7	1 med-fat meat
Cheese Cubes, Natural	8 pieces	120	<1	10	75	6	30	210	0	8	1 high-fat meat
Cheese Cubes, Natural 2% Reduced-Fat	7 pieces	90	<1	6	56	4	20	270	0	8	1 med-fat meat
Cheese Spread, Pimento	2 Tbsp	80	3	6	68	4	25	140	0	2	1 med-fat meat

CHEESE, COTTAGE CHEESE, CREAM CHEESE

	Serving	Calories	Carb. (g)	Fat (g)	% Cal. Fat	Sat. Fat (g)	Chol. (mg)	Sod. (mg)	Fib. (g)	Prot. (g)	Servings/ Exchanges
Cheez Whiz Cheese Sauce	2 Tbsp	90	4	7	70	2	5	520	0	3	1 med-fat meat
Cheez Whiz Mild Salsa Con Queso Cheese Sauce	2 Tbsp	90	4	7	70	3	15	500	0	3	1 med-fat meat
Classic Melts Four Cheese Shredded Cheese	1/4 cup	100	2	8	72	5	30	380	0	5	1 high-fat meat
Colby	1 oz	110	<1	9	74	6	30	180	0	7	1 high-fat meat
Colby, Natural 2% Reduced-Fat	1 oz	80	0	6	68	4	20	220	0	7	1 med-fat meat
Colby & Monterey Jack, Shredded	1/4 cup	100	1	8	72	5	25	190	0	6	1 high-fat meat
Cracker Barrel, Spreadable Sharp Cheddar	2 Tbsp	80	<1	8	90	5	20	180	0	3	1 high-fat meat
Cream Cheese, Neufchatel, Philadelphia	1 oz	70	<1	6	77	4	20	120	0	3	1 med-fat meat

Food	Serving										
Cream Cheese, Philadelphia Brick	1 oz	100	<1	10	90	6	30	90	0	2	2 fat
Cream Cheese, Philadelphia Brick, Fat-Free	1 oz	30	2	0	0	0	<5	200	0	4	1 very lean meat
Cream Cheese, Philadelphia Soft	2 Tbsp	90	2	9	90	5	35	130	0	2	2 fat
Cream Cheese, Philadelphia Soft, Chive & Onion	2 Tbsp	90	2	9	90	5	35	160	0	2	2 fat
Cream Cheese, Philadelphia Soft, Fat-Free	2 Tbsp	30	1	0	0	0	<5	200	0	5	1 very lean meat
Cream Cheese, Philadelphia Soft, Light	2 Tbsp	60	2	5	75	3	15	150	0	3	1 fat
Cream Cheese, Philadelphia Soft, Honey Nut	2 Tbsp	90	4	8	80	5	30	125	0	1	2 fat

CHEESE, COTTAGE CHEESE, CREAM CHEESE

	Serving	Calories	Carb. (g)	Fat (g)	% Cal. Fat	Sat. Fat (g)	Chol. (mg)	Sod. (mg)	Fib. (g)	Prot. (g)	Servings/ Exchanges
Cream Cheese, Philadelphia Soft, Pineapple	2 Tbsp	90	4	7	70	5	30	115	0	1	2 fat
Cream Cheese, Philadelphia Soft, Salmon	2 Tbsp	80	2	8	90	5	30	220	0	2	2 fat
Cream Cheese, Philadelphia Soft, Strawberry	2 Tbsp	90	5	8	80	5	30	120	0	1	2 fat
Cream Cheese, Philadelphia Swirls, Triple Berries 'n Cream	2 Tbsp	90	4	8	78	5	30	115	0	1	2 fat
Cream Cheese, Philadelphia Whipped	2 Tbsp	60	1	6	90	4	20	90	0	1	1 fat
Easy Cheese Cheddar Cheese Snack	2 Tbsp	90	2	6	67	3	20	410	0	5	1 med-fat meat
Easy Cheese Cheddar 'n Bacon Cheese Snack	2 Tbsp	90	2	6	67	3	20	430	0	5	1 med-fat meat

Mexican Cheddar Jack, Shredded 2% Reduced-Fat	1/4 cup	110	1	9	73	5	25	190	0	6	1 high-fat meat
Mexican Four Cheese, Shredded	1/4 cup	80	<1	5	56	4	15	240	0	7	1 med-fat meat
Monterey Jack	1 oz	110	0	9	74	6	30	190	0	6	1 high-fat meat
Monterey Jack, Natural 2% Reduced-Fat	1 oz	80	<1	6	68	4	20	240	0	7	1 med-fat meat
Monterey Jack, Shredded	1/4 cup	100	<1	8	72	6	<1	170	0	6	1 high-fat meat
Monterey Jack & Jalapeño Pepper	1 oz	110	<1	9	74	6	30	190	0	7	1 high-fat meat
Mozzarella, 2% Natural, Shredded	1/4 cup	70	<1	4	51	3	15	200	8	9	1 med-fat meat
Mozzarella, Part-Skim, Shredded	1/4 cup	80	5	4	45	4	15	200	0	7	1 med-fat meat
Mozzarella, Part-Skim	1 oz	80	<1	6	68	4	15	200	0	7	1 med-fat meat
Parmesan, Grated	2 tsp	20	0	2	90	1	<5	85	0	2	free

CHEESE, COTTAGE CHEESE, CREAM CHEESE

	Serving	Calories	Carb. (g)	Fat (g)	% Cal. Fat	Sat. Fat (g)	Chol. (mg)	Sod. (mg)	Fib. (g)	Prot. (g)	Servings/ Exchanges
Parmesan & Romano, Grated	2 tsp	20	0	2	90	1	<5	85	0	2	free
Singles American 2% Reduced-Fat	3/4-oz slice	45	2	3	60	2	10	270	0	4	1 lean meat
Singles American Pasteurized Processed Cheese	3/4-oz slice	60	2	5	75	3	15	270	0	4	1 med-fat meat
Singles Fat-Free Pasteurized Processed American Cheese Slice	3/4-oz slice	30	2	0	0	0	<5	250	0	4	1 very lean meat
Singles Fat-Free Pasteurized Processed Sharp Cheddar Cheese	2/3-oz slice	30	2	0	0	0	<5	280	0	5	1 very lean meat

Food	Serving	Cal.								Protein	Exchanges
Singles Fat-Free Pasteurized Processed Mozzarella Cheese	3/4-oz slice	30	2	0	0	0	<5	270	0	5	1 very lean meat
Singles Pasteurized Processed Swiss Cheese Food	3/4-oz slice	70	1	5	64	4	15	320	0	4	1 med-fat meat
Singles Pasteurized Processed White American Cheese	3/4-oz slice	60	2	5	75	3	20	280	0	4	1 med-fat meat
String-Ums 2% Milk String Cheese	1 stick	80	<1	5	50	3	15	220	0	8	1 med-fat meat
Swiss Cheese, Shredded	1/3 cup	100	<1	8	72	5	25	45	0	7	1 high-fat meat
Velveeta Cheese Spread	1 oz	80	3	6	68	4	20	440	0	5	1 med-fat meat
Velveeta Cheese Spread, Mexican, Mild, or Hot	1 oz	80	3	6	68	4	25	400	0	5	1 med-fat meat

CHEESE, COTTAGE CHEESE, CREAM CHEESE

	Serving	Calories	Carb. (g)	Fat (g)	% Cal. Fat	Sat. Fat (g)	Chol. (mg)	Sod. (mg)	Fib. (g)	Prot. (g)	Servings/ Exchanges
Velveeta Light Processed Cheese	1 oz	60	4	3	45	2	15	420	0	5	1 lean meat
Lifetime											
Cheddar, Low-Fat	1 oz	55	1	5	42	1	10	200	1	7	1 med-fat meat
Cheddar, Fat-Free, Shredded	1/4 cup	45	2	0	0	0	<5	310	0	8	1 very lean meat
Jalapeño Jack, Fat-Free	1 oz	40	1	0	0	0	<5	220	0	8	1 very lean meat
Sargento Bistro Blends											
Cheddar Salsa with tomato & Jalapeño Peppers	1/4 cup	110	2	9	73	5	25	190	0	7	1 high-fat meat
Mozzarella & Asiago with Roasted Garlic	1/4 cup	80	2	5	63	4	15	270	0	7	1 med-fat meat
Mozzarella with Sun-Dried Tomatoes & Basil	1/4 cup	90	1	6	67	5	20	220	0	7	1 med-fat meat

Shamrock

Cottage Cheese, 4% Traditional	1/2 cup	110	5	5	41	3	20	430	0	13	2 lean meat
Cottage Cheese, Apple Cinnamon	5.5 oz	120	10	2	15	2	10	460	<1	13	2 very lean meat, 1/2 carb
Cottage Cheese, Fat-Free	1/2 cup	80	4	0	0	0	5	420	0	14	2 very lean meat
Cottage Cheese, Lowfat 2%	1/2 cup	100	5	2	20	2	10	430	0	13	2 very lean meat
Cottage Cheese, Mixed Berry	5.5 oz	180	28	2	10	2	10	420	<1	13	2 very lean meat, 2 carb
Cottage Cheese, Peach	5.5 oz	180	27	2	10	2	10	420	0	13	2 very lean meat, 2 carb
Cottage Cheese, Strawberry Banana	5.5 oz	120	10	2	15	2	10	430	<1	13	2 very lean meat, 1/2 carb

Smart Balance

Cheddar, Par Skim	1 oz	80	<1	5	63	2	5	260	0	7	1 med-fat meat
Mozzarella, Part Skim, Shredded	1 oz	80	<1	5	63	2	5	260	0	7	1 med-fat meat

COMBINATION FOODS

	Serving	Calories	Carb. (g)	Fat (g)	% Cal. Fat	Sat. Fat (g)	Chol. (mg)	Sod. (mg)	Fib. (g)	Prot. (g)	Servings/Exchanges
Beef Burgundy	1 cup	285	10	11	35	3	91	110	2	34	1/2 carb, 5 lean meat
Beef Stroganoff & Noodles	1 cup	342	21	20	53	8	73	454	2	20	1 1/2 carb, 2 med-fat meat, 2 fat
Beef with Macaroni & Tomato Sauce, Homemade	1 cup	254	26	10	35	4	39	862	3	16	2 carb, 2 med-fat meat
Burrito, Bean	1	224	36	7	28	4	2	493	4	7	2 1/2 carb, 1 fat
Burrito, Beef	1	262	30	11	38	6	32	746	<1	13	2 carb, 1 med-fat meat, 1 fat
Cabbage Rolls, Stuffed	8 oz	179	23	6	30	1	11	551	4	8	1 1/2 carb, 1 med-fat meat, 1 fat
Chicken & Noodles, Homemade	1 cup	367	26	19	47	6	96	600	2	22	2 carb, 2 med-fat meat, 2 fat
Chicken a la King, Homemade	1 cup	468	12	34	44	13	186	760	1	27	1 carb, 3 med-fat meat, 4 fat
Chicken Tetrazzini	1 cup	372	28	20	48	7	50	813	2	19	2 carb, 2 med-fat meat, 2 fat

Food	Serving										Exchanges
Chilis Rellenos	1	425	7	35	74	17	165	620	1	23	1/2 carb, 3 med-fat meat, 4 fat
Chili Con Carne with Beans & Rice	1 cup	297	46	8	24	4	25	1162	6	11	3 carb, 2 fat
Chili Con Carne, without Beans	1 cup	350	21	19	49	7	81	1407	4	25	1 1/2 carb, 3 med-fat meat, 1 fat
Chimichanga, Beef & Bean	1	249	26	12	43	3	24	242	3	11	2 carb, 1 med-fat meat, 1 fat
Chop Suey, Shrimp, with Noodles	1 cup	277	22	12	39	2	122	937	2	21	1 1/2 carb, 2 med-fat meat
Chop Suey & Noodles, Beef	1 cup	425	31	25	53	5	46	818	3	22	2 carb, 2 med-fat meat, 3 fat
Chow Mein, Beef, No Noodles	1 cup	275	12	16	52	4	54	774	2	22	1 carb, 3 med-fat meat
Chow Mein, Shrimp, with Noodles	1 cup	277	22	12	39	2	122	937	2	21	1 1/2 carb, 2 med-fat meat
Corndog	1	460	56	19	37	5	79	973	NA	17	4 carb, 1 med-fat meat, 3 fat
Corned Beef Hash, Canned	1 cup	398	24	25	57	12	73	1188	1	19	1 1/2 carb, 2 med-fat meat, 3 fat

COMBINATION FOODS

	Serving	Calories	Carb. (g)	Fat (g)	% Cal. Fat	Sat. Fat (g)	Chol. (mg)	Sod. (mg)	Fib. (g)	Prot. (g)	Servings/ Exchanges
Curry, Beef	1 cup	437	13	32	66	7	70	1323	3	27	1 carb, 3 med-fat meat, 3 fat
Eggplant Parmesan	1 cup	320	17	22	62	10	57	683	3	15	1 carb, 2 med-fat meat, 2 fat
Enchilada, Beef & Cheese	1	323	31	18	50	9	40	1319	NA	12	2 carb, 1 med-fat meat, 3 fat
Enchilada, Chicken	1	195	16	9	42	4	36	312	2	13	1 carb, 2 med-fat meat
Fajita, Chicken	1	405	50	13	29	3	41	439	4	22	3 carb, 2 med-fat meat, 1 fat
Goulash, Beef, with Noodles	1 cup	341	23	14	37	4	88	457	2	30	1 1/2 carb, 3 med-fat meat
Lasagna	8 oz	302	27	12	36	NA	34	885	NA	22	2 carb, 2 med-fat meat
Macaroni & Cheese	1 cup	228	26	10	39	4	NA	730	NA	9	2 carb, 2 med-fat meat
Meat Loaf, Beef & 1/3 Pork	1 slice	205	5	14	61	5	84	381	<1	15	2 med-fat meat, 1 fat
Meat Tamale	1	183	16	10	49	4	24	229	3	7	1 carb, 1 med-fat meat, 1 fat
Meat Tortellini	1 cup	372	33	15	36	5	238	797	1	25	2 carb, 3 med-fat meat
Moo Goo Gai Pan	1 cup	281	12	20	64	5	39	327	3	15	2 vegetable, 2 med-fat meat, 2 fat
Pepper, Stuffed Green Bell	1	229	20	12	47	5	34	201	2	11	1 carb, 1 vegetable, 2 med-fat meat, 2 fat

Food	Serving										Exchanges
Pizza, Cheese, Thin Crust	1/4 of 10-inch	317	28	17	48	7	20	770	NA	14	2 carb, 2 med-fat meat, 1 fat
Pizza, Meat, Thin Crust	1/4 of 10-inch	368	29	21	51	7	29	1000	NA	15	2 carb, 2 med-fat meat, 2 fat
Pot Pie	7 oz	450	35	28	56	NA	34	778	NA	13	2 carb, 2 med-fat meat, 4 fat
Quesadilla	1	199	21	10	45	4	14	255	1	6	1 1/2 carb, 2 fat
Quiche Lorraine	1/8 pie	508	20	39	69	18	205	549	<1	20	1 carb, 3 med-fat meat, 5 fat
Ravioli, Cheese with Tomato Sauce	1	336	38	14	38	6	160	1541	2	14	2 1/2 carb, 1 med-fat meat, 2 fat
Salad, Carrot Raisin	1/2 cup	202	21	14	62	2	10	117	2	1	1/2 fruit, 2 vegetable, 3 fat
Salad, Chef-Style	1 1/2 cup	267	5	16	54	8	140	743	NA	26	1 vegetable, 3 med-fat meat
Salad, Egg	1/2 cup	293	2	28	86	6	287	333	0	8	1 med-fat meat, 5 fat
Salad, Potato, No Egg	1/2 cup	134	16	7	47	1	5	345	2	2	1 carb, 1 fat
Salad, Seafood	1/2 cup	166	3	12	65	2	64	274	<1	13	2 med-fat meat
Salad, Shrimp	1/2 cup	141	3	9	57	2	103	196	<1	13	2 med-fat meat
Salad, Three-Bean	1/2 cup	70	7	4	51	<1	0	257	2	2	1/2 carb, 1 fat
Salad, Tuna	1/2 cup	192	10	10	47	2	13	412	0	16	1/2 carb, 2 med-fat meat
Salad, Waldorf	1/2 cup	201	6	20	90	2	10	118	1	2	1/2 fruit, 4 fat

COMBINATION FOODS

	Serving	Calories	Carb. (g)	Fat (g)	% Cal. Fat	Sat. Fat (g)	Chol. (mg)	Sod. (mg)	Fib. (g)	Prot. (g)	Servings/Exchanges
Salmon Patty/Cake	4.5 oz	261	14	16	55	4	57	657	1	16	1 carb, 2 med-fat meat, 1 fat
Shepherd's Pie, Beef	1 cup	287	31	10	31	3	41	702	3	18	2 carb, 2 med-fat meat
Sloppy Joe Gravy/Sauce, Beef	1 cup	380	24	23	54	9	81	1246	3	21	1 1/2 carb, 2 med-fat meat, 3 fat
Spaghetti with Meatballs	1 cup	258	29	10	35	2	NA	1220	NA	12	2 carb, 2 med-fat meat
Shrimp, Stuffed	1 cup	276	9	14	46	3	221	694	<1	28	1/2 carb, 4 lean meat
Shrimp with Noodles & Cheese Sauce	1 cup	350	24	15	39	6	220	698	2	28	1 1/2 carb, 3 med-fat meat
Souffle, Cheese, Homemade	1 cup	197	6	14	64	6	194	299	<1	12	2 med-fat meat, 1 fat
Souffle, Spinach	1 cup	219	3	18	74	7	184	763	3	12	2 med-fat meat, 2 fat
Sukiyaki	1 cup	175	6	8	41	3	154	762	1	19	1/2 carb, 3 lean meat
Swedish Meatballs with Cream Sauce	1 cup	404	17	23	51	10	162	1157	<1	31	1 carb, 4 med-fat meat, 1 fat

Food	Serving										Exchanges
Sweet & Sour Pork with Rice	1 cup	269	40	6	20	2	29	906	1	13	2 1/2 carb, 1 med-fat meat
Taco, Chicken	1	173	9	8	42	3	45	106	1	15	1/2 carb, 2 med-fat meat
Tostada, Bean & Cheese	1	223	27	10	40	5	30	543	7	10	2 carb, 1 med-fat meat, 1 fat
Tostada, Bean & Chicken	1	248	18	11	40	5	53	434	3	20	1 carb, 2 med-fat meat
Tuna-Noodle Casserole	9 oz	259	34	8	28	NA	NA	1043	NA	13	2 carb, 2 med-fat meat
Turkey-Noodle Casserole	1 cup	326	29	13	36	4	84	732	2	23	2 carb, 2 med-fat meat, 2 fat
Veal Parmigiana	1 cup	350	15	20	51	8	138	755	1	27	1 strch, 3 med-fat meat

Brands

Armour Lunch Makers

Food	Serving										Exchanges
Cracker Crunchers Bologna	1	410	48	20	44	9	45	830	1	9	3 carb, 4 fat
Loco Nachos	1	380	60	14	34	3	20	760	2	2	4 carb, 3 fat
Pepperoni Pizza	1	430	69	13	28	5	25	660	1	8	4 1/2 carb, 3 fat

Betty Crocker

Food	Serving										Exchanges
Chicken Helper, Cheddar & Broccoli	1 cup	310	27	10	29	3	65	790	1	27	2 carb, 3 lean meat

COMBINATION FOODS

	Serving	Calories	Carb. (g)	Fat (g)	% Cal. Fat	Sat. Fat (g)	Chol. (mg)	Sod. (mg)	Fib. (g)	Prot. (g)	Servings/ Exchanges
Chicken Helper, Chicken & Stuffing	1 cup	290	27	9	28	2	60	820	1	25	2 carb, 3 lean meat
Chicken Helper, Chicken Fried Rice	1 cup	250	23	9	32	2	115	670	1	22	1 1/2 carb, 3 lean meat
Chicken Helper, Fettuccine Alfredo	1 cup	270	27	8	27	3	55	800	1	24	2 carb, 3 lean meat
Hamburger Helper, Beef Taco	1 cup	280	29	11	35	4	50	890	1	18	2 carb, 2 med-fat meat
Hamburger Helper, Cheeseburger Macaroni	1 cup	350	34	15	38	6	50	890	1	21	2 carb, 2 med-fat meat, 1 fat
Hamburger Helper, Cheesy Enchilada	1 cup	360	38	15	38	5	60	740	<1	21	2 1/2 carb, 2 med-fat meat, 1 fat
Hamburger Helper, Cheesy Hashbrowns	1 cup	400	36	20	45	6	55	540	2	21	2 1/2 carb, 2 med-fat meat, 2 fat

Food	Serving										Exchanges
Hamburger Helper, Fettuccine Alfredo	1 cup	300	24	14	40	5	55	870	0	20	2 carb, 2 med-fat meat, 1 fat
Hamburger Helper, Lasagna	1 cup	280	26	11	35	4	55	900	1	20	2 carb, 2 med-fat meat
Hamburger Helper, Double Cheese Pizza	1 cup	320	32	12	34	5	55	960	1	21	2 carb, 2 med-fat meat
Hamburger Helper, Potato Stroganoff	1 cup	290	1	14	41	60	23	830	20	18	1 1/2 carb, 2 med-fat meat
Hamburger Helper, Rice Oriental	1 cup	300	31	11	33	4	55	980	0	19	2 carb, 2 med-fat meat
Hamburger Helper, Stroganoff	1 cup	320	26	14	41	5	60	870	1	23	2 carb, 2 med-fat meat, 1 fat
Suddenly Salad, Caesar	1 cup	250	34	10	36	2	0	650	1	6	2 carb, 2 fat
Suddenly Salad, Classic Pasta	1 cup	240	37	8	30	1	0	860	2	6	2 1/2 carb, 2 fat
Suddenly Salad, Ranch & Bacon	3/4 cup	330	31	20	55	3	15	360	1	7	2 carb, 4 fat

COMBINATION FOODS

	Serving	Calories	Carb. (g)	Fat (g)	% Cal. Fat	Sat. Fat (g)	Chol. (mg)	Sod. (mg)	Fib. (g)	Prot. (g)	Servings/Exchanges
Tuna Helper, Creamy Pasta	1 cup	290	30	13	41	4	10	890	1	13	2 carb, 1 med-fat meat, 1 fat
Tuna Helper, Fettuccine Alfredo	1 cup	300	29	14	43	4	20	960	1	12	2 carb, 2 med-fat meat, 1 fat
Tuna Helper, Tetrazzini	1 cup	280	31	11	36	3	10	910	1	15	2 carb, 2 med-fat meat
Tuna Helper, Tuna Melt	1 cup	300	30	13	37	4	20	920	1	12	2 carb, 1 med-fat meat, 1 fat
Campbell's SpaghettiOs											
RavioliOs	1 cup	290	39	10	31	4	20	1160	3	12	2 1/2 carb, 1 med-fat meat, 1 fat
SpaghettiOs Original	1 cup	180	37	1	6	<1	10	890	3	6	2 1/2 carb
SpaghettiOs with Meatballs	1 cup	240	32	8	29	4	25	890	3	11	2 carb, 2 fat
SpaghettiOs with Meat Sauce	1 cup	170	31	2	12	1	10	890	3	8	2 carb
Chef Boyardee											
Beefaroni	1 cup	260	33	10	35	5	25	990	3	10	2 carb, 1 med-fat meat, 1 fat
Cheese Nacho Twistaroni	1 cup	230	36	6	22	3	15	1230	0	8	2 1/2 carb, 1 fat
Hormel Kid's Kitchen											
Beans & Wieners	7.5 oz	320	37	13	34	5	35	760	7	13	2 1/2 carb, 1 med-fat meat, 2 fat

Food	Serving										Exchanges
Cheezy Mac 'n Cheese	7.5 oz	270	32	11	37	6	35	710	1	12	2 carb, 1 med-fat meat, 1 fat
Mac & Beef	7.5 oz	170	24	5	29	3	20	800	2	8	1 1/2 carb, 1 med-fat meat
Oscar Mayer Lunchables											
Cracker Snackers Ham & American	1	430	54	17	37	8	50	1110	<1	15	3 1/2 carb, 1 med-fat meat, 2 fat
Cracker Snackers Turkey & Cheddar	1	430	65	14	28	7	50	1120	0	12	4 carb, 3 fat
Lunchables Nachos	1	540	78	23	39	7	15	860	<1	7	5 carb, 5 fat
Lunchables Pepperoni Flavored Sausage	1	450	66	14	29	7	35	840	1	16	4 1/2 carb, 1 med-fat meat, 2 fat
Lunchables Beef Tacos	1	470	70	13	26	6	40	1180	2	20	4 1/2 carb, 1 med-fat meat, 2 fat
Lunchables Mega Cracker Combo Ham & Cheddar	1	630	81	26	37	10	55	1710	2	19	5 1/2 carb, 1 med-fat meat, 4 fat
Lunchables Mega Deep Dish Pizza	1	630	90	21	29	8	35	1220	2	23	6 carb, 1 med-fat meat, 3 fat

DIPS, SPREADS, SALSA

Brands

	Serving	Calories	Carb. (g)	Fat (g)	% Cal. Fat	Sat. Fat (g)	Chol. (mg)	Sod. (mg)	Fib. (g)	Prot. (g)	Servings/Exchanges
Alouette											
Vegetable & Herb Spreadable Cheese, All Varieties	2 Tbsp	60–70	1	6–7	90	3–4	15–30	80–160	0	1–2	1 fat
Arriba!											
Fire Roasted Salsa, All Varieties	2 Tbsp	10	0	0	0	0	125	2	0	0	free
Athenos											
Hummus, All Varieties	2 Tbsp	50–60	5	3	45	0	0	180–270	1	2	1 fat
Best Food/Hellman's											
Honey Mustard Madness Dippin' Sauce	1 Tbsp	40	4	3	68	0	<5	190	0	0	1 fat

Rockin' Ranch Dippin' Sauce	1 Tbsp	50	0	6	100	1	5	0	0	0	1 fat
Totally BBQ Dippin' Sauce	1 Tbsp	30	5	1	30	1	0	180	0	0	1/2 carb

Cantare Foods

Olive Tapenade	2 Tbsp	70	2	5	64	5	0	310	0	1	1 fat

Dean's

French Onion or Ranch Dip	2 Tbsp	50–60	2	4–5	75	0–1	0	150	0	1	1 fat
Guacamole Dip	2 Tbsp	90	1	9	90	3	5	190	0	1	2 fat
IMO Ranch Dip	2 Tbsp	110	2	11	90	2	10	160	0	1	2 fat

Fritos

Chili Cheese Dip	2 Tbsp	45	3	3	60	1	<5	310	0	1	1 fat
Hot Bean Dip	2 Tbsp	40	5	1	23	0	0	210	1	2	1/2 carb
Jalapeño Cheddar Flavor Cheese Dip	2 Tbsp	50	4	4	72	1	5	300	0	1	1 fat
Original Flavor Bean Dip	2 Tbsp	40	5	1	23	0	0	170	1	2	1/2 carb

DIPS, SPREADS, SALSA

	Serving	Calories	Carb. (g)	Fat (g)	% Cal. Fat	Sat. Fat (g)	Chol. (mg)	Sod. (mg)	Fib. (g)	Prot. (g)	Servings/ Exchanges
Guiltless Gourmet											
Roasted Red Pepper Salsa	2 Tbsp	10	2	0	0	0	0	120	0	0	free
Southwestern Grill Salsa	2 Tbsp	10	2	0	0	0	0	150	0	0	free
Spicy Black Bean Dip	2 Tbsp	30	5	0	0	0	0	100	1	2	free
Herdez											
Salsa Casera	2 tsp	10	1	0	0	0	0	270	0	0	free
Salsa Verde	2 tsp	10	1	0	0	0	0	310	0	0	free
K.C. Masterpiece											
Cool BBQ Dip & Top	1 Tbsp	50	3	4	72	1	<5	125	0	0	1 fat
Honey Dijon Dip & Top	1 Tbsp	45	3	3	60	0	<5	220	0	0	1 fat
Kaukauna/WisPride											
Garden Vegetable Cream Cheese Spread	2 Tbsp	90	2	8	80	5	25	190	0	2	2 fat
Lite Sharp Cheddar Cold Pack Cheese Food	2 Tbsp	70	5	3	39	2	15	190	0	5	1 lean meat

Nacho Cheese Dip	2 Tbsp	80	3	6	68	2	10	330	0	2	1 fat
Port Wine Cold Pack Cheese Food	2 Tbsp	90	3	7	70	3	20	210	0	5	1 high-fat meat
Salsa Con Queso	2 Tbsp	70	5	4	51	3	10	250	0	1	1 fat
Sharp Cheddar Cold Pack Cheese Food	2 Tbsp	90	3	7	70	3	20	210	0	5	1 high-fat meat
Kraft											
American Cheese Spread	2 Tbsp	80	2	6	68	4	20	420	0	4	1 med. fat meat
Bacon Cheese Spread	2 Tbsp	90	1	8	80	5	25	570	0	5	1 high-fat meat
Bacon and Cheddar Dip	2 Tbsp	60	3	5	75	3	<5	180	0	1	1 fat
Cheddar 'n Bacon Cheese Spread	2 Tbsp	90	2	7	70	4	25	140	0	5	1 high-fat meat
Cheez Whiz Light	2 Tbsp	80	6	3	35	2	20	500	0	6	1 lean meat
Cheez Whiz Medium Salsa Con Queso	2 Tbsp	90	4	7	70	3	15	500	0	3	2 fat
Cheez Whiz Original	2 Tbsp	90	4	7	70	2	10	490	0	3	2 fat

DIPS, SPREADS, SALSA

	Serving	Calories	Carb. (g)	Fat (g)	% Cal. Fat	Sat. Fat (g)	Chol. (mg)	Sod. (mg)	Fib. (g)	Prot. (g)	Servings/ Exchanges
Creamy Ranch Dip	2 Tbsp	60	3	4	60	3	0	190	0	1	1 fat
French Onion Dip/Green Onion Dip	2 Tbsp	60	3–4	4	60	3	0	190–210	0	1	1 fat
Nabisco Easy Cheese Cheddar Cheese Spread	2 Tbsp	80	2	6	68	4	20	430	0	5	1 med-fat meat
Nabisco Easy Cheese Nacho Cheese Spread	2 Tbsp	90	3	7	70	4	25	480	0	5	1 med-fat meat
Olive & Pimento Cheese Spread	2 Tbsp	80	3	7	79	4	25	220	0	2	2 fat
Pimento Cheese Spread	2 Tbsp	80	3	6	68	4	25	170	0	2	2 fat
Pineapple Cheese Spread	2 Tbsp	70	4	5	64	3	25	120	0	2	1 fat
Roka Blue Cheese Spread	2 Tbsp	80	2	7	79	4	30	290	0	3	2 fat
Sharp Old English Cheese Spread	2 Tbsp	90	1	8	80	5	25	520	0	5	1 high-fat meat

La Victoria

Salsa, All Varieties	2 Tbsp	10	1-2	0	0	0	0	115-140	0	0 free

Litehouse

Fat-Free Caramel Apple Dip	2 Tbsp	110	28	0	0	0	0	160	0	1 2 carb
Lite Ranch Veggie Dip	2 Tbsp	70	3	6	77	1	10	125	0	1 1 fat
Premium Caramel Apple Dip	2 Tbsp	120	20	5	38	4	0	115	0	1 1 carb, 1 fat
Ranch Veggie Dip	2 Tbsp	120	1	13	98	1	10	180	0	1 3 fat
Spinach Veggie Dip	2 Tbsp	110	2	11	90	1	10	240	0	1 2 fat

Maria's Dip

Dill	2 Tbsp	80	2	8	90	3	20	290	0	1 2 fat
French Onion	2 Tbsp	80	2	8	90	3	20	290	0	1 2 fat
Guacamole Dip	2 Tbsp	90	1	9	90	2	4	190	0	1 2 fat
Lite Ranch	2 Tbsp	80	2	8	90	3	NA	260	0	1 2 fat
Spinach	2 Tbsp	85	3	8	85	3	20	260	0	1 2 fat

DIPS, SPREADS, SALSA

	Serving	Calories	Carb. (g)	Fat (g)	% Cal. Fat	Sat. Fat (g)	Chol. (mg)	Sod. (mg)	Fib. (g)	Prot. (g)	Servings/ Exchanges
Newman's Own											
Bandito Salsa	2 Tbsp	10	2	0	0	0	0	105	1	0	free
Peach Salsa	2 Tbsp	25	6	0	0	0	0	90	1	0	1/2 carb
Pineapple Salsa	2 Tbsp	15	3	0	0	0	0	90	1	0	free
Roasted Garlic Salsa	2 Tbsp	10	2	0	0	0	0	150	1	1	free
Old El Paso											
Thick 'n Chunky Salsa	2 Tbsp	10	3	0	0	0	0	230	0	0	free
Old Wisconsin											
Black Pepper Spreadable Pate	2 oz	210	3	18	77	7	75	530	0	8	1 high-fat meat, 2 fat
Onion & Parsley Spreadable Pate	2 oz	210	3	18	77	7	75	530	0	8	1 high-fat meat, 2 fat

Ortega											
Thick & Chunky Salsa	2 Tbsp	10	2	0	0	0		210	0	0	free
Pace											
Salsa, All Varieties	2 Tbsp	10–15	2–3	0	0	0		200–230	0	0	free
Salsa Con Queso	2 Tbsp	45	4	3	60	1		240	0	0	1 fat
Rojo's											
Guacamole	2 Tbsp	57	3	5	72	1	0	147	2	1	1 fat
Zesty Garlic Salsa	2 Tbsp	10	2	0	0	0		150	0	0	free
Rondele											
French Onion Spreadable Cheese	2 Tbsp	100	1	9	80	6	30	180	0	2	2 fat
Lite Garlic & Herbs Spreadable Cheese	2 Tbsp	60	2	5	75	3	20	190	0	3	1 fat
Ruffles											
French Onion Dip	2 Tbsp	50	2	5	90	2	<5	230	0	1	1 fat
Ranch Dip	2 Tbsp	60	1	5	75	2	<5	240	0	1	1 fat

DIPS, SPREADS, SALSA

	Serving	Calories	Carb. (g)	Fat (g)	% Cal. Fat	Sat. Fat (g)	Chol. (mg)	Sod. (mg)	Fib. (g)	Prot. (g)	Servings/ Exchanges
The Laughing Cow											
Light Creamy Swiss Spreadable Cheese Wedges	1 wedge	35	1	2	51	1	10	260	0	3	1 fat
Original Creamy Swiss Spreadable Cheese Wedges	1 wedge	50	1	4	70	2	15	250	0	2	1 fat
T. Marzetti's											
Blue Cheese Veggie Dip	2 Tbsp	180	1	19	94	3	15	220	0	1	4 fat
Dill Veggie Dip	2 Tbsp	140	2	14	93	3	25	190	0	1	3 fat
Fat-Free Ranch Veggie Dip	2 Tbsp	35	6	0	0	0	0	320	0	1	1/2 carb
French Onion Veggie Dip	2 Tbsp	130	2	13	92	3	25	220	0	1	3 fat
Light Ranch Veggie Dip	2 Tbsp	80	6	6	75	1	10	400	0	0	1/2 carb, 1 fat

Old Fashioned Caramel Apple Dip	2 Tbsp	150	23	6	67	2	4	90	0	1	1 1/2 carb, 1 fat
Peanut Butter Caramel Apple Dip	2 Tbsp	130	16	7	46	1	0	160	1	3	1 carb, 1 fat
Ranch Veggie Dip	2 Tbsp	130	2	13	92	3	25	220	0	1	3 fat
Spinach Veggie Dip	2 Tbsp	140	1	14	86	3	25	240	0	1	3 fat
Tostitos											
Salsa, All Varieties	2 Tbsp	10–15	2–3	0	0	0	0	230–280	0–1	0	free

EGGS, EGG DISHES, EGG PRODUCTS

	Serving	Calories	Carb. (g)	Fat (g)	% Cal. Fat	Sat. Fat (g)	Chol. (mg)	Sod. (mg)	Fib. (g)	Prot. (g)	Servings/ Exchanges
1-Egg Omelet, Plain	1	93	<1	7	68	2	214	165	0	6	1 med-fat meat
1-Egg Omelet, Spanish	1	125	7	9	65	2	126	251	2	5	1 vegetable, 1 med-fat meat, 1 fat
1-Egg Omelet with Cheese & Ham	1	142	<1	11	70	4	231	368	0	10	1 med-fat meat, 1 fat
1-Egg Omelet with Chicken	1	149	<1	10	60	3	287	222	0	13	2 med-fat meat
1-Egg Omelet with Fish	1	132	<1	9	61	3	267	277	0	10	2 med-fat meat
1-Egg Omelet with Mushroom	1	91	1	7	69	2	204	158	<1	6	1 med-fat meat
1-Egg Omelet with Onion, Pepper, Tomato, Mushroom	1	125	7	9	65	2	126	251	2	5	1 vegetable, 1 med-fat meat, 1 fat

Food	Serving										Exchange
1-Egg Omelet with Sausage & Mushroom	1	172	1	13	68	4	254	454	<1	11	2 med-fat meat, 1 fat
Deviled Egg	1/2 egg	95	2	7	66	2	201	201	<1	7	1 med-fat meat
Deviled Egg	1/2 egg	63	<1	5	71	1	121	94	0	4	1 med-fat meat
Egg, Boiled/Cooked	1 extra large	90	<1	6	60	2	246	72	0	7	1 med-fat meat
Egg, Boiled/Cooked	1 jumbo	99	<1	7	64	2	271	79	0	8	1 med-fat meat
Egg, Boiled/Cooked	1 large	78	<1	5	58	2	212	62	0	6	1 med-fat meat
Egg, Boiled/Cooked	1 medium	68	<1	5	66	1	187	55	0	6	1 med-fat meat
Egg, Boiled/Cooked	1 small	57	<1	4	63	1	157	46	0	5	1 med-fat meat
Egg, Fried in Margarine	1 large	92	<1	7	68	2	211	162	0	6	1 high-fat meat
Egg, Scrambled, Plain	1	101	1	7	62	2	215	171	0	7	2 med-fat meat
Egg Substitute	1/4 cup	35	2	0	0	0	0	110	0	7	1 very lean meat
Egg Whites	2	34	<1	0	0	0	0	110	0	7	1 very lean meat
Souffle, Cheese	1 cup	197	6	14	64	6	194	299	<1	12	1/2 reduced-fat milk, 1 med-fat meat, 1 fat

EGGS, EGG DISHES, EGG PRODUCTS

	Serving	Calories	Carb. (g)	Fat (g)	% Cal. Fat	Sat. Fat (g)	Chol. (mg)	Sod. (mg)	Fib. (g)	Prot. (g)	Servings/ Exchanges
Souffle, Spinach	1 cup	218	3	18	74	7	184	763	3	12	1/2 reduced-fat milk, 1 med-fat meat, 2 fat
Brands											
Fleischmann's											
Egg Beaters	1/4 cup	30	1	0	0	0	0	115	0	6	1 very lean meat
Egg Beaters, Cheese & Chive	1/4 cup	35	1	1	26	1.5	<5	210	0	6	1 very lean meat
Egg Beaters, Garden Vegetable	1/4 cup	30	1	0	0	0	0	160	0	6	1 very lean meat
Egg Beaters, Southwestern	1/4 cup	30	1	0	0	0	0	180	0	6	1 very lean meat
Egg Whites	3 Tbsp	25	0	0	0	0	0	75	0	5	1 very lean meat
Morningstar Farms											
Better'n Eggs	1/4 cup	20	0	0	0	0	0	90	0	5	1 very lean meat

	Scramblers	**Papetti Foods** All Whites	Better'n Eggs
	1/4 cup	3 Tbsp	1/4 cup
	35	25	30
	0	0	1
	0	0	0
	0	0	0
	0	0	0
	35	75	115
	0	0	0
	6	5	6
	1 very lean meat	1 very lean meat	1 very lean meat

ETHNIC FOODS

ALASKA NATIVE

	Serving	Calories	Carb. (g)	Fat (g)	% Cal. Fat	Sat. Fat (g)	Chol. (mg)	Sod. (mg)	Fib. (g)	Prot. (g)	Servings/Exchanges
Beach Asparagus	1 cup	15	2	<1	0	NA	0	23	NA	1	free
Caribou, Cooked	1 oz	47	0	1	<1	<1	31	17	0	8	1 very lean meat
Dried Fish/King Salmon	1/2 oz	60	0	5	75	NA	NA	NA	0	7	1 med-fat meat
Fiddlehead Fern, Raw	1 cup	34	5	<1	0	NA	0	84	NA	3	1 vegetable
Gumboots/Leathery Chiton	2 oz	46	0	<1	0	NA	NA	NA	0	10	1 very lean meat
Halibut, Cooked	1 oz	39	0	<1	0	<1	12	20	0	8	1 very lean meat
Herring Eggs, Plain	1/2 cup	48	4	<1	0	NA	NA	52	0	8	1 very lean meat
Highbush Cranberries	1 1/4 cup	58	15	<1	0	NA	0	1	NA	<1	1 fruit
Hooligan, Smoked	1 oz	86	0	7	73	NA	NA	NA	0	6	1 high-fat meat
Huckleberries	1 cup	56	13	<1	0	NA	0	15	NA	<1	1 fruit
Moose, Cooked	1 oz	38	0	<1	0	<1	22	19	0	8	1 very lean meat
Muktuk with Skin and Fat	1x1x2 inches	138	0	12	78	NA	NA	NA	0	8	1 high-fat meat, 1 fat

Food	Serving										Exchanges
Muskrat, Cooked	1 oz	67	0	3	40	0	34	27	0	9	1 lean meat
Pike, Cooked	1 oz	33	0	<1	0	0	14	13	0	7	1 very lean meat
Pilot Bread	1 4-inch round	104	18	2	17	NA	NA	142	NA	2	1 strch
Salmon, Sockeye, Cooked	1 oz	60	0	3	45	<1	24	18	0	8	1 lean meat
Salmonberries	1 1/2 cup	55	13	<1	0	NA	0	52	NA	1	1 fruit
Seal Meat, Raw	1 oz	41	0	<1	0	<1	NA	NA	0	9	1 very lean meat
Seal Oil	1 tsp	45	0	5	100	<1	8	NA	0	0	1 fat
Seaweed, Dried Black	1 cup	39	<1	0	NA	NA	0	40	NA	4	1 vegetable
Sour Dock, Cooked	1/2 cup	19	4	<1	0	NA	0	NA	NA	1	1 vegetable
Venison, Cooked	1 oz	44	0	<1	0	<1	31	15	0	9	1 very lean meat
Walrus, Raw	1 oz	56	0	4	64	<1	22	NA	0	5	1 lean meat
Whale, Bonehead, Raw	1 oz	37	0	<1	0	<1	NA	17	0	7	1 very lean meat
Willow Greens, Cooked	1/2 cup	28	6	<1	0	NA	0	NA	NA	2	1 vegetable

CAJUN & CREOLE

Food	Serving										Exchanges
Alligator, Cooked	1 oz	42	0	0.5	12	<1	19	22	0	9	1 very lean meat

ETHNIC FOODS

	Serving	Calories	Carb. (g)	Fat (g)	% Cal. Fat	Sat. Fat (g)	Chol. (mg)	Sod. (mg)	Fib. (g)	Prot. (g)	Servings/ Exchanges
Beef Tasso	1 oz	47	0	1	19	0.5	12	NA	0	8	1 very lean meat
Café au Lait	8 oz	76	6	4	47	3	17	59	0	4	1/2 whole milk
Couche-couche, No Fat Added	1/2 cup	82	17	<1	0	NA	0	4	1	3	1 strch
Cracklins	1/4 cup	131	0	11	76	4	19	362	0	7	1 high-fat meat, 1 fat
Crawfish, Cooked	2 oz	46	0	0.5	12	<1	81	107	0	10	1 very lean meat
Cushaw Squash	1/2 cup	41	9	0.5	12	<1	0	2	3	1	1 vegetable
Dewberries/Blackberries	3/4 cup	60	15	<1	0	0	0	0	6	<1	1 fruit
Dove, Cooked	1 oz	62	0	4	58	1	33	82	0	7	1 med-fat meat
Frog Legs, Steamed	2 legs (1 1/2 oz)	45	0	<1	0	NA	31	36	0	10	1 very lean meat
Goat, Baked or Roasted	1 oz	45	0	2	40	<1	38	96	0	7	1 lean meat
Guinea, Flesh Only, Cooked	1 oz	42	0	1	21	<1	24	26	0	8	1 very lean meat

Hogshead Cheese	1/4 cup	77	0	6	70	2	29	455	0	6	1 med-fat meat
Kumquats	5	60	16	0	0	0	0	6	4	1	1 fruit
Lamb, Cooked	1 oz	83	0	6	65	3	28	20	0	7	1 med-fat meat
Mirliton/Chayote, Cooked	1/2 cup	24	5	0.5	21	0	0	1	3	<1	1 vegetable
Muscadines (Scuppernongs)	17	60	15	0.5	8	0	0	2	<1	<1	1 fruit
Passionfruit (Maypops)	3	52	13	0	0	0	0	17	1	1	1 fruit
Peas, Crowder, Purple Hull	1/2 cup	92	15	<1	0	<1	0	8	4	7	1 strch
Persimmons (Japanese)	1/2 of 2 1/2 inch	59	16	0	0	0	0	1	1	0.5	1 fruit
Pickled Pigs Feet	1/2 foot	88	0	7	72	2	40	402	0	6	1 high-fat meat
Pork Sausage, Cooked	1 oz	105	0	9	77	3	24	367	0	6	1 high-fat meat
Pumpkin, Cooked	1/2 cup	20	5	0	0	0	0	1	2	<1	1 vegetable
Remoulade Sauce	1 Tbsp	52	<1	6	100	2	7	54	0	<1	1 fat
Salt Pork or Fatback	1/2-inch cube	45	0	5	100	2	5	80	0	<1	1 fat
Satsuma/Mandarin	2 small	62	16	0	0	0	0	1	1	<1	1 fruit

ETHNIC FOODS

	Serving	Calories	Carb. (g)	Fat (g)	% Cal. Fat	Sat. Fat (g)	Chol. (mg)	Sod. (mg)	Fib. (g)	Prot. (g)	Servings/ Exchanges
Shrimp, Dried	36	55	0.5	1	16	<1	79	77	0	11	2 very lean meat
Smoked Beef Sausage	1 oz	89	<1	8	81	3	19	321	0	4	1 high-fat meat
Smoked Pork Sausage	1 oz	110	0	9	74	3	19	426	0	6	1 high-fat meat
Squab, Flesh Only, Cooked	1 oz	60	0	3	45	<1	38	22	0	7	1 lean meat
Tongue, Beef, Cooked	1 oz	80	0	6	68	3	30	17	0	6	1 med-fat meat
Tripe, Cooked	2 oz	57	0	1	16	<1	54	41	0	11	2 very lean meat
Turtle, Cooked	1 1/2 oz	57	0	2	32	<1	26	170	0	10	1 lean meat
CHINESE AMERICAN											
Amaranth/Chinese Spinach, Cooked	1/2 cup	14	3	<1	0	0	0	14	NA	1	1 vegetable
Amaranth/Chinese Spinach, Raw	1 cup	7	1	<1	0	0	0	6	NA	<1	1 vegetable
Arrowheads/Fresh Corn, Large	1	25	5	<1	0	NA	NA	6	NA	1	1 vegetable

Food	Serving										Exchange
Baby Corn, Canned	1/2 cup	13	2	<1	0	NA	0	730	NA	2	1 vegetable
Bamboo Shoots, Canned	1/2 cup	13	2	<1	0	0	0	5	<1	1	1 vegetable
Beef Jerky	1/2 oz	57	2	4	63	2	7	310	<1	5	1 lean meat
Beef Tongue	1 oz	81	<1	6	67	3	30	17	0	6	1 med-fat meat
Bitter Melon/Bitter Gourds Balsam-Pear Pods	1 cup	16	3	<1	0	0	0	5	3	<1	1 vegetable
Bok Choy/Chinese Cabbage/Pakchoi	1/2 cup	9	2	<1	0	0	0	46	<1	1	1 vegetable
Carambola/Star Fruit, Medium	2	60	14	<1	0	0	0	4	5	1	1 fruit
Cellophane/Mung Bean Noodles, Cooked	1/2 cup	67	16	NA	NA	0	0	2	<1	NA	1 strch
Cha Shu Bun, Frozen, Steamed	2	360	50	13	33	5	20	410	1	8	2 strch, 3 fat
Chayote, Raw	1 cup	32	7	<1	0	0	0	5	4	1	1 vegetable
Chinese Banana, Dwarf	1	72	18	<1	0	NA	0	18	NA	2	1 fruit

ETHNIC FOODS

	Serving	Calories	Carb. (g)	Fat (g)	% Cal. Fat	Sat. Fat (g)	Chol. (mg)	Sod. (mg)	Fib. (g)	Prot. (g)	Servings/ Exchanges
Chinese Celery, Raw	1 cup	26	5	<1	0	0	0	116	0	2	1 vegetable
Chinese Eggplant, Purple, Cooked	1/2 cup	17	4	<1	0	NA	0	NA	2	<1	1 vegetable
Chinese Eggplant, White, Cooked	1/2 cup	20	5	<1	0	NA	0	NA	2	<1	1 vegetable
Chinese Sausage	1 oz	100	2	8	72	3	NA	246	NA	6	1 high-fat meat
Chinese/Black Mushrooms, Medium, Dried	2	21	5	<1	0	0	0	1	<1	<1	1 vegetable
Chinese/Peking/Pe-tsai/ Napa Cabbage, Raw	1 cup	12	3	<1	0	0	0	1	<1	<1	1 vegetable
Choy Sum/Chinese Flowering Cabbage	1 cup	9	2	NA	NA	NA	0	NA	NA	1	1 vegetable
Coconut Milk	1 Tbsp	35	<1	4	100	3	0	2	<1	2	1 fat

Food	Serving									Exchange
Coriander, Raw	1 cup	3	<1	0	0	0	4	<1		free
Dried Mung Beans/Green Beans, Cooked	1/2 cup	106	19	<1	0	<1	2	8	7	1 strch, 1 very lean meat
Dried Red Beans, Cooked	1/3 cup	99	19	<1	0	0	6	1	6	1 strch, 1 very lean meat
Garland Chrysanthemum, Raw	1 cup	4	1	0	0	NA	13	NA	<1	free
Ginger Root, Raw	1/4 cup	17	4	<1	0	NA	3	NA	<1	free
Ginkgo Seeds, Canned	1/2 cup	86	~7	1	10	0	238	7	2	1 strch
Guava, Medium	1 1/2	69	16	<1	0	<1	4	7	1	1 fruit
Hairy Melon/Hairy Cucumber, Raw	1 cup	22	5	NA	NA	NA	NA	2	1	1 vegetable
Kumquat, Medium	5	30	16	<1	0	0	6	6	<1	1 fruit
Leeks, Cooked	1/2 cup	16	4	<1	0	0	5	<1	<1	1 vegetable
Litchi/Lychee, Canned	1/2 cup	57	15	<1	0	NA	27	<1	<1	1 fruit
Litchi/Lychee, Raw	10	63	16	<1	0	<1	1	1	<1	1 fruit
Longan, Canned	3/4 cup	68	18	<1	0	0	54	NA	<1	1 fruit

ETHNIC FOODS

	Serving	Calories	Carb. (g)	Fat (g)	% Cal. Fat	Sat. Fat (g)	Chol. (mg)	Sod. (mg)	Fib. (g)	Prot. (g)	Servings/ Exchanges
Longan, Raw	30	58	15	<1	0	0	0	0	1	1	1 fruit
Lotus Root	10 slices	45	14	<1	0	<1	0	33	4	2	1 strch
Luffa, Angled, Raw	1 cup	30	7	<1	0	NA	0	2	NA	1	1 vegetable
Luffa, Smooth/Sponge, Raw	1 cup	34	8	<1	0	NA	0	6	NA	2	1 vegetable
Mango, Small	1/2 cup	68	18	<1	0	<1	0	2	2	<1	1 fruit
Moon Cake, Plain Lotus Seed Paste	1/4	169	24	8	43	NA	2	NA	<1	2	1 1/2 carb, 2 fat
Mung Bean Sprouts, Seed Attached, Raw	1 cup	31	6	<1	0	0	0	6	2	3	1 vegetable
Mustard Greens, Cooked	1/2 cup	11	2	<1	0	0	0	11	1	2	1 vegetable
Mustard Greens, Salted	2 Tbsp	14	4	<1	0	NA	0	NA	NA	<1	free
Oriental Radish/Daikon, Raw	1 cup	16	4	<1	0	0	0	18	1	<1	1 vegetable

Food	Serving										Exchange
Papaya, Medium	1/2	59	15	<1	0	<1	0	5	3	<1	1 fruit
Peapods/Sugar Peas, Cooked	1/2 cup	34	6	<1	0	0	0	3	2	3	1 vegetable
Pepper, Chili, Raw	1 cup	60	14	<1	0	0	0	11	2	3	3 vegetable
Persimmon	1/2	59	16	<1	0	0	0	1	3	<1	1 fruit
Pummelo	3/4 cup	58	14	<1	0	NA	0	1	<1	1	1 fruit
Rice Noodles, Fresh	1/2 cup	99	23	<1	0	0	0	NA	NA	1	1 1/2 strch
Rice Vermicelli, Cooked	1/2 cup	56	13	0	0	0	0	NA	NA	1	1 strch
Salted Duck Egg	1	137	<1	7	46	NA	NA	NA	0	10	1 high-fat meat
Scallop, Dried, Large	1	44	1	<1	0	NA	NA	NA	NA	9	1 very lean meat
Sesame Paste	2 tsp	60	2	5	75	1	0	12	<1	2	2 fat
Sesame Seeds, Whole, Dried	1 Tbsp	52	2	5	87	<1	0	1	1	2	2 fat
Shrimp, Dried, Medium	10	40	2	<1	0	0	NA	NA	NA	7	1 very lean meat
Soybean Milk, Unsweetened	1 cup	81	4	5	56	<1	0	29	3	7	1 med-fat meat

ETHNIC FOODS

	Serving	Calories	Carb. (g)	Fat (g)	% Cal. Fat	Sat. Fat (g)	Chol. (mg)	Sod. (mg)	Fib. (g)	Prot. (g)	Servings/ Exchanges
Soybean Sprouts, Seed Attached, Raw	1 cup	86	7	5	52	<1	0	10	<1	9	1 vegetable, 1 med-fat meat
Soybeans, Cooked	3 Tbsp	56	3	3	48	<1	0	0	2	5	1 lean meat
Squid, Raw	2 oz	52	2	<1	0	<1	132	26	0	9	1 very lean meat
Straw Mushrooms, Canned	1/2 cup	20	4	<1	0	NA	0	172	NA	2	1 vegetable
Sweet Rice Dough Ball	3	220	29	10	41	6	0	0	1	3	2 carb, 2 fat
Taro, Cooked	1/2 cup	94	23	<1	0	<1	0	10	3	<1	1 1/2 strch
Tofu/Soybean Curd	4 oz, 1/2 cup	91	2	6	59	<1	0	8	1	10	1 med-fat meat
Tripe, Beef, Raw	2 oz	56	0	2	32	1	54	26	0	8	1 lean meat
Turnip, Raw	1 cup	35	8	<1	0	0	0	87	2	1	1 vegetable
Water Chestnuts, Chinese	1/2 cup	66	15	<1	0	0	0	9	2	<1	1 strch
Watercress, Raw	1 cup	4	<1	0	0	0	0	14	<1	<1	free
Winter Melon/Wax Gourd/ Chinese Preserving Melon	1 cup	17	4	<1	0	0	0	147	4	<1	1 vegetable

Won Ton, Cantonese Style	5	83	13	<1	0	0	0	850	2	6	1 strch
Yard-Long Beans, Cooked	1/2 cup	24	5	<1	0	0	0	2	NA	1	1 vegetable
Yard-Long Beans, Raw	1 cup	43	8	<1	0	<1	0	4	NA	3	1 vegetable

FILIPINO AMERICAN

Bamboo Shoots, Canned	1/2 cup	13	2	<1	0	<1	0	5	1	1	1 vegetable
Banana Squash, Cooked	1/2 cup	24	6	<1	0	<1	0	2	1	<1	1 vegetable
Banana Sauce	1 tsp	11	3	NA	NA	NA	0	NA	0	0	free
Banana, Native, Small	1	46	12	<1	0	<1	0	0	<1	<1	1 fruit
Beef Shank, Lean, Cooked	1 oz	57	0	2	22	32	<1	18	0	10	1 lean meat
Beef Tongue	1 oz	80	<1	6	30	68	3	17	0	6	1 med-fat meat
Bitter Melon, Cooked	1/2 cup	12	3	<1	0	0	NA	4	NA	<1	1 vegetable
Bottle Gourd, Cooked	1/2 cup	9	2	<1	0	0	NA	NA	<1	<1	free
Cassava Tuber, Cooked	1/2 cup	60	15	<1	0	<1	0	4	<1	<1	1 strch
Ceylon Moss Bar, Dried	1/4	8	2	0	0	0	0	3	<1	<1	free
Chayote, Cooked	1/2 cup	19	4	<1	0	0	0	1	<1	<1	1 vegetable
Chicken Gizzard, Cooked	1 oz	43	<1	1	21	55	<1	19	0	8	1 lean meat

ETHNIC FOODS

	Serving	Calories	Carb. (g)	Fat (g)	% Cal. Fat	Sat. Fat (g)	Chol. (mg)	Sod. (mg)	Fib. (g)	Prot. (g)	Servings/ Exchanges
Chinese Celery, Raw	1 cup	32	5	2	56	NA	NA	48	<1	3	1 vegetable
Chinese Sausage	1 oz	100	2	8	72	3	30	249	NA	6	1 high-fat meat
Chinese Spinach, Raw	1 cup	7	1	<1	0	<1	0	5	NA	<1	free
Clam, Cooked	3, 1oz	42	2	<1	0	0	19	32	0	7	1 lean meat
Coconut Milk, Canned	1 Tbsp	35	<1	4	100	3	0	2	0	<1	1 fat
Corned Beef, Canned	1 oz	71	0	4	51	2	24	285	0	8	1 med-fat meat
Cracklings, Crushed	2 Tbsp	42	0	3	64	<1	9	3	0	4	1 fat
Fish Sauce	1 Tbsp	4	0	<1	0	NA	NA	1088	0	<1	free
Guava, Raw	1 1/2	61	14	<1	0	<1	0	3	7	1	1 fruit
Horseradish Leaves, Cooked	1/2 cup	13	2	<1	0	NA	0	2	NA	1	1 vegetable
Indian Sardines, Dried	1 oz	57	0	1	16	NA	NA	NA	0	11	1 lean meat
Jicama, Cooked	1/2 cup	19	4	0	0	0	0	2	<1	<1	1 vegetable
Long-Jawed Anchovy, Dried	2 Tbsp	64	0	1	14	NA	NA	26	0	12	1 lean meat

Food	Serving										Exchanges
Mango, Small	1/2	61	18	<1	0	<1	0	2	3	<1	1 fruit
Mung Bean Noodles, Cooked	3/4 cup	73	18	0	0	0	0	9	NA	0	1 strch
Mung Beans, Cooked	1/3 cup	71	13	<1	0	<1	0	1	NA	5	1 strch
Native Sausage, Raw	1 oz	167	<1	17	92	NA	NA	NA	0	3	1 high-fat meat, 1 fat
Oriental Radish/Daikon, Raw	1 cup	16	2	0	0	0	0	9	NA	<1	free
Oyster, Cooked, Medium	1	41	3	1	22	<1	38	53	0	5	1 lean meat
Papaya, Unripe, Cooked	1/2 cup	20	5	<1	0	NA	0	3	<1	1	1 vegetable
Papaya, Yellow, Raw, Cubed	1 cup	54	14	<1	0	<1	0	4	2	<1	1 fruit
Peapods, Cooked	1/2 cup	34	6	<1	0	<1	0	3	1	3	1 vegetable
Plantain, Cooked, Sliced	1/2 cup	89	24	<1	0	NA	0	4	2	<1	1 1/2 strch
Pummelo	3/4 cup	62	15	<1	0	NA	0	0	2	1	1 fruit
Rice Sticks/Noodles, Cooked	3/4 cup	91	19	1	10	NA	0	1	<1	1	1 strch

ETHNIC FOODS

	Serving	Calories	Carb. (g)	Fat (g)	% Cal. Fat	Sat. Fat (g)	Chol. (mg)	Sod. (mg)	Fib. (g)	Prot. (g)	Servings/Exchanges
Sausage, Simulated	1 oz	72	3	5	63	<1	0	251	0	5	1 med-fat meat
Sesame Seeds, Dried	1 Tbsp	52	2	5	87	<1	0	1	<1	2	1 fat
Shrimp, Fermented, Small	1 Tbsp	12	0	<1	0	<1	0	734	<1	3	free
Soy Bean Curd/Tofu	1/2 cup	94	2	6	57	<1	0	9	2	10	1 med-fat meat
Spanish Sausage	1 oz	125	NA	11	79	4	30	367	0	7	1 high-fat meat, 1 fat
Swamp Cabbage, Cooked	1/2 cup	9	<1	<1	0	NA	0	63	<1	1	free
Taro, Cooked	1/3 cup	62	15	<1	0	<1	0	6	NA	<1	1 strch
Watermelon Seeds, Dried	1 Tbsp	38	1	3	71	<1	0	6	<1	2	1 fat
Yard-Long Beans, Cooked	1/2 cup	24	5	<1	0	<1	0	2	NA	1	1 vegetable
HMONG											
Asian Pear	1	51	13	<1	0	0	0	0	4	<1	1 fruit
Bamboo Shoots, Canned	1/2 cup	13	2	<1	0	<1	0	4	<1	1	1 vegetable
Beef Tallow	1 tsp	39	0	4	92	2	5	0	0	0	1 fat
Bitter Melon, Raw	1 cup	16	3	<1	0	0	0	5	3	<1	1 vegetable

Food	Serving										Exchanges
Cellophane/Mung Bean Noodles, Cooked	1/2 cup	67	16	NA	NA	0	0	2	<1	NA	1 strch
Chicken Fat	1 tsp	39	0	4	92	1	4	0	0	0	1 fat
Chitterlings, Boiled	2 Tbsp	42	0	4	86	1	20	6	0	1	1 fat
Coconut Cream, Canned	1 Tbsp	36	2	3	75	3	0	10	<1	<1	1 fat
Coconut Milk, Canned	1 Tbsp	30	<1	3	90	3	0	2	0	<1	1 fat
Coconut Milk, Raw	1 Tbsp	35	<1	4	100	3	0	2	<1	<1	1 fat
Coconut, Raw	2 Tbsp	35	2	3	77	3	0	2	<1	<1	1 fat
Condensed Milk, Sweetened	2 Tbsp	123	21	3	22	2	13	46	0	3	1 1/2 carb, 1 fat
Coriander/Chinese Parsley, Raw	1 cup	3	<1	<1	0	0	0	4	<1	<1	free
Cucuzzi Squash, Cooked	1/2 cup	23	5	<1	0	0	0	14	1	<1	1 vegetable
Fish Sauce	1 Tbsp	6	<1	0	0	0	0	1390	0	<1	free
Guava, Medium	1	69	16	<1	0	<1	0	4	7	1	1 fruit
Jackfruit	1/2 cup	78	20	<1	0	0	0	2	1	1	1 fruit

ETHNIC FOODS

	Serving	Calories	Carb. (g)	Fat (g)	% Cal. Fat	Sat. Fat (g)	Chol. (mg)	Sod. (mg)	Fib. (g)	Prot. (g)	Servings/ Exchanges
Leeks, Cooked	1/2 cup	16	4	<1	0	0	0	6	NA	<1	1 vegetable
Luffa Gourd/Squash, Raw	1 cup	30	7	<1	0	NA	0	6	NA	2	1 vegetable
Mango, Small	1/2	68	18	<1	0	<1	0	2	2	<1	1 fruit
Mung Bean Sprouts with Seeds, Cooked	1/2 cup	13	3	<1	0	0	0	6	<1	1	1 vegetable
Mustard Greens	1/2 cup	10	2	<1	0	0	0	11	1	2	1 vegetable
Papaya, Medium	1/2	59	15	<1	0	<1	9	4	3	<1	1 fruit
Peas, Podded, Cooked	1/2 cup	24	6	<1	0	0	0	3	2	3	1 vegetable
Peas, Podded, Raw	1/2 cup	26	5	<1	0	0	0	3	2	2	1 vegetable
Pheasant, No Skin, Raw	1 oz	38	0	1	0	<1	19	10	0	7	1 very lean meat
Pig's Feet	1/2 foot	68	0	4	53	1.5	35	11	0	7	1 med-fat meat
Pork Lard	1 tsp	39	0	4	92	2	4	0	0	0	1 fat
Pork, Ground	1 oz	84	0	6	64	2	27	21	0	7	1 high-fat meat
Pumpkin Blossom, Cooked	1 cup	20	4	<1	0	0	0	8	1	2	free
Pumpkin, Cooked	1/2 cup	24	6	<1	0	0	0	2	1	<1	1 vegetable

Food	Serving										Exchanges
Rice Noodles, Fresh	1/2 cup	99	23	<1	0	0	0	NA	<1	1	1 strch
Squirrel, Roasted	1 oz	49	0	1	18	<1	34	34	0	9	1 very lean meat
Tofu/Soybean Curd	4 oz, 1/2 cup	94	2	6	57	<1	0	9	2	10	1 med-fat meat
Venison	1 oz	45	0	<1	0	<1	32	15	0	9	1 very lean meat
Vinespinach, Raw	1 cup	11	2	<1	0	0	0	13	0	1	free
Yard-Long Beans, Cooked	1/2 cup	102	18	<1	0	<1	0	4	NA	7	1 strch, 1 very lean meat

INDIAN & PAKISTANI

Food	Serving										Exchanges
Aviyal	1/2 cup	81	14	2	22	1	NA	412	NA	2	1 strch
Brinjal, Cooked	1/2 cup	13	3	0	0	0	0	1	1	0	1 vegetable
Chai Masala	1/2 cup	14	3	0	0	0	0	0	NA	1	free
Chicken Tikka	3 1-inch pieces	54	0	2	33	<1	23	156	0	9	1 lean meat
Chickpeas, Cooked	1/2 cup	134	23	2	13	<1	0	6	4	7	1 1/2 strch, 1 lean meat
Coconut, Fresh, Shredded	3 Tbsp	53	2	5	85	4	0	3	1	1	1 fat
Coriander, Fresh	1/2 cup	2	0	0	0	0	0	2	<1	0	free
Cucumber Raita	1/2 cup	21	3	0	22	0	0	22	NA	1	1 vegetable

ETHNIC FOODS

	Serving	Calories	Carb. (g)	Fat (g)	% Cal. Fat	Sat. Fat (g)	Chol. (mg)	Sod. (mg)	Fib. (g)	Prot. (g)	Servings/ Exchanges
Dhakla, Khaman	1-inch square	104	12	5	43	0	NA	539	NA	5	1 strch, 1 fat
Dhansak	1/2 cup	104	15	4	35	0.5	NA	137	NA	4	1 strch, 1 fat
Fresh Shredded Coconut	3 Tbsp	53	2	5	85	4	0	3	1	1	1 fat
Ghee	1 tsp	45	0	5	100	3	20	0	0	0	1 fat
Ginger, Fresh	1/4 cup	17	4	<1	0	0	0	3	0.5	0	free
Green Plantain, Cooked	1/3 cup	60	16	<1	0	0	0	3	1	0	1 strch
Guava, Medium, Raw	1 1/2	61	14	<1	0	<1	0	3	7	1	1 fruit
Idli	3 inch	70	12	0	0	0	0	12	NA	2	1 strch
Jheera Pani	1/2 cup	16	3	0.5	31	0.5	NA	104	NA	1	free
Karela, Cooked	1/2 cup	12	3	0	0	0	0	4	1	1	1 vegetable
Lassi	1 cup	90	13	0	0	0	4	128	0	10	1 skim milk
Mango, Small, Raw	1/2	68	18	<1	0	0	0	2	2	1	1 fruit
Matki Usual	1/2 cup	104	10	6	52	4	0	192	NA	3	1 strch, 1 fat
Mung Bean Sprouts, Cooked	1/2 cup	13	3	<1	0	0	0	6	0.5	1	1 vegetable

Mung Dhal, Cooked	1/2 cup	107	19	<1	0	<1	0	2	8	7	1 strch, 1 very lean meat
Naan	1/4 8 × 2-inch piece	75	13	2	24	<1	9	90	<1	2	1 strch
Phulka/Chappathi	6 inch	68	15	<1	0	<1	0	179	2	3	1 strch
Okra, Cooked	1/2 cup	34	8	0	0	0	0	3	3	2	1 vegetable
Paneer	1 oz	103	12	3	26	2	NA	246	0	8	1 2% milk
Pesrattu	9 inch	127	14	5	35	1	NA	372	NA	5	1 strch, 1 fat
Poha	1/2 cup	140	18	6	39	1	NA	405	NA	2	1 strch, 1 fat
Puri	5 inch	128	16	7	49	<1	0	1	2	3	1 strch. 1 fat
Rasam	1 cup	22	2	1	41	<1	NA	255	NA	1	free
Sambar	1/2 cup	88	6	1	10	0	NA	263	NA	5	1 strch
Tandoori Chicken	1 oz	75	2	4	48	1	NA	152	NA	8	1 med-fat meat
Tomato, Dhal	1/2 cup	132	18	3	20	2	NA	262	NA	7	1 strch, 1 lean meat
Toor Dhal, Cooked	1/2 cup	103	20	<1	0	<1	0	4	5	6	1 strch, 1 very lean meat

JEWISH

Bagel	1/2	78	15	<1	0	<1	0	151	<1	3	1 strch

ETHNIC FOODS

	Serving	Calories	Carb. (g)	Fat (g)	% Cal. Fat	Sat. Fat (g)	Chol. (mg)	Sod. (mg)	Fib. (g)	Prot. (g)	Servings/ Exchanges
Beef Brisket	1 oz	52	1	2	35	<1	16	28	0	6	1 lean meat
Beef Tongue	1 oz	80	<1	6	68	3	30	17	0	6	1 med-fat meat
Bialy	1/2	69	16	0	0	0	0	167	1	7	1 strch
Blintzes	2 1/4 oz	80	13	2	23	<1	118	135	0	6	1 carb
Borekas	1/2 pie	114	15	11	87	5	45	191	<1	5	1 strch, 2 fat
Borscht	1/2 cup	26	5	<1	0	<1	0	473	1	2	1 vegetable
Bulgur, Cooked	1/2 cup	76	17	<1	0	0	0	5	4	3	1 strch
Bulke Roll	1/2 roll	78	15	<1	0	NA	0	137	<1	4	1 strch
Challah	1 oz	81	14	2	22	<1	15	139	<1	3	1 strch
Chicken Liver	1 oz	45	<1	2	40	<1	179	15	0	7	1 lean meat
Chickpeas	1/2 cup	135	23	2	13	<1	0	6	6	7	1 1/2 strch, 1 very lean meat
Corned Beef	1 oz	71	<1	5	63	2	28	321	0	5	1 med-fat meat
Couscous	1/2 cup	88	18	<1	0	0	0	4	1	3	1 strch
Cream Cheese	1 Tbsp	51	<1	5	88	3	16	43	0	1	1 fat

Food	Serving										Exchanges
Farfel	1/2 cup	73	15	<1	0	0	0	0	0	<1	2	1 strch
Flanken, Raw	1 oz	51	0	3	53	1	15	20	0	6	1 lean meat
Gefilte Fish	2 pieces	71	6	2	25	<1	25	440	0	8	1/2 carb, 1 very lean meat
Herring in Wine Sauce	1/4 cup	90	7	4	40	1	25	420	0	5	1/2 carb, 1 med-fat meat
Herring, Pickled	1 oz	74	3	5	61	<1	4	247	0	4	1 med-fat meat
Horseradish, Root	1 Tbsp	7	2	<1	0	0	0	47	<1	<1	free
Kasha, Cooked	1/2 cup	77	17	<1	0	<1	0	3	2	3	1 strch
Kasha, Dry	2 Tbsp	71	15	<1	0	<1	0	2	2	2	1 strch
Kichlach	2-3	106	15	4	34	<1	42	13	<1	3	1 carb, 1 fat
Knishes	1 1/2 oz	114	15	5	39	<1	35	162	1	3	1 strch, 1 fat
Kreplach	2 oz	128	13	4	28	1	62	70	<1	10	1 carb, 1 lean meat
Kugel	1/2 cup	113	17	2	16	<1	31	277	<1	7	1 carb
Leckach	1 oz	84	16	2	21	<1	13	43	<1	1	1 strch
Lentils, Cooked	1/2 cup	115	20	<1	0	0	0	2	8	9	1 strch, 1 very lean meat
Lox	1 oz	33	0	1	27	<1	7	567	0	5	1 very lean meat
Matzoh	3/4 oz	84	18	<1	0	0	0	0	<1	2	1 strch

ETHNIC FOODS

	Serving	Calories	Carb. (g)	Fat (g)	% Cal. Fat	Sat. Fat (g)	Chol. (mg)	Sod. (mg)	Fib. (g)	Prot. (g)	Servings/ Exchanges
Matzoh Ball	3 balls	212	16	13	55	4	127	678	<1	6	1 carb, 2 1/2 fat
Matzoh Meal	2 Tbsp	65	0	<1	0	0	0	0	<1	2	1 strch
Pastrami	1 oz	99	<1	8	73	3	26	348	0	5	1 high-fat meat
Pickles, Dill, Large	1 1/2	36	8	<1	0	<1	0	2596	2	1	1 vegetable
Potato Flour	2 Tbsp	71	14	<1	0	<1	0	11	1	1	1 strch
Potato Pancakes, Medium	1	124	13	7	51	1	13	232	<1	3	1 strch, 1 fat
Pumpernickel Bread	1 oz	71	14	<1	0	<1	0	190	2	3	1 strch
Rye Bread	1 oz	73	14	<1	0	<1	0	187	2	2	1 strch
Sablefish	1 oz	73	0	6	74	1	18	209	0	5	1 med-fat meat
Salmon, Canned	1 oz	39	0	2	46	<1	16	157	0	6	1 lean meat
Sardines, Medium, Canned in Oil, Drained	2	60	0	3	45	<1	41	145	0	7	1 lean meat
Schmaltz	1 tsp	38	0	4	95	1	4	0	0	0	1 fat
Smelt	1 oz	35	0	<1	0	<1	26	22	0	6	1 very lean meat
Sour Cream	2 Tbsp	52	<1	5	87	3	11	13	0	<1	1 fat

Split Peas, Cooked	1/2 cup	116	21	<1	0	0	0	2	8	8	1 1/2 strch, 1 very lean meat
Sweet Wine	4 oz	173	13	0	0	0	0	10	0	2	1 carbohydrate
Tzimmes	1/4 cup	88	21	<1	0	0	0	118	2	1	1 1/2 strch
Whitefish, Smoked	1 oz	31	0	<1	0	0	9	289	0	7	1 very lean meat

MEXICAN AMERICAN

Avocado, Medium	1/8	40	2	4	90	<1	0	3	<1	<1	1 fat
Bolillo, Large	1/4	82	16	<1	0	<1	0	183	<1	3	1 strch
Chayote, Boiled, Drained	1/2 cup	19	4	<1	0	0	0	1	2	<1	1 vegetable
Chorizo	1 oz	129	<1	11	77	4	25	351	0	7	1 high-fat meat, 1 fat
Corn Tortilla	6 inch	58	12	<1	0	<1	0	42	1	2	1 strch
Corn Tortilla, Fat Added	6 inch	102	12	6	53	<1	0	42	1	2	1 strch, 1 fat
Flour Tortilla	6 inch	104	18	2	17	<1	0	153	1	3	1 strch
Flour Tortilla, Fat Added	6 inch	148	18	7	43	1	0	153	1	3	1 strch, 1 fat
Frijoles Cocidos	1/2 cup	117	22	<1	0	<1	0	2	7	7	1 strch, 1 very lean meat
Frijoles Refritos, Fat Added	1/2 cup	161	22	5	28	<1	0	378	7	7	1 strch, 1 very lean meat, 1 fat
Jicama, Raw	1 cup	49	12	<1	0	0	0	5	6	<1	2 vegetable

ETHNIC FOODS

	Serving	Calories	Carb. (g)	Fat (g)	% Cal. Fat	Sat. Fat (g)	Chol. (mg)	Sod. (mg)	Fib. (g)	Prot. (g)	Servings/ Exchanges
Mango, Small, Raw	1/2	68	18	<1	0	<1	0	2	2	<1	1 fruit
Menudo	1 cup	170	1	9	37	4	NA	950	NA	20	3 lean meat
Nopales, Cooked	1/2 cup	11	3	0	0	0	0	15	2	1	1 vegetable
Nopales, Raw	1 cup	14	3	<1	0	<1	0	19	2	1	1 vegetable
Pan Dulce	5 inch	458	59	21	41	NA	NA	389	NA	8	4 carb, 4 fat
Papaya, Raw, Cubed	1 cup	55	14	<1	0	<1	0	4	3	<1	1 fruit
Peppers, Hot Green Chili, Chopped, Raw	1 cup	60	14	<1	0	0	0	11	2	3	2 vegetable
Queso Anejo	1 oz	106	1	9	76	5	30	321	0	6	1 high-fat meat
Queso Asadero	1 oz	101	<1	8	71	5	30	186	0	6	1 high-fat meat
Queso Chihuahua	1 oz	106	2	8	68	5	30	175	0	6	1 high-fat meat
Queso Fresco	1 oz	83	NA	7	76	4	NA	200	0	6	1 med-fat meat
Salsa De Chili	1/4 cup	14	3	<1	0	0	0	166	1	<1	free
Taco Shell	2 6-inch	122	16	6	44	<1	0	95	2	2	1 strch, 1 fat

Verdolagas, Cooked	1/2 cup	10	2	<1	0	0	0	26	1	<1	1 vegetable

NAVAJO

Blue Corn Mush	3/4 cup	94	21	<1	0	NA	0	32	NA	3	1 strch
Corn Hominy, Steamed	1/2 cup	70	13	1	13	<1	0	18	3	2	1 strch
Flour Tortilla	1/4 8-inch	87	19	<1	0	NA	0	211	1	3	1 strch
Mutton, Lean and Fat, Cooked	1 oz	96	0	9	84	NA	NA	NA	0	4	1 high-fat meat
Mutton, Lean, Cooked	1 oz	55	0	3	46	1	21	10	0	8	1 lean meat
Piñon Nuts, in Shell	1 Tbsp, 25	60	<1	6	90	<1	0	7	1	1	1 fat

PLAINS INDIAN

Beans, Dried, Cooked	1/2 cup	117	22	<1	0	<1	0	1	7	7	1 1/2 strch, 1 very lean meat
Beef Fat, Raw	1 tsp	38	0	4	95	2	5	0	0	0	1 fat
Biscuit Mix, Dry	1/4 cup	129	19	5	35	1	19	383	<1	2	1 strch, 1 fat
Buffalo/Bison	1 oz	40	0	<1	0	<1	23	16	0	8	1 very lean meat
Chicken with Skin, Fried	1 oz	76	<1	4	47	1	26	24	0	8	1 med-fat meat
Commodity Meat, Luncheon	1 oz	97	1	9	84	NA	NA	420	NA	3	1 high-fat meat

ETHNIC FOODS

	Serving	Calories	Carb. (g)	Fat (g)	% Cal. Fat	Sat. Fat (g)	Chol. (mg)	Sod. (mg)	Fib. (g)	Prot. (g)	Servings/ Exchanges
Cracklings	1/3 oz	57	0	5	79	2	9	18	0	2	1 fat
Dry Meat	1 oz	47	<1	1	19	<1	12	984	0	8	1 very lean meat
Eggs, Dried Powdered	3 Tbsp	81	0	7	78	2	351	12	0	4	1 med-fat meat
Elk, Roasted	1 oz	41	0	<1	0	<1	0	17	0	9	1 very lean meat
Huckleberries	1 cup	56	13	<1	0	NA	NA	15	NA	<1	1 fruit
Indian Corn, Dried	1/4 cup	132	26	2	14	NA	NA	37	<1	4	2 strch
Kidney, Raw	1 oz	30	<1	<1	0	<1	81	51	0	5	1 very lean meat
Lemon, Raw, Peeled	1	17	5	<1	0	NA	0	1	0	<1	free
Liver, Beef	1 oz	46	1	1	20	<1	110	20	0	7	1 lean meat
Pheasant, Skinless	1 oz	38	0	1	24	<1	0	10	0	7	1 very lean meat
Pilot Bread	4-inch piece	104	18	2	17	NA	NA	142	NA	2	1 strch
Potatoes, Fried	1/2 cup	163	17	11	61	4	NA	19	2	2	1 strch, 2 fat
Short Ribs	1 oz	83	0	5	54	2	0	16	0	9	1 med-fat meat
Sweetbreads, Breaded, Fried	1 oz	108	1	8	67	3	NA	126	0	7	1 high-fat meat

Food	Serving										Exchange
Venison	1 oz	45	0	<1	0	32		15	0	9	1 very lean meat
White Fish, Dry Heat Cooked	1 oz	49	0	2	37	<1	22	19	0	7	1 lean meat
Wild Rice, Zizania Aquatica	1/2 cup	82	17	<1	0	0	0	3	<1	3	1 strch

SOUTHERN & SOUL

Food	Serving										Exchange
Fatback, Raw	1/4 oz	58	0	6	93	2	4	1	0	0	1 fat
Ham Hock	1 oz	90	2	7	70	2	18	383	0	6	1 high-fat meat
Hog Jowl	1 oz	54	0	5	83	2	9	7	0	2	1 fat
Hog Maw	1 oz	45	0	3	60	NA	55	15	0	5	1 lean meat
Hominy	3/4 cup	86	17	1	10	<1	0	252	3	2	1 strch
Kale, Cooked	1/2 cup	21	4	0	0	0	0	15	1	1	1 vegetable
Muscadines	17	60	15	0.5	8	0	0	2	1	<1	1 fruit
Lard	1 tsp	38	0	4	100	2	4	0	0	0	1 fat
Opossum	1 oz	63	0	3	43	NA	23	27	0	9	1 lean meat
Oxtail	1 oz	72	0	4	50	1	30	20	0	9	1 med-fat meat
Pig Ear	1 oz or 1/4 ear	47	0	3	57	NA	26	48	0	5	1 lean meat

ETHNIC FOODS

	Serving	Calories	Carb. (g)	Fat (g)	% Cal. Fat	Sat. Fat (g)	Chol. (mg)	Sod. (mg)	Fib. (g)	Prot. (g)	Servings/ Exchanges
Pig Foot	1/2 foot	68	0	4	53	2	35	58	0	7	1 med-fat meat
Pig Tail	1 oz or 1/3 tail	113	0	10	80	4	37	48	0	5	1 high-fat meat
Poke Salad, Cooked	1/2 cup	16	3	0	0	0	0	NA	1	2	1 vegetable
Pork Brains	1 oz	39	0	3	69	0.5	727	26	0	4	1 lean meat
Pork Cracklings	1 Tbsp	57	0	5	79	2	9	18	0	2	1 fat
Pork Neck Bones	1 oz	66	0	4	55	2	24	20	0	7	1 med-fat meat
Pork Skin (Rind), Fried	1 cup	68	0	4	53	2	17	231	0	8	1 med-fat meat
Pork Tongue	1 oz or 1/3 tongue	77	0	5	58	2	42	31	0	7	1 med-fat meat
Sousemeat (Headcheese)	1 oz	60	0	5	75	1	23	357	0	5	1 med-fat meat
Succotash	1/2 cup	79	17	1	11	0	0	38	5	4	1 strch
Tripe	2 oz	56	0	2	32	1	54	26	0	8	1 lean meat

FAST FOODS

ARBY'S

Roast Beef Sandwiches

	Serving	Calories	Carb. (g)	Fat (g)	% Cal. Fat	Sat. Fat (g)	Chol. (mg)	Sod. (mg)	Fib. (g)	Prot. (g)	Servings/Exchanges
Beef 'n Cheddar	1	440	44	21	41	7	50	1270	2	22	3 carb, 2 med-fat meat, 2 fat
Big Montana	1	590	41	29	44	14	115	2080	3	47	3 carb, 5 med-fat meat, 1 fat
Giant Roast Beef	1	450	41	19	38	9	75	1440	2	32	3 carb, 3 med-fat meat, 1 fat
Junior Roast Beef	1	270	34	9	33	4	30	740	2	16	2 carb, 2 med-fat meat
Regular Roast Beef	1	320	34	13	34	6	45	950	2	21	2 carb, 2 med-fat meat, 1 fat
Super Roast Beef	1	440	48	19	39	7	45	1130	3	22	3 carb, 2 med-fat meat, 2 fat

Other Sandwiches

	Serving	Calories	Carb. (g)	Fat (g)	% Cal. Fat	Sat. Fat (g)	Chol. (mg)	Sod. (mg)	Fib. (g)	Prot. (g)	Servings/Exchanges
Chicken Bacon 'n Swiss	1	550	49	27	44	7	70	1640	2	31	3 carb, 3 med-fat meat, 2 fat
Chicken Breast Fillet	1	500	48	25	44	4	55	1220	3	25	3 carb, 2 med-fat meat, 3 fat
Chicken Fingers	4 pack	640	42	38	55	8	70	1590	3	31	3 carb, 3 med-fat meat, 5 fat
Roast Chicken Club	1	470	39	25	49	7	65	1320	2	27	2 1/2 carb, 3 med-fat meat, 2 fat

FAST FOODS

	Serving	Calories	Carb. (g)	Fat (g)	% Cal. Fat	Sat. Fat (g)	Chol. (mg)	Sod. (mg)	Fib. (g)	Prot. (g)	Servings/Exchanges
Market Fresh Sandwiches											
Chicken Salad	1	770	78	38	44	9	75	1240	9	30	5 carb, 2 med-fat meat, 6 fat
Roast Beef & Swiss	1	780	74	39	45	12	90	1740	6	37	5 carb, 3 med-fat meat, 5 fat
Roast Ham & Swiss	1	700	74	31	39	7	85	2140	5	36	5 carb, 3 med-fat meat, 3 fat
Roast Turkey & Swiss	1	720	74	27	35	6	90	1790	5	45	5 carb, 4 med-fat meat, 1 fat
Roast Turkey, Ranch & Bacon	1	830	75	38	41	10	110	2260	5	49	5 carb, 5 med-fat meat, 3 fat
Ultimate BLT	1	780	75	46	53	9	50	1570	6	23	5 carb, 1 med-fat meat, 8 fat
Market Fresh Wraps											
Chicken Club	1	680	52	38	51	14	100	1800	31	43	3 1/2 carb, 5 med-fat meat, 3 fat
Roast Turkey Ranch & Bacon	1	710	48	39	49	11	110	2420	30	51	3 carb, 6 med-fat meat, 2 fat
Southwest Chicken	1	550	45	30	49	9	75	1690	30	35	3 carb, 4 med-fat meat, 2 fat
Ultimate BLT	1	650	48	47	65	11	50	1730	31	25	3 carb, 2 med-fat meat, 7 fat

Market Fresh Salads

Chicken Club	1	530	32	33	57	10	210	1120	5	30	2 carb, 4 med-fat meat, 3 fat
Martha's Vineyard	1	250	23	8	28	4.5	60	490	4	26	1 1/2 carb, 3 lean meat
Santa Fe	1	520	40	29	50	9	60	1120	5	27	2 1/2 carb, 2 med-fat meat, 4 fat

Salad Dressing

Buttermilk Ranch	1 pkg	330	4	34	91	5	30	660	0	1	7 fat
Light Buttermilk Ranch	1 pkg	110	13	6	55	1	0	470	<1	1	1 carb, 1 fat
Raspberry Vinaigrette	1 pkg	170	16	12	65	2	0	340	0	0	1 carb, 2 fat
Santa Fe Ranch	1 pkg	300	4	31	93	5	20	690	0	1	6 fat

Premium Potatoes

Cheddar Cheese Sauce	1 pkg	60	4	5	67	1	0	360	0	1	1 fat
Curly Fries (Small)	1 order	340	39	18	47	3	0	790	4	4	2 1/2 carb, 4 fat
Curly Fries (Medium)	1 order	410	47	22	49	3	0	950	5	5	3 carb, 4 fat
Curly Fries (Large)	1 order	630	73	34	48	5	0	1480	7	8	5 carb, 7 fat
Homestyle Fries (Small)	1 order	300	44	13	37	2	0	550	3	3	3 carb, 3 fat
Homestyle Fries (Medium)	1 order	380	55	16	37	3	0	690	4	4	3 1/2 carb, 3 fat

FAST FOODS

	Serving	Calories	Carb. (g)	Fat (g)	% Cal. Fat	Sat. Fat (g)	Chol. (mg)	Sod. (mg)	Fib. (g)	Prot. (g)	Servings/ Exchanges
Homestyle Fries (Large)	1 order	570	82	24	37	4	0	1030	6	6	5 1/2 carb, 5 fat
Potato Cakes	2	250	26	15	56	2	0	390	2	2	2 carb, 3 fat
Sidekickers											
Jalapeño Bites (Regular)	5	310	29	19	55	7	30	530	2	5	2 carb, 4 fat
Jalapeño Bites (Large)	10	610	58	37	54	14	55	1050	4	11	6 carb, 7 fat
Mozzarella Sticks (Regular)	4	430	38	23	47	10	45	1370	2	18	2 1/2 carb, 2 med-fat meat, 2 fat
Mozzarella Sticks (Large)	8	850	76	45	48	19	90	2740	4	36	5 carb, 3 med-fat meat, 6 fat
Onion Petals (Regular)	1 order	330	35	19	52	3	0	330	2	4	2 carb, 4 fat
Onion Petals (Large)	1 order	830	88	48	53	7	0	830	5	10	6 carb, 10 fat
Desserts											
Apple Turnover	1	250	35	10	36	3	0	200	2	4	2 carb, 2 fat
Cherry Turnover	1	250	35	10	36	3	0	200	2	4	2 carb, 2 fat

FAST FOODS 181

BOSTON MARKET

Individual Meals

Item	Amount	Cal	Fat					Sodium			Exchanges
1/2 Chicken Spicy Tuscan Rotisserie Chicken	10.2 oz	630	8	34	49	10	295	1370	1	72	1/2 carb, 10 lean meat
1/2 Sweet Garlic Rotisserie Chicken with Skin	9.9 oz	590	4	33	51	10	290	1010	0	70	10 lean meat
1/4 Dark Spicy Tuscan Rotisserie Chicken	4.7 oz	340	4	22	59	6	160	680	1	31	4 med-fat meat
1/4 Dark Sweet Garlic Rotisserie Chicken, No Skin	3.4 oz	190	1	10	47	3	115	440	0	22	3 lean meat
1/4 Dark Sweet Garlic Rotisserie Chicken, with Skin	4.4 oz	320	2	21	59	6	155	500	0	30	4 med-fat meat
1/4 White Spicy Tuscan Rotisserie Chicken	5.6 oz	200	4	5	20	1	95	700	1	37	5 very lean meat

FAST FOODS

	Serving	Calories	Carb. (g)	Fat (g)	% Cal. Fat	Sat. Fat (g)	Chol. (mg)	Sod. (mg)	Fib. (g)	Prot. (g)	Servings/ Exchanges
1/4 White Sweet Garlic Rotisserie Chicken, No Skin or Wing	5 oz	170	2	4	21	1	85	480	0	33	5 very lean meat
1/4 White Sweet Garlic Rotisserie Chicken, with Skin & Wing	5.4 oz	280	2	12	39	4	135	510	0	40	6 lean meat
Crispy-Baked Country Chicken with Gravy	7.4 oz	440	33	23	47	5	35	970	5	26	2 carb, 3 med-fat meat, 2 fat
Double-Sauced Angus Meatloaf	2 slices	510	22	34	61	15	140	890	2	32	1 1/2 carb, 4 med-fat meat, 2 fat
Double-Sauced Angus Meatloaf & Beef Gravy	2 slices	580	27	39	62	16	140	1270	2	33	2 carb, 4 med-fat meat, 3 fat
Double-Sauced Angus Meatloaf & Chunky Tomato	11 oz	550	30	34	56	15	140	1270	3	33	2 carb, 4 med-fat meat, 2 fat

Hand Carved Honey Glazed Ham	5 oz	210	10	8	33	3	75	1460	0	24	1/2 carb, 3 lean meat
Hand Carved Rotisserie Turkey	5 oz	170	3	1	6	0	100	850	0	36	5 very lean meat
North Atlantic Baked Cod	8.8 oz	330	11	16	45	9	130	430	0	37	1 carb, 5 lean meat
Pastry Top Chicken Pot Pie	15 oz	750	57	46	55	14	110	1530	2	26	4 carb, 2 med-fat meat, 7 fat

Hot Side

Butternut Squash	3.9 oz	150	25	6	33	4	20	560	6	2	1 1/2 carb, 1 fat
Creamed Spinach	6.5 oz	260	11	20	70	13	55	740	2	9	1 carb, 1 med-fat meat, 3 fat
Garlic Dill New Potatoes	4.7 oz	130	25	3	15	0	0	150	2	3	1 1/2 carb, 1 fat
Green Bean Casserole	6.1 oz	80	9	5	50	1.5	5	670	2	1	1 vegetable, 1 fat
Green Beans	3 oz	70	6	4	57	0.5	0	250	2	1	1 vegetable, 1 fat
Homestyle Mashed Potatoes	6.2 oz	210	30	9	38	5	25	590	2	4	2 carb, 2 fat
Homestyle Mashed Potatoes with Gravy	7.2 oz	230	32	9	35	5	25	780	3	4	2 carb, 2 fat

FAST FOODS

	Serving	Calories	Carb. (g)	Fat (g)	% Cal. Fat	Sat. Fat (g)	Chol. (mg)	Sod. (mg)	Fib. (g)	Prot. (g)	Servings/ Exchanges
Hot Cinnamon Apples	6.5 oz	250	56	5	16	0.5	0	45	3	0	4 carb, 1 fat
Macaroni & Cheese	6.9 oz	280	33	11	36	6	30	890	1	13	2 carb, 1 med-fat meat, 1 fat
Penne Pasta	5.4 oz	240	29	9	33	5	10	680	2	10	2 carb, 1 med-fat meat, 1 fat
Poultry Gravy	1 oz	15	2	0.5	30	0	0	180	0	0	free
Sauteed Spinach	6.1 oz	90	8	5	50	3	15	550	5	6	1 vegetable, 1 fat
Savory Stuffing	4.7 oz	190	27	8	37	2	5	620	2	4	2 carb, 2 fat
Squash Casserole	6.7 oz	330	20	24	67	13	70	1110	3	7	1 carb, 1 med-fat meat, 4 fat
Steamed Vegetable Medley	3.6 oz	30	6	0	0	0	0	135	2	2	1 vegetable
Sweet Corn	5.2 oz	180	30	4	27	0.5	0	170	2	5	2 carb, 1 fat
Sweet Potato Casserole	6.5 oz	280	39	13	43	5	10	190	2	3	2 1/2 carb, 3 fat
Cold Sides											
Caesar Side Salad	4.3 oz	300	13	26	77	4.5	15	690	<1	5	1 carb, 5 fat
Cranberry Individuals	2.5 oz	130	25	2	13	0	0	0	<1	1	1 1/2 carb

	Amount										Exchanges/Choices
Garden Fresh Coleslaw	15.3 oz	310	29	22	65	3	20	230	10	7	2 carb, 4 fat
Seasonal Fruit Salad	6.2 oz	70	16	0	0	0	0	15	1	1	1 fruit
Sandwiches											
Chicken Carver with Cheese & Sauce	11.3 oz	670	68	33	43	7	90	420	5	38	4 1/2 carb, 4 med-fat meat, 3 fat
Meatloaf Carver with Cheese	13.1 oz	1070	102	55	47	23	190	1480	7	57	7 carb, 5 med-fat meat, 6 fat
Turkey Carver with Cheese & Sauce	11.3 oz	690	68	29	38	7	130	690	5	49	4 1/2 carb, 7 lean meat
Salads & Soups											
Asian Rotisserie Chicken Salad with Dressing & Noodles	22.4 oz	540	57	15	26	3	85	1880	8	41	4 carb, 4 med-fat meat
Caesar Salad Entrée	9.6 oz	470	17	40	77	9	35	1070	3	14	1 carb, 2 med-fat meat, 6 fat
Hearty Chicken Noodle Soup	6.8 oz	100	8	5	40	2	30	500	0	6	1/2 carb, 1 med-fat meat

FAST FOODS

	Serving	Calories	Carb. (g)	Fat (g)	% Cal. Fat	Sat. Fat (g)	Chol. (mg)	Sod. (mg)	Fib. (g)	Prot. (g)	Servings/ Exchanges
Rotisserie Chicken Caesar Salad	14.5 oz	640	19	44	63	11	120	1530	3	46	1 carb, 6 med-fat meat, 3 fat
Tortilla Soup with Toppings	6.6 oz	170	18	8	41	3	25	1060	2	8	1 carb, 1 med-fat meat, 1 fat
Desserts											
Apple Pie	1 slice	550	66	31	51	8	0	240	3	4	4 1/2 carb, 6 fat
Chocolate Brownie	5.1 oz	580	88	23	36	5	95	350	6	9	6 carb, 5 fat
Chocolate Cake	5.7 oz	650	86	32	45	8	60	320	2	4	6 carb, 6 fat
Cornbread	1.6 oz	120	21	4	25	1	5	220	0	1	1 1/2 carb, 1 fat
BURGER KING											
Original WHOPPER											
Original WHOPPER	1	700	52	42	53	13	85	1020	4	31	3 1/2 carb, 3 med-fat meat, 5 fat
Original WHOPPER, Low Carb	1	280	3	20	64	9	75	290	<1	22	3 med-fat meat, 1 fat

Food											Exchanges
Original WHOPPER with Cheese	1	800	53	49	55	18	110	1450	4	35	3 1/2 carb, 4 med-fat meat, 6 fat
Original WHOPPER with Cheese, Low Carb	1	370	5	28	68	14	95	720	<1	27	4 med-fat meat, 2 fat
Original Double WHOPPER	1	970	52	61	57	22	160	1110	4	52	3 1/2 carb, 6 med-fat meat, 6 fat
Original Double WHOPPER, Low Carb	1	540	3	40	67	18	150	380	<1	43	6 med-fat meat, 2 fat
Original Double WHOPPER with Cheese	1	1060	53	69	58	27	185	1540	4	56	3 1/2 carb, 7 med-fat meat, 7 fat
Original Double WHOPPER with Cheese, Low Carb	1	630	5	47	68	23	170	810	<1	48	7 med-fat meat, 2 fat
Original WHOPPER JR.	1	390	31	22	51	7	45	550	2	17	2 carb, 2 med-fat meat, 2 fat
Original WHOPPER JR., Low Carb	1	140	1	10	64	4.5	40	140	0	11	2 med-fat meat

FAST FOODS

	Serving	Calories	Carb. (g)	Fat (g)	% Cal. Fat	Sat. Fat (g)	Chol. (mg)	Sod. (mg)	Fib. (g)	Prot. (g)	Servings/Exchanges
Original WHOPPER JR. with Cheese	1	430	32	26	53	9	55	770	2	19	2 carb, 2 med-fat meat, 3 fat
Fire-Grilled Burgers											
Hamburger	1	310	30	13	39	5	40	550	1	17	2 carb, 2 med-fat meat, 1 fat
Cheeseburger	1	350	31	17	43	8	50	770	1	19	2 carb, 2 med-fat meat, 1 fat
Double Hamburger	1	440	30	23	48	10	75	600	1	28	2 carb, 3 med-fat meat, 2 fat
Double Cheeseburger	1	530	32	31	53	15	100	1030	2	32	2 carb, 4 med-fat meat, 2 fat
Bacon Cheeseburger	1	390	31	20	46	9	60	990	1	22	2 carb, 2 med-fat meat, 2 fat
Bacon Double Cheeseburger	1	570	32	34	54	17	110	1250	2	35	2 carb, 4 med-fat meat, 3 fat
Angus Steak Burger	1	570	62	22	35	8	180	1270	3	33	4 carb, 3 med-fat meat, 1 fat
Angus Steak Burger, Low Carb	1	260	2	18	62	7	180	490	<1	24	3 med-fat meat
Angus Bacon & Cheese	1	710	64	33	42	15	215	1990	3	41	4 carb, 4 med-fat meat, 3 fat

Angus Bacon & Cheese, Low Carb	1	410	4	29	63	14	215	1210	<1	32	5 med-fat meat, 1 fat

Chicken, Fish & Veggie

Chicken WHOPPER	1	570	48	25	40	4.5	75	1410	4	38	3 carb, 4 med-fat meat, 1 fat
Chicken WHOPPER, Low Carb	1	160	3	3.5	19	1	60	850	1	30	4 med-fat meat, 2 fat
Original Chicken Sandwich	1	560	52	28	46	6	60	1270	3	25	3 1/2 carb, 2 med-fat meat, 4 fat
Tendercrisp Chicken Sandwich	1	780	70	45	51	7	55	1730	6	27	4 1/2 carb, 2 med-fat meat, 7 fat
Chicken Tenders	4 piece	170	10	9	53	2.5	25	420	0	11	1/2 carb, 2 med-fat meat
Chicken Tenders	6 piece	250	15	14	52	4	35	630	<1	16	1 carb, 2 med-fat meat, 1 fat
Chicken Tenders	8 piece	340	20	19	50	5	50	840	<1	22	1 carb, 3 med-fat meat, 1 fat
BK Big Fish Sandwich	1	630	69	30	43	5	55	1340	4	23	4 1/2 carb, 1 med-fat meat, 5 fat
BK Veggie Burger	1	420	46	16	36	3	10	1090	7	23	3 carb, 2 med-fat meat, 1 fat

Side Orders

French Fries (Small)	1 order	230	29	11	43	3	0	410	2	3	2 carb, 2 fat

FAST FOODS

	Serving	Calories	Carb. (g)	Fat (g)	% Cal. Fat	Sat. Fat (g)	Chol. (mg)	Sod. (mg)	Fib. (g)	Prot. (g)	Servings/ Exchanges
French Fries (Medium)	1 order	260	46	18	44	5	0	640	4	4	3 carb, 4 fat
French Fries (Large)	1 order	500	63	25	44	7	0	880	5	6	4 carb, 5 fat
French Fries (King)	1 order	600	76	30	45	8	0	1070	6	7	5 carb, 6 fat
Onion Rings (Small)	1 order	180	22	9	44	2	0	260	2	2	1 1/2 carb, 2 fat
Onion Rings (Medium)	1 order	320	40	16	44	4	0	460	3	4	2 1/2 carb, 3 fat
Onion Rings (Large)	1 order	480	60	23	44	6	0	690	5	7	4 carb, 5 fat
Mott's Strawberry Flavored Applesauce	1	90	23	0	0	0	0	0	<1	0	1 1/2 carb
Dipping Sauces											
BBQ Dipping Sauce	1	35	9	0	0	0	0	390	0	0	1/2 carb
Honey Flavored Dipping Sauce	1	90	23	0	0	0	0	0	0	0	1 1/2 carb
Honey Mustard Dipping Sauce	1	90	9	6	67	1	10	150	0	0	1/2 carb, 1 fat

Sweet & Sour Dipping Sauce	1	40	10	0	0	0		65	0	0	1/2 carb
Ranch Dipping Sauce	1	140	1	15	93	2.5	5	95	NA	1	3 fat
Zesty Onion Ring Dipping Sauce	1	150	3	15	93	2.5	15	210	<1	0	3 fat

Salads (without Dressing or Toast)

Side Garden Salad	1	20	4	0	0	0	0	15	<1	1	1 vegetable
Fire-Grilled Chicken Caesar Salad	1	190	9	7	32	3	50	900	1	25	2 vegetable, 3 lean meat
Fire-Grilled Shrimp Caesar Salad	1	180	9	10	50	3	120	880	2	20	2 vegetable, 2 med-fat meat
Tendercrisp Chicken Caesar Salad	1	390	25	22	51	5	40	1160	4	24	1 1/2 carb, 3 med-fat meat, 1 fat
Tendercrisp Chicken Garden Salad	1	410	28	22	49	5	40	1170	5	25	2 carb, 3 med-fat meat, 1 fat

FAST FOODS

	Serving	Calories	Carb. (g)	Fat (g)	% Cal. Fat	Sat. Fat (g)	Chol. (mg)	Sod. (mg)	Fib. (g)	Prot. (g)	Servings/ Exchanges
Fire-Grilled Chicken Garden Salad	1	210	12	7	29	3	50	910	2	26	1 carb, 3 lean meat
Fire-Grilled Shrimp Garden Salad	1	200	12	10	45	3	120	900	3	21	1 carb, 3 lean meat
Salad Dressing & Toppings											
Creamy Garlic Caesar	2 oz	130	7	11	77	2	20	710	0	2	1/2 carb, 2 fat
Fat-Free Honey Mustard	2 oz	70	18	0	0	0	0	230	0	0	1 carb
Garden Ranch	2 oz	120	7	10	75	1.5	20	610	0	1	1/2 carb, 2 fat
Garlic Parmesan Toast	1	70	9	2.5	29	0	0	120	0	2	1/2 carb, 1 fat
Sweet Onion Vinaigrette	2 oz	100	8	8	70	1	0	960	0	0	1/2 carb, 2 fat
Tomato Balsamic Vinaigrette	2 oz	110	9	9	73	1	0	760	0	0	1/2 carb, 2 fat
Desserts											
Dutch Apple Pie	1	300	45	13	40	3	0	270	1	2	3 carb, 3 fat

Hershey's Sundae Pie	1	300	31	18	53	10	10	190	1	3	2 carb, 4 fat

Breakfast

Croissan'wich with Bacon, Egg & Cheese	1	340	26	20	53	7	200	920	<1	14	2 carb, 1 med-fat meat, 3 fat
Croissan'wich with Egg & Cheese	1	300	26	17	50	6	195	700	<1	12	2 carb, 1 med-fat meat, 2 fat
Croissan'wich with Ham, Egg & Cheese	1	340	26	18	47	6	210	1470	<1	17	2 carb, 2 med-fat meat, 2 fat
Croissan'wich with Sausage & Cheese	1	410	24	29	66	11	45	830	1	13	1 1/2 carb, 1 med-fat meat, 5 fat
Croissan'wich with Sausage, Egg & Cheese	1	500	26	36	66	12	220	1060	1	18	2 carb, 2 med-fat meat, 5 fat
French Toast	5	390	46	20	46	4.5	0	440	2	6	4 carb, 4 fat
Hash Browns (Small)	1	230	23	15	57	4	0	450	2	2	1 1/2 carb, 3 fat
Hash Browns (Medium)	1	390	38	25	59	7	0	760	4	3	2 1/2 carb, 5 fat

FAST FOODS

	Serving	Calories	Carb. (g)	Fat (g)	% Cal. Fat	Sat. Fat (g)	Chol. (mg)	Sod. (mg)	Fib. (g)	Prot. (g)	Servings/ Exchanges
Drinks											
Chocolate Milkshake (Small)	1	410	65	13	29	8	50	300	<1	7	4 carb, 3 fat
Chocolate Milkshake (Medium)	1	600	97	18	27	11	70	470	2	10	6 1/2 carb, 4 fat
Chocolate Milkshake (Large)	1	850	133	27	28	17	105	620	2	15	9 carb, 5 fat
Vanilla Milkshake (Small)	1	400	57	15	33	9	60	240	0	8	4 carb, 3 fat
Vanilla Milkshake (Medium)	1	540	76	20	33	13	80	320	0	11	5 carb, 4 fat
Vanilla Milkshake (Large)	1	800	113	29	34	19	120	480	<1	16	7 1/2 carb, 6 fat
CARL'S JR.											
Sandwiches											
Famous Star Hamburger	1	590	50	32	49	9	70	910	3	24	3 carb, 2 med-fat meat, 4 fat
Famous Star with Cheese	1	650	51	37	52	12	85	1170	3	28	3 1/2 carb, 3 med-fat meat, 4 fat

Food	Serving										Exchanges
Super Star Hamburger	1	790	52	47	53	14	130	980	3	41	3 1/2 carb, 4 med-fat meat, 5 fat
Super Star with Double Cheese	1	920	53	57	55	21	160	1490	3	48	3 1/2 carb, 5 med-fat meat, 6 fat
Sourdough Bacon Cheeseburger	1	550	41	29	51	14	85	500	2	31	3 carb, 3 med-fat meat, 3 fat
Double Sourdough Bacon Cheeseburger	1	920	45	59	59	24	170	1020	2	52	3 carb, 6 med-fat meat, 6 fat
Western Bacon Cheeseburger	1	660	64	30	41	12	85	1410	2	32	4 carb, 3 med-fat meat, 3 fat
Hamburger	1	280	36	9	29	4	35	480	1	14	2 1/2 carb, 1 med-fat meat, 1 fat
Charbroiled BBQ Chicken Sandwich	1	370	47	4	9	1	60	1070	4	35	3 carb, 4 very lean meat
Charbroiled Chicken Club Sandwich	1	550	43	23	38	7	95	1330	4	42	3 carb, 4 med-fat meat
Charbroiled Santa Fe Chicken Sandwich	1	610	43	32	48	8	100	1440	4	38	3 carb, 4 med-fat meat, 2 fat

FAST FOODS

	Serving	Calories	Carb. (g)	Fat (g)	% Cal. Fat	Sat. Fat (g)	Chol. (mg)	Sod. (mg)	Fib. (g)	Prot. (g)	Servings/ Exchanges
Carl's Ranch Crispy Chicken Sandwich	1	660	72	31	42	7	70	1180	3	24	5 carb, 1 med-fat meat, 5 fat
Carl's Bacon Swiss Crispy Chicken Sandwich	1	750	91	28	33	11	80	1900	3	31	6 carb, 2 med-fat meat, 4 fat
Spicy Chicken Sandwich	1	480	48	26	48	5	40	1220	2	14	3 carb, 1 med-fat meat, 4 fat
Carl's Catch Fish Sandwich	1	560	58	27	45	7	80	990	2	19	4 carb, 1 med-fat meat, 4 fat
The Six Dollar Burger	1	1000	72	62	56	25	135	1690	6	39	5 carb, 3 med-fat meat, 9 fat
The Western Bacon Six Dollar Burger	1	1060	79	61	52	27	135	2180	2	45	5 carb, 4 med-fat meat, 10 fat
Chili Burger	1	690	57	35	46	15	110	1400	5	39	4 carb, 4 med-fat meat, 3 fat
Sides											
French Fries (Small)	1 order	290	37	14	41	3	0	170	3	5	2 1/2 carb, 3 fat
French Fries (Medium)	1 order	460	59	22	43	5	0	280	5	7	4 carb, 4 fat
French Fries (Large)	1 order	620	80	29	45	8	0	380	7	10	5 carb, 6 fat

Chicken Breast Strips	3 piece	380	27	21	53	4	55	1360	1	22	2 carb, 2 med-fat meat, 2 fat
Chicken Stars	6 piece	270	15	17	56	5	40	500	0	14	1 carb, 2 med-fat meat, 1 fat
Chili Cheese Fries	1 order	920	89	51	50	16	65	1030	9	29	6 carb, 2 med-fat meat, 8 fat
CrissCut Fries	- order	410	43	24	54	5	0	950	4	5	3 carb, 5 fat
Hash Brown Nuggets	1 order	330	32	21	58	5	0	470	3	3	2 carb, 4 fat
Onion Rings	1 order	440	53	22	43	5	0	700	3	7	3 1/2 carb, 4 fat
Zucchini	1 order	320	31	19	53	5	0	860	2	6	2 carb, 4 fat

Baked Potatoes

Bacon & Cheese	1	620	71	29	42	8	40	1160	7	22	5 carb, 1 med-fat meat, 5 fat
Broccoli & Cheese	1	510	71	21	37	5	15	941	7	12	5 carb, 4 fat
Plain Potato	1	280	63	0	0	0	0	30	7	7	4 carb
Plain Potato with Margarine	1	380	63	12	29	2	0	140	7	7	4 carb, 2 fat

Salads

Charbroiled Chicken Salad-To-Go	1	330	17	7	21	4	75	880	5	34	1 carb, 4 very lean meat

FAST FOODS

	Serving	Calories	Carb. (g)	Fat (g)	% Cal. Fat	Sat. Fat (g)	Chol. (mg)	Sod. (mg)	Fib. (g)	Prot. (g)	Servings/Exchanges
Garden Salad-To-Go	1	120	5	3	21	2	5	230	2	3	1 vegetable, 1 fat
Buffalo Ranch Chicken Salad	1	380	42	16	39	3	35	1180	6	19	3 carb, 2 med-fat meat, 1 fat
Breakfast											
Sourdough Breakfast Sandwich No Meat	1	410	39	19	41	9	255	510	2	21	2 1/2 carb, 2 med-fat meat, 2 fat
Sourdough Breakfast Sandwich with Bacon	1	470	39	24	47	11	305	680	2	25	2 1/2 carb, 3 med-fat meat, 2 fat
Sourdough Breakfast Sandwich with Ham	1	450	40	20	40	9	270	950	2	28	2 1/2 carb, 3 med-fat meat, 1 fat
Sourdough Breakfast Sandwich with Sausage	1	610	39	37	54	16	290	1040	2	28	2 1/2 carb, 3 med-fat meat, 4 fat
Croissant Sunrise Sandwich No Meat	1	360	28	21	53	8	245	470	0	13	2 carb, 1 med-fat meat, 3 fat

Croissant Sunrise Sandwich with Bacon	1	410	29	25	56	9	255	610	0	16	2 carb, 1 med-fat meat, 4 fat
Croissant Sunrise Sandwich with Sausage	1	550	31	40	65	14	285	970	0	21	2 carb, 2 med-fat meat, 6 fat
Breakfast Burrito	1	560	37	32	50	11	495	980	1	29	2 1/2 carb, 3 med-fat meat, 3 fat
Scrambled Egg Breakfast-Sausage	1	900	72	56	57	15	525	1480	5	27	5 carb, 2 med-fat meat, 9 fat
Breakfast Quesadilla	1	390	38	18	41	5	285	920	2	17	2 1/2 carb, 2 med-fat meat, 2 fat
French Toast Dips	5 piece	450	59	20	40	6	5	570	0	10	4 carb, 4 fat
CINNABON											
Caramel Pecanbon	1	1100	141	56	46	NA	NA	NA	8	NA	9 carb, 11 fat
CinnabonStix	5 sticks	350	54	11	28	NA	NA	NA	<1	NA	3 1/2 carb, 2 fat
Cinnapack (6-pack to go box)	1/2 roll	440	59	20	41	NA	NA	NA	4	NA	4 carb, 4 fat
Classic Cinnabon	1	730	114	24	30	NA	NA	NA	2	NA	7 1/2 carb, 5 fat
Minibon	1	300	45	11	33	NA	NA	NA	<1	NA	3 carb, 2 fat

FAST FOODS

DAIRY QUEEN

Burgers

	Serving	Calories	Carb. (g)	Fat (g)	% Cal. Fat	Sat. Fat (g)	Chol. (mg)	Sod. (mg)	Fib. (g)	Prot. (g)	Servings/Exchanges
DQ Homestyle Burger	1	290	29	12	38	5	45	630	2	17	2 carb, 2 med-fat meat
DQ Homestyle Cheeseburger	1	340	29	17	44	8	55	850	2	20	2 carb, 2 med-fat meat, 1 fat
DQ Homestyle Double Cheeseburger	1	540	30	31	52	16	115	1130	2	35	2 carb, 4 med-fat meat, 2 fat
DQ Homestyle Bacon Double Cheeseburger	1	610	31	36	52	18	130	1380	2	41	2 carb, 5 med-fat meat, 2 fat
DQ Ultimate Burger	1	670	29	43	58	19	135	1210	2	40	2 carb, 5 med-fat meat, 4 fat
FlameThrower Burger	1	810	27	60	67	22	160	1390	2	43	2 carb, 5 med-fat meat, 7 fat
Classic GrillBurger	1	540	41	30	50	11	65	990	2	27	3 carb, 3 med-fat meat, 3 fat
Classic GrillBurger with Cheese	1	610	41	36	54	15	85	1110	2	31	3 carb, 3 med-fat meat, 4 fat

	Serving	Calories	Carb. (g)	Fat (g)	% Fat Cal.	Sat. Fat (g)	Chol. (mg)	Sodium (mg)	Fiber (g)	Prot. (g)	Exchanges
1/2 lb. GrillBurger	1	800	41	50	56	21	130	1230	2	47	3 carb, 5 med-fat meat, 5 fat
1/2 lb. GrillBurger with Cheese	1	930	41	60	58	27	160	1380	2	56	3 carb, 7 med-fat meat, 5 fat
Bacon Cheese GrillBurger	1	710	40	45	58	19	105	1430	1	36	2 1/2 carb, 4 med-fat meat, 5 fat
Mushroom Swiss GrillBurger	1	700	37	47	60	16	90	890	1	30	2 1/2 carb, 3 med-fat meat, 6 fat
Hot Dogs											
Hot Dog	1	240	19	14	50	5	25	730	1	9	1 carb, 1 med-fat meat, 2 fat
Chili 'N' Cheese Dog	1	330	22	21	58	9	45	1090	2	14	1 1/2 carb, 1 med-fat meat, 3 fat
Sandwiches/Baskets											
Crispy Chicken Sandwich	1	590	50	34	53	6	40	1100	5	21	3 carb, 2 med-fat meat, 5 fat
Grilled Chicken Sandwich	1	340	26	16	44	3	55	1000	2	22	2 carb, 2 med-fat meat, 1 fat
Chicken Strip Basket	4 piece	920	92	49	48	9	40	2090	7	32	6 carb, 2 med-fat meat, 8 fat
Salads (No Dressing)											
Crispy Chicken Salad	1	350	21	20	51	6	40	620	6	21	1 1/2 carb, 2 med-fat meat, 2 fat
Grilled Chicken Salad	1	240	12	10	38	5	65	950	4	26	1 carb, 3 lean meat

FAST FOODS

	Serving	Calories	Carb. (g)	Fat (g)	% Cal. Fat	Sat. Fat (g)	Chol. (mg)	Sod. (mg)	Fib. (g)	Prot. (g)	Servings/ Exchanges
Side Salad	1	60	6	3	42	2	5	60	2	3	1 vegetable, 1 fat
Fries/Onion Rings											
French Fries (Small)	1	300	45	12	37	3	0	700	3	3	3 carb, 2 fat
French Fries (Medium)	1	380	56	15	37	3	0	880	4	4	4 carb, 3 fat
French Fries (Large)	1	480	72	19	35	4	0	1140	5	5	5 carb, 4 fat
Onion Rings	1 order	470	45	30	57	6	0	740	3	6	3 carb, 6 fat
Cones											
DQ Vanilla Soft Serve	1/2 cup	140	22	4.5	29	3	15	70	0	3	1 1/2 carb, 1 fat
DQ Chocolate Soft Serve	1/2 cup	150	22	5	30	4	15	75	0	4	1 1/2 carb, 1 fat
Vanilla Cone (Small)	1	230	38	7	26	5	20	115	0	6	2 1/2 carb, 1 fat
Vanilla Cone (Medium)	1	330	53	9	27	6	30	160	0	8	3 1/2 carb, 2 fat
Vanilla Cone (Large)	1	480	76	15	27	9	45	230	0	11	5 carb, 3 fat
Dipped Cone (Small)	1	340	42	17	44	9	20	130	1	6	3 carb, 3 fat
Dipped Cone (Medium)	1	490	59	24	45	13	30	190	1	8	4 carb, 5 fat

Dipped Cone (Large)	1	710	85	36	46	17	45	250	0	12	5 1/2 carb, 7 fat

Malts, Shakes, and Misty Slush

Chocolate Malt (Small)	1	640	111	16	23	11	55	340	1	15	7 1/2 carb, 3 fat
Chocolate Malt (Medium)	1	870	153	22	23	14	70	450	2	20	10 carb, 4 fat
Chocolate Malt (Large)	1	1320	222	35	23	22	110	670	2	29	15 carb, 7 fat
Chocolate Shake (Small)	1	560	93	15	25	10	50	280	1	13	6 carb, 3 fat
Chocolate Shake (Medium)	1	760	129	20	24	13	70	370	2	17	8 1/2 carb, 4 fat
Chocolate Shake (Large)	1	1140	186	33	26	21	105	550	2	26	12 carb, 7 fat
Misty Slush (Small)	1	220	56	0	0	0	0	20	0	0	4 carb
Misty Slush (Medium)	1	290	74	0	0	0	0	30	0	0	5 carb

MooLatte Frozen Blended Coffee

Cappuccino MooLatte	1	490	68	18	33	14	30	170	0	7	4 1/2 carb, 4 fat
French Vanilla MooLatte	1	570	87	18	28	14	30	170	0	7	6 carb, 4 fat
Mocha MooLatte	1	590	80	23	36	15	30	210	1	8	5 carb, 5 fat

Sundaes

Chocolate Sundae (Small)	1	280	49	7	21	5	20	140	0	5	3 carb, 1 fat

FAST FOODS

	Serving	Calories	Carb. (g)	Fat (g)	% Cal. Fat	Sat. Fat (g)	Chol. (mg)	Sod. (mg)	Fib. (g)	Prot. (g)	Servings/ Exchanges
Chocolate Sundae (Medium)	1	400	71	10	23	6	30	210	0	8	5 carb, 2 fat
Chocolate Sundae (Large)	1	580	100	15	24	10	45	260	1	11	6 1/2 carb, 3 fat
Royal Treats											
Banana Split	1	510	96	12	20	8	30	180	3	8	6 1/2 carb, 2 fat
Brownie Earthquake	1	740	112	27	32	16	50	350	0	10	7 1/2 carb, 5 fat
Peanut Buster Parfait	1	730	99	31	38	17	35	400	2	16	6 1/2 carb, 6 fat
Strawberry Shortcake	1	430	70	14	28	9	60	360	1	7	4 1/2 carb, 3 fat
Triple Chocolate Utopia	1	770	96	39	45	17	55	390	5	12	6 1/2 carb, 8 fat
Novelties											
Buster Bar	1	500	45	28	50	15	15	230	2	11	3 carb, 6 fat
Chocolate Dilly Bar	1	220	25	13	55	10	15	85	0	3	1 1/2 carb, 3 fat
DQ Fudge Bar (No-Sugar-Added)	1	50	13	0	0	0	0	70	0	4	1 carb
DQ Sandwich	1	200	31	6	30	3	10	140	1	4	2 carb, 1 fat

DQ Vanilla Orange Bar (No-Sugar-Added)	1	60	17	0	0	0	0	40	0	2	1 carb
Lemon DQ Freez'r	1/2 cup	80	20	0	0	0		10	0	0	1 carb
StarKiss	1	80	21	0	0	0		10	0	0	1 1/2 carb
Blizzard Treats											
Oreo Cookies Blizzard (Small)	1	570	83	21	33	10	40	430	<1	11	5 1/2 carb, 4 fat
Oreo Cookies Blizzard (Medium)	1	700	103	26	34	12	45	560	1	13	7 carb, 5 fat
Oreo Cookies Blizzard (Large)	1	1010	148	37	34	18	70	770	2	19	10 carb, 7 fat
Chocolate Chip Cookie Dough Blizzard (Small)	1	720	105	28	39	14	50	370	0	12	7 carb, 6 fat
Chocolate Chip Cookie Dough Blizzard (Medium)	1	1030	150	40	35	20	70	520	0	17	10 carb, 8 fat

FAST FOODS

	Serving	Calories	Carb. (g)	Fat (g)	% Cal. Fat	Sat. Fat (g)	Chol. (mg)	Sod. (mg)	Fib. (g)	Prot. (g)	Servings/ Exchanges
Chocolate Chip Cookie Dough Blizzard (Large)	1	1320	193	52	36	26	90	670	0	21	13 carb, 10 fat
DQ Cake											
DQ 8-inch Round Cake	1/8 Cake	370	56	13	30	8	25	280	<1	7	4 carb, 3 fat
DOMINO'S											
Classic Hand Tossed, 14-Inch Large											
Cheese	1 slice	256	38	8	28	3	12	536	2	10	2 1/2 carb, 2 fat
Pepperoni	1 slice	305	38	12	35	5	22	718	2	12	2 1/2 carb, 1 med-fat meat, 1 fat
Sausage	1 slice	320	39	14	39	5	24	744	2	13	2 1/2 carb, 1 med-fat meat, 2 fat
Ham & Pineapple	1 slice	275	40	9	30	4	17	653	2	12	2 1/2 carb, 1 med-fat meat, 1 fat
Green Pepper, Onion, Mushroom	1 slice	263	39	8	27	3	12	537	2	11	2 1/2 carb, 1 med-fat meat, 1 fat
Beef	1 slice	312	38	13	38	5	23	690	2	13	2 1/2 carb, 1 med-fat meat, 1 fat
Vegi Feast	1 slice	300	40	11	33	5	18	678	3	13	2 1/2 carb, 1 med-fat meat, 1 fat

Ultimate Deep Dish, 14-Inch Large

Cheese	1 slice	336	41	15	40	5	16	782	2	13	3 carb, 1 med-fat meat, 2 fat
Pepperoni	1 slice	385	41	20	47	7	26	964	2	15	3 carb, 1 med-fat meat, 3 fat
Sausage	1 slice	400	42	21	47	7	27	990	3	15	3 carb, 1 med-fat meat, 3 fat
Ham & Pineapple	1 slice	355	42	16	41	6	21	900	2	14	3 carb, 1 med-fat meat, 2 fat
Green Pepper, Onion, Mushroom	1 slice	343	42	15	39	5	16	783	3	13	3 carb, 1 med-fat meat, 2 fat
Beef	1 slice	392	41	20	46	7	26	937	2	15	3 carb, 1 med-fat meat, 3 fat
Vegi Feast	1 slice	380	43	18	43	7	21	924	3	15	3 carb, 1 med-fat meat, 3 fat

Crunchy Thin Crust, 14-Inch Large

Cheese	1 slice	188	19	10	48	4	13	409	1	7	1 carb, 1 med-fat meat, 1 fat
Pepperoni	1 slice	237	19	15	57	6	24	591	1	10	1 carb, 1 med-fat meat, 2 fat
Sausage	1 slice	252	20	16	57	6	25	616	2	10	1 carb, 1 med-fat meat, 2 fat
Ham & Pineapple	1 slice	207	21	11	48	4	18	523	1	9	1 1/2 carb, 1 med-fat meat, 1 fat
Green Pepper, Onion, Mushroom	1 slice	201	21	10	45	4	13	410	2	8	1 1/2 carb, 1 med-fat meat, 1 fat

FAST FOODS

	Serving	Calories	Carb. (g)	Fat (g)	% Cal. Fat	Sat. Fat (g)	Chol. (mg)	Sod. (mg)	Fib. (g)	Prot. (g)	Servings/ Exchanges
Beef	1 slice	243	19	15	56	6	24	563	1	10	1 carb, 1 med-fat meat, 2 fat
Vegi Feast	1 slice	231	21	14	55	5	19	551	2	10	1 1/2 carb, 1 med-fat meat, 2 fat
Side Dishes											
Breadsticks	1	115	12	6	47	1	0	122	0	2	1 carb, 1 fat
Cheesy Bread	1	123	13	7	51	2	6	162	0	4	1 carb, 1 fat
Marinara Dipping Sauce	1 container	25	5	0	0	0	0	263	0	1	free
Garlic Sauce	1 container	440	0	49	100	10	0	380	0	0	10 fat
Cinna Stix	1	123	15	6	44	1	0	111	1	2	1 carb, 1 fat
Sweet Icing	1 container	250	57	3	11	3	0	0	0	0	4 carb, 1 fat
Barbeque Buffalo Wings	1	50	2	3	54	0.5	26	176	0	6	1 med-fat meat
Hot Buffalo Wings	1	45	1	3	60	0.5	26	255	0	5	1 med-fat meat
Pizza Buffalo Chicken Kickers	1	47	3	2	38	0.5	9	163	0	4	1 med-fat meat
Blue Cheese Dipping Sauce	1 container	223	1	24	97	4	20	417	0	1	5 fat

Hot Dipping Sauce	1 container	15	4	0	0	0	0	1820	0	0	free
Ranch Dipping Sauce	1 container	197	2	21	96	3	9	380	0	1	4 fat

DUNKIN DONUTS

Donuts

Apple Crumb	1	230	34	10	39	3	0	270	1	3	2 carb, 2 fat
Bavarian Creme	1	210	30	9	39	2	0	270	1	3	2 carb, 2 fat
Blueberry Cake	1	290	35	16	50	3.5	10	400	1	3	2 carb, 3 fat
Boston Kreme	1	240	36	9	34	2	0	280	1	3	2 1/2 carb, 2 fat
Chocolate Frosted Cake	1	360	40	20	50	5	25	350	1	4	2 1/2 carb, 4 fat
Chocolate Glazed Cake	1	290	33	16	50	3.5	0	370	1	3	2 carb, 3 fat
Chocolate Kreme Filled	1	270	35	13	43	3	0	260	1	3	2 carb, 3 fat
Glazed	1	180	25	8	40	1.5	0	250	1	3	1 1/2 carb, 2 fat
Glazed Cake	1	350	41	19	49	5	25	340	1	4	3 carb, 4 fat
Jelly Filled	1	210	32	8	34	1.5	0	280	1	3	2 carb, 2 fat
Maple Frosted	1	210	30	9	39	2	0	260	1	3	2 carb, 2 fat
Powdered Cake	1	330	36	19	52	5	25	330	1	4	2 1/2 carb, 4 fat

FAST FOODS

	Serving	Calories	Carb. (g)	Fat (g)	% Cal. Fat	Sat. Fat (g)	Chol. (mg)	Sod. (mg)	Fib. (g)	Prot. (g)	Servings/ Exchanges
Sugar Raised	1	170	22	8	42	1.5	0	250	1	3	1 1/2 carb, 2 fat
Whole-Wheat Glazed Cake	1	310	32	19	55	4	0	380	2	4	2 carb, 4 fat
Fancies											
Apple Fritter	1	300	41	14	42	3	0	360	1	4	3 carb, 4 fat
Coffee Roll	1	270	33	14	47	3	0	340	1	4	2 carb, 3 fat
Éclair	1	270	39	11	37	2.5	0	290	1	3	2 1/2 carb, 2 fat
Glazed Fritter	1	260	31	14	48	3	0	330	1	4	2 carb, 3 fat
Munchkins											
Glazed	5	200	27	9	41	2	0	220	1	3	2 carb, 2 fat
Glazed Cake	3	280	38	13	42	3	20	190	1	3	2 1/2 carb, 3 fat
Jelly Filled	5	210	30	9	38	2	0	240	1	3	2 carb, 2 fat
Plain Cake	4	270	27	16	53	4	25	240	1	3	2 carb, 3 fat
Danish											
Apple Danish	1	250	36	10	36	2.5	5	220	0	4	2 1/2 carb, 2 fat

Cheese Danish	1	270	32	14	47	4.5	15	210	0	4	2 carb, 3 fat
Strawberry Cheese Danish	1	250	33	12	43	3.5	10	200	0	4	2 carb, 2 fat

Muffins

Banana Walnut	1	540	73	23	38	6	75	550	3	10	5 carb, 5 fat
Blueberry	1	490	75	18	33	6	75	630	2	8	3 carb, 4 fat
Chocolate Chip	1	590	85	23	35	10	75	570	3	9	5 1/2 carb, 5 fat
Cranberry Orange	1	460	71	16	31	5	70	530	3	8	5 carb, 3 fat
Honey Bran Raisin	1	490	81	14	26	3.5	60	510	5	10	5 1/2 carb, 3 fat
Reduced-Fat Blueberry	1	450	74	13	26	3.5	70	650	2	9	5 carb, 3 fat

Scones

Maple Walnut	1	470	62	22	42	5	40	320	1	6	4 carb, 4 fat
Raspberry White Chocolate	1	450	59	22	44	7	40	330	2	6	4 carb, 4 fat

Bagels

Blueberry	1	350	69	3	8	0.5	0	630	2	11	4 1/2 strch, 1 fat
Everything	1	430	75	7	15	0.5	0	780	3	17	5 strch, 1 fat
Plain	1	360	69	3	8	0.5	0	780	2	14	4 1/2 strch, 1 fat

FAST FOODS

	Serving	Calories	Carb. (g)	Fat (g)	% Cal. Fat	Sat. Fat (g)	Chol. (mg)	Sod. (mg)	Fib. (g)	Prot. (g)	Servings/ Exchanges
Wheat	1	350	66	4.5	12	1	0	650	4	13	4 1/2 strch, 1 fat
Cream Cheese											
Lite Cream Cheese	2 oz	110	6	9	74	7	30	230	0	4	1/2 carb, 2 fat
Plain Cream Cheese	2 oz	190	4	17	81	13	55	190	0	4	3 fat
Strawberry Cream Cheese	2 oz	190	9	17	81	9	45	150	0	4	1/2 carb, 3 fat
Sandwiches											
Bagel Egg Bacon Cheese Sandwich	1	500	71	13	23	6	135	1410	2	26	5 strch, 2 med-fat meat, 1 fat
Bagel Ham Cheese Sandwich	1	500	70	11	20	5	145	1450	2	29	4 1/2 strch, 2 med-fat meat
Biscuit Egg Cheese Sandwich	1	360	31	20	50	7	125	1190	1	14	2 strch, 2 med-fat meat, 2 fat
Croissant Egg Ham Cheese Sandwich	1	470	38	27	52	9	150	940	0	20	2 1/2 strch, 2 med-fat meat, 3 fat

English Muffin Bacon Egg Cheese Sandwich	1	310	35	11	32	5	135	1230	1	18	2 strch, 2 med-fat meat
English Muffin Egg Cheese Sandwich	1	270	35	8	27	4.5	125	1030	1	15	2 strch, 1 med-fat meat, 1 fat

Beverages

Coffee Coolatta with 2% milk	16 oz	190	41	2	9	1.5	10	80	0	4	3 carb
Coffee Coolatta with cream	16 oz	350	40	22	57	14	75	65	0	3	2 1/2 carb, 4 fat
Coffee Coolatta with skim milk	16 oz	170	41	0	0	0	0	80	0	4	3 carb
Coffee Coolatta with whole milk	16 oz	210	42	4	17	2.5	15	80	0	4	3 carb, 1 fat
Cappuccino	10 oz	80	7	4.5	51	2.5	20	70	0	4	1/2 carb, 1 fat
Caramel Swirl Latte	10 oz	230	36	6	23	3.5	25	140	0	8	2 1/2 carb, 1 fat
Espresso	2 oz	0	0	0	0	0	0	5	0	0	free
Latte	10 oz	120	10	6	45	3.5	25	95	0	6	1/2 carb, 1 fat

FAST FOODS

	Serving	Calories	Carb. (g)	Fat (g)	% Cal. Fat	Sat. Fat (g)	Chol. (mg)	Sod. (mg)	Fib. (g)	Prot. (g)	Servings/ Exchanges
Orange Mango Coolatta	16 oz	270	66	0	0	0	0	25	2	1	4 1/2 carb
EINSTEIN BROS.											
Bagels											
Asiago Cheese	1	360	71	3	7	1.5	5	570	2	13	5 strch, 1 fat
Chocolate Chip	1	370	76	3	8	2	0	500	3	11	5 strch, 1 fat
Chopped Garlic	1	380	79	3	3	1	0	680	4	13	5 strch, 1 fat
Chopped Onion	1	330	71	1	3	0	0	500	2	11	5 strch
Cinnamon Raisin Swirl	1	350	78	1	3	0	0	490	2	11	5 strch
Cinnamon Sugar	1	330	74	1	3	0	0	490	2	10	5 strch
Dark Pumpernickel	1	320	68	1	3	0	0	730	3	11	4 1/2 strch
Egg	1	340	69	3	9	1	35	510	2	11	4 1/2 strch, 1 fat
Everything	1	340	75	2	5	0	0	820	2	13	5 strch
Honey Whole-Wheat	1	320	71	1	3	0	0	470	3	10	5 strch
Low Carb 9 Grain	1	210	28	3.5	14	1	0	650	10	25	2 strch, 2 very lean meat

Lower Carb 9 Grain, Plain	1	310	29	13	39	7	30	730	10	27	2 strch, 3 med-fat meat
Nutty Banana	1	360	74	3	8	1	0	510	2	11	5 strch, 1 fat
Plain	1	320	71	1	3	0	0	520	2	11	5 strch
Potato	1	350	69	4.5	11	1	0	590	2	10	4 1/2 strch, 1 fat
Power Bagel with Peanut Butter	1	750	92	34	41	6	0	780	7	27	6 strch, 1 med-fat meat, 6 fat
Sesame	1	380	75	5	12	1	0	680	3	11	5 strch, 1 fat
Sundried Tomato	1	320	69	1	4	0	0	520	3	11	4 1/2 strch
Wild Blueberry	1	350	77	1	3	0	0	510	3	11	5 strch
Top Shelf Bagels											
Roasted Red Pepper & Pesto	1	410	73	7	15	3	15	710	2	17	5 strch, 1 fat
Six Cheese	1	390	72	6	13	3	15	650	2	16	5 strch, 1 fat
Spicy Nacho	1	450	77	9	18	5	20	890	3	17	5 strch, 2 fat
Spinach Florentine	1	410	72	7	17	4	20	620	3	17	5 strch, 1 fat

FAST FOODS

Cream Cheese

	Serving	Calories	Carb. (g)	Fat (g)	% Cal. Fat	Sat. Fat (g)	Chol. (mg)	Sod. (mg)	Fib. (g)	Prot. (g)	Servings/ Exchanges
Whipped Blueberry	2 Tbsp	70	6	5	66	3.5	15	50	0	1	1/2 carb, 1 fat
Whipped Garden Vegetable	2 Tbsp	60	3	5	75	3.5	15	100	0	1	1 fat
Whipped Honey Almond Reduced-Fat	2 Tbsp	70	6	5	64	3	15	45	0	1	1/2 carb, 1 fat
Whipped Maple Raisin Walnut	2 Tbsp	60	4	5	75	3.5	15	45	0	1	1 fat
Whipped Plain	2 Tbsp	70	1	7	86	4.5	20	65	0	1	1 fat
Whipped Plain Reduced-Fat	2 Tbsp	60	2	5	75	3.5	15	85	0	1	1 fat
Whipped Pumpkin	2 Tbsp	100	6	8	70	6	25	80	0	1	1/2 carb, 2 fat
Whipped Strawberry	2 Tbsp	70	5	5	64	3.5	15	50	0	1	1 fat
Whipped Sundried Tomato & Basil	2 Tbsp	60	2	5	75	3.5	15	100	0	1	1 fat

Roll-Ups

Albuquerque Turkey	1	790	81	39	44	15	85	2040	5	31	5 1/2 carb, 2 med-fat meat, 6 fat
Thai Vegetable	1	630	97	21	30	2	0	1310	5	24	6 1/2 carb, 1 vegetable, 4 fat
Thai Vegetable with Chicken	1	670	99	18	25	1	40	1850	4	27	6 1/2 carb, 1 med-fat meat, 3 fat

Salads

Asian Chicken Salad	14.5 oz	550	88	9	15	1.5	55	1610	5	29	6 carb, 2 med-fat meat
Caesar Salad	9.5 oz	650	— 25	51	71	10	35	1380	2	12	1 1/2 carb, 1 med-fat meat, 9 fat
Chicken Caesar Salad	12.5 oz	750	26	53	64	11	90	1850	2	33	2 carb, 4 med-fat meat, 7 fat
Chicken Salad on Greens	10.5 oz	210	11	9	38	2	55	640	3	19	2 vegetable, 3 lean meat
Egg Salad	4 oz	200	5	17	75	4	310	340	0	9	1 med-fat meat, 2 fat
Mixed Greens	3.5 oz	220	13	18	73	3	0	380	1	2	3 vegetable, 4 fat
Roasted Corn Salad	3 oz	90	13	3	28	0	0	150	4	2	1 carb, 1 fat
Traditional Potato Salad	1/2 cup	290	21	21	66	3	15	600	2	3	1 1/2 carb, 3 fat
Tuna Salad on Greens	10.5 oz	170	10	5	29	1	35	520	3	20	2 carb, 2 lean meat

Sandwiches

Chicago Bagel Dog, Asiago	1	740	78	34	40	15	80	1360	2	29	5 carb, 2 med-fat meat, 5 fat

FAST FOODS

	Serving	Calories	Carb. (g)	Fat (g)	% Cal. Fat	Sat. Fat (g)	Chol. (mg)	Sod. (mg)	Fib. (g)	Prot. (g)	Servings/Exchanges
Chicago Chili Cheese Bagel Dog	1	810	83	38	42	17	105	1550	4	33	5 1/2 carb, 2 med-fat meat, 6 fat
Chicken Salad	1	500	78	10	18	2	55	1160	4	28	5 carb, 2 med-fat meat
Denver Omelet Breakfast Panini	1	740	70	33	41	13	310	1380	3	42	4 1/2 carb, 2 med-fat meat, 5 fat
Egg Salad	1	560	79	18	29	4.5	315	860	3	20	5 carb, 1 med-fat meat, 3 fat
Egg, Homestyle Sausage	1	550	74	14	22	5	295	1000	2	33	5 carb, 2 med-fat meat, 1 fat
Egg, Original	1	480	74	10	19	4	270	680	2	23	5 carb, 1 med-fat meat, 1 fat
Egg, Salmon & Shmear	1	650	82	22	31	12	310	1040	3	31	5 1/2 carb, 2 med-fat meat, 2 fat
Ham	1	450	74	6	11	1.5	45	1390	3	26	5 carb, 2 lean meat
Hummus & Feta	1	540	89	13	22	4	15	880	5	18	6 carb, 3 fat
Roast Beef	1	460	76	4	8	1.5	45	880	3	31	5 carb, 2 lean meat
Reuben Deli	1	660	83	19	26	6	65	2590	4	39	5 1/2 carb, 3 med-fat meat, 1 fat
Tasty Turkey	1	570	83	15	23	9	80	1420	4	31	5 1/2 carb, 2 med-fat meat, 1 fat

The Veg Out	1	490	77	13	22	7	30	850	3	17	5 carb, 3 fat
Tuna Salad	1	470	77	6	13	1.5	35	1040	4	29	5 carb, 2 lean meat
Turkey Pastrami Deli	1	440	76	2	3	0	40	1610	3	31	5 carb, 2 very lean meat

Paninis

Cali Club	1	730	90	24	29	9	75	2340	9	47	6 carb, 4 med-fat meat, 1 fat
Cuban Ham	1	700	68	31	40	11	90	2010	4	40	4 1/2 carb, 4 med-fat meat, 2 fat
Taos Turkey	1	740	93	25	30	9	80	2140	9	45	6 carb, 4 med-fat meat, 1 fat
Ultimate Toasted Cheese	1	900	96	44	44	24	110	1910	7	39	6 1/2 carb, 3 med-fat meat, 6 fat

Soups

Broccoli, Sharp Cheddar	6 oz	230	13	15	61	8	40	490	1	8	1 carb, 1 med-fat meat, 2 fat
Chicken & Wild Rice	6 oz	190	29	3.5	18	0.5	15	1440	2	10	2 carb, 1 fat
Chicken Noodle	6 oz	220	17	9	36	2.5	60	980	2	16	1 carb, 2 med-fat meat
Clam Chowda	6 oz	160	11	11	63	6	35	480	0	5	1 carb, 2 fat
Low-Fat Minestrone	6 oz	150	27	4.5	27	0.5	0	1220	3	6	2 carb, 1 fat
Tomato Bisque	6 oz	190	23	10	47	3.5	15	1390	3	5	1 1/2 carb, 2 fat
Tortilla Soup	6 oz	90	14	2.5	28	0	0	1530	2	2	1 carb, 1 fat

FAST FOODS

	Serving	Calories	Carb. (g)	Fat (g)	% Cal. Fat	Sat. Fat (g)	Chol. (mg)	Sod. (mg)	Fib. (g)	Prot. (g)	Servings/ Exchanges
Turkey Chili	6 oz	140	14	4.5	29	1	20	930	2	10	1 carb, 1 med-fat meat
HARDEE'S											
Sandwiches											
1/3 lb. Thickburger	1	850	54	57	60	22	105	1470	3	30	3 1/2 carb, 3 med-fat meat, 8 fat
1/3 lb. Cheeseburger	1	680	51	39	51	19	90	1320	3	30	3 1/2 carb, 3 med-fat meat, 4 fat
1/3 lb. Mushroom 'n Swiss Thickburger	1	720	48	42	53	21	100	1570	2	35	3 carb, 4 med-fat meat, 4 fat
1/3 lb. Bacon Cheese Thickburger	1	910	50	63	63	24	115	1490	3	33	3 carb, 3 med-fat meat, 10 fat
1/3 lb. Chili Cheese Thickburger	1	870	55	54	55	26	135	1840	4	41	3 1/2 carb, 5 med-fat meat, 6 fat
1/3 lb. Low Carb Thickburger	1	420	5	32	67	12	115	1010	2	30	4 med-fat meat, 2 fat
1/2 lb. Six Dollar Burger	1	1120	72	73	59	30	150	1870	5	42	5 carb, 4 med-fat meat, 11 fat

Item	Amount										Exchanges
1/2 lb. Grilled Sourdough Thickburger	1	1100	61	74	60	30	155	1430	5	47	4 carb, 5 med-fat meat, 10 fat
2/3 lb. Bacon Cheese Thickburger	1	1340	60	96	65	40	205	2110	5	56	4 carb, 6 med-fat meat, 13 fat
2/3 lb. Double Thickburger	1	1230	53	90	66	38	195	2090	3	52	3 1/2 carb, 6 med-fat meat, 12 fat
Charbroiled Chicken Sandwich	1	590	53	26	39	7	80	1180	4	36	3 1/2 carb, 4 med-fat meat, 1 fat
Big Chicken Sandwich	1	770	73	36	43	8	95	2000	4	39	5 carb, 3 med-fat meat, 4 fat
Spicy Chicken Sandwich	1	430	46	22	47	5	40	1190	2	14	3 carb, 1 med-fat meat, 3 fat
Regular Roast Beef	1	330	29	16	45	7	40	860	2	19	2 carb, 2 med-fat meat, 1 fat
Big Roast Beef	1	470	38	23	45	10	60	1290	2	29	2 1/2 carb, 3 med-fat meat, 2 fat
Hot Ham 'n Cheese	1	420	39	18	40	10	55	1600	2	30	2 1/2 carb, 3 med-fat meat, 1 fat
Big Hot Ham 'n Cheese	1	570	59	23	35	12	70	2020	3	37	4 carb, 4 med-fat meat, 1 fat
Hot Dog	1	420	22	30	64	12	55	1200	1	16	1 1/2 carb, 2 med-fat meat, 4 fat
Chicken Strips	3 piece	380	27	21	50	4	55	1360	1	22	2 carb, 2 med-fat meat, 2 fat

FAST FOODS

	Serving	Calories	Carb. (g)	Fat (g)	% Cal. Fat	Sat. Fat (g)	Chol. (mg)	Sod. (mg)	Fib. (g)	Prot. (g)	Servings/Exchanges
Chicken Strips	5 piece	630	45	34	49	6	90	2260	2	37	3 carb, 4 med-fat meat, 3 fat
Fried Chicken & Sides											
Fried Chicken Breast	1	370	29	15	35	4	75	1190	0	29	2 carb, 3 med-fat meat
Fried Chicken Wing	1	200	23	8	35	2	30	740	0	10	1 1/2 carb, 1 med-fat meat, 1 fat
Fried Chicken Thigh	1	330	30	15	39	4	60	1000	0	19	2 carb, 2 med-fat meat, 1 fat
Fried Chicken Leg	1	170	15	7	35	2	45	570	0	13	1 carb, 1 med-fat meat
French Fries (Small)	1 order	390	51	19	44	4	0	240	4	6	3 1/2 carb, 4 fat
French Fries (Medium)	1 order	520	67	24	42	5	0	320	5	8	4 1/2 carb, 5 fat
French Fries (Large)	1 order	610	78	28	43	6	0	370	6	10	5 carb, 6 fat
Chili Cheese Fries	1 order	700	67	39	50	13	50	780	7	22	4 1/2 carb, 1 med-fat meat, 7 fat
Crispy Curls (Small)	1 order	340	43	17	44	4	0	840	4	4	3 carb, 3 fat
Crispy Curls (Medium)	1 order	410	52	20	44	5	0	1020	4	5	3 1/2 carb, 4 fat
Crispy Curls (Large)	1 order	480	60	23	44	6	0	1190	5	6	4 carb, 5 fat
Coleslaw (Small)	1 order	170	20	10	53	2	10	140	2	1	1 carb, 2 fat

Mashed Potatoes (Small)	1 order	90	17	2	17	0	0	410	0	1	1 carb

Breakfast

Made from Scratch Biscuit	1	370	35	23	57	5	0	890	0	5	2 carb, 5 fat
Bacon Biscuit	1	560	37	38	61	11	225	1360	0	16	2 1/2 carb, 1 med-fat meat, 7 fat
Sausage Biscuit	1	530	36	38	64	10	30	1240	0	11	2 1/2 carb, 1 med-fat meat, 7 fat
Country Ham Biscuit	1	440	36	26	55	6	35	1710	0	14	2 1/2 carb, 1 med-fat meat, 4 fat
Chicken Fillet Biscuit	1	600	50	34	52	7	55	1680	1	24	3 carb, 2 med-fat meat, 5 fat
Country Steak Biscuit	1	620	44	41	60	11	35	1360	0	16	3 carb, 1 med-fat meat, 7 fat
Smoked Sausage Biscuit	1	620	37	46	66	15	40	1680	0	15	2 1/2 carb, 1 med-fat meat, 8 fat
Sausage & Egg Biscuit	1	610	36	44	64	11	235	1290	0	17	2 1/2 carb, 2 med-fat meat, 7 fat
Bacon, Egg & Cheese Biscuit	1	560	37	38	61	11	225	1360	0	16	2 1/2 carb, 1 med-fat meat, 7 fat
Biscuit 'n Gravy	1	530	47	34	58	8	10	1550	0	8	3 carb, 7 fat
Low Carb Breakfast Bowl	1	620	6	50	73	21	325	1380	2	36	1/2 carb, 5 med-fat meat, 5 fat
Sunrise Croissant with Ham	1	430	28	26	53	10	250	1050	0	23	2 carb, 2 med-fat meat, 3 fat

FAST FOODS

	Serving	Calories	Carb. (g)	Fat (g)	% Cal. Fat	Sat. Fat (g)	Chol. (mg)	Sod. (mg)	Fib. (g)	Prot. (g)	Servings/ Exchanges
Sunrise Croissant with Bacon	1	450	28	29	58	12	240	900	0	19	2 carb, 2 med-fat meat, 4 fat
Frisco Breakfast Sandwich	1	360	38	13	31	5	230	670	2	24	2 1/2 carb, 2 med-fat meat, 1 fat
Tortilla Scrambler	1	310	18	19	55	7	230	570	0	15	1 carb, 1 med-fat meat, 3 fat
Pancakes	3	300	55	5	15	1	25	830	2	8	3 1/2 carb, 1 fat
IN-N-OUT BURGER											
Hamburger with Onion	1	390	39	19	44	5	40	650	3	16	2 1/2 carb, 2 med-fat meat, 2 fat
Hamburger (Protein Style)	1	240	11	17	63	4	40	370	3	13	2 vegetable, 2 med-fat meat, 1 fat
Cheeseburger with Onion	1	480	39	27	50	10	60	1000	3	22	2 1/2 carb, 2 med-fat meat, 3 fat
Cheeseburger (Protein Style)	1	330	11	25	67	9	60	720	3	18	2 vegetable, 2 med-fat meat, 3 fat
Double-Double with Onion	1	670	39	41	55	18	120	1440	3	37	2 1/2 carb, 4 med-fat meat, 4 fat
Double-Double (Protein Style)	1	520	11	39	67	17	120	1160	3	33	2 vegetable, 4 med-fat meat, 4 fat

	1 order	400	54	18	40	5	0	245	2	7	3 1/2 carb, 4 fat
French Fries	1 order	400	54	18	40	5	0	245	2	7	3 1/2 carb, 4 fat
Chocolate Shake	15 oz	690	83	36	46	24	95	350	0	9	5 1/2 carb, 7 fat
Strawberry Shake	15 oz	690	91	33	43	22	85	280	0	9	6 carb, 7 fat
Vanilla Shake	15 oz	680	78	37	49	25	90	390	0	9	5 carb, 7 fat

JACK IN THE BOX

Burgers

Hamburger	1	310	30	14	40	5	45	590	0	17	2 carb, 2 med-fat meat, 1 fat
Hamburger with Cheese	1	355	31	18	44	7	55	770	0	19	2 carb, 2 med-fat meat, 1 fat
Hamburger Deluxe	1	370	32	21	50	6	50	545	0	17	2 carb, 2 med-fat meat, 2 fat
Hamburger Deluxe with Cheese	1	460	34	28	53	10	75	915	0	21	2 carb, 2 med-fat meat, 4 fat
Bacon Bacon Cheeseburger	1	780	50	50	57	19	90	1545	2	33	3 carb, 3 med-fat meat, 7 fat
Jumbo Jack	1	600	52	35	52	12	45	935	2	20	3 1/2 carb, 2 med-fat meat, 5 fat
Junior Bacon Cheeseburger	1	525	32	36	61	9.5	70	880	0	21	2 carb, 2 med-fat meat, 5 fat

FAST FOODS

	Serving	Calories	Carb. (g)	Fat (g)	% Cal. Fat	Sat. Fat (g)	Chol. (mg)	Sod. (mg)	Fib. (g)	Prot. (g)	Servings/Exchanges
Sourdough Jack	1	715	36	51	64	18	75	1165	2	26	2 1/2 carb, 3 med-fat meat, 7 fat
Ultimate Cheeseburger	1	945	52	65	61	27	120	1525	2	39	3 1/2 carb, 4 med-fat meat, 9 fat
Bacon Ultimate Cheeseburger	1	1025	53	71	61	29	135	1985	2	46	3 1/2 carb, 5 med-fat meat, 9 fat
Turkey Jack	1	635	55	33	46	11	110	1745	2	34	4 carb, 3 med-fat meat, 3 fat
Chicken & Fish											
Chicken Breast Strips	1 order	630	39	38	52	8	90	1470	3	35	2 1/2 carb, 4 med-fat meat, 4 fat
Chicken Fajita Pita	1	315	33	9	25	4	65	1080	0	22	2 carb, 2 med-fat meat
Chicken Sandwich	1	390	39	21	47	4	35	730	1	15	2 1/2 carb, 1 med-fat meat, 3 fat
Jack's Spicy Chicken	1	615	62	31	44	6	50	1090	3	24	4 carb, 2 med-fat meat, 4 fat
Sourdough Grilled Chicken Club	1	505	35	27	48	7	75	1220	2	29	2 carb, 3 med-fat meat, 2 fat
Fish & Chips	1	840	69	56	60	11	55	1600	4	16	4 1/2 carb, 1 med-fat meat, 10 fat

Tacos & Snacks

Taco	1	160	15	8	43	3	15	270	2	5	1 carb, 2 fat
Monster Taco	1	240	20	14	54	5	20	390	3	8	1 carb, 1 med-fat meat, 2 fat
Chicken Monster Taco	1	180	18	8	39	3	15	320	2	9	1 carb, 1 med-fat meat, 1 fat
Bacon Cheddar Potato Wedges	1 order	620	45	41	59	15	55	1300	5	18	3 carb, 1 med-fat meat, 7 fat
Egg Roll	1	175	26	6	34	2	5	470	2	5	2 carb, 1 fat
Stuffed Jalapeños	3	230	22	13	48	6	20	690	2	7	1 1/2 carb, 3 fat

Sandwiches

Deli Trio Pannido	1	645	53	34	50	9	95	2530	2	30	3 1/2 carb, 3 med-fat meat, 4 fat
Ham & Turkey Pannido	1	610	54	29	43	7	110	1785	2	36	3 1/2 carb, 4 med-fat meat, 2 fat
Ultimate Club Sandwich	1	630	52	29	42	9	105	1985	2	36	3 1/2 carb, 4 med-fat meat, 2 fat

Salads

Asian Chicken Salad	1	595	58	33	48	5	25	1315	8	20	6 carb, 1 med-fat meat, 5 fat
Chicken Club Salad	1	825	34	62	67	13	95	2065	5	34	2 carb, 4 med-fat meat, 8 fat
Side Salad	1	155	16	8	48	3	10	290	0	5	1 carb, 1 fat

FAST FOODS

	Serving	Calories	Carb. (g)	Fat (g)	% Cal. Fat	Sat. Fat (g)	Chol. (mg)	Sod. (mg)	Fib. (g)	Prot. (g)	Servings/ Exchanges
Southwest Chicken Salad	1	735	46	44	52	10	95	2155	4	27	3 carb, 3 med-fat meat, 6 fat
Fries & Rings											
French Fries (Small)	1	330	44	16	42	4	0	550	3	3	3 carb, 3 fat
French Fries (Medium)	1	410	55	20	44	5	0	690	4	4	4 carb, 4 fat
French Fries (Large)	1	580	77	28	43	6	0	960	6	6	5 carb, 6 fat
Onion Rings	1	500	51	30	54	6	0	420	3	6	3 1/2 carb, 6 fat
Seasoned Curly Fries (Small)	1	270	30	15	52	3	0	590	3	4	2 carb, 3 fat
Seasoned Curly Fries (Medium)	1	400	45	23	50	5	0	890	5	6	3 carb, 5 fat
Seasoned Curly Fries (Large)	1	550	60	31	51	6	0	1200	6	8	4 carb, 6 fat
Breakfast											
Breakfast Jack	1	305	34	14	39	4	205	715	0	13	2 carb, 1 med-fat meat, 2 fat

Item	Amount									Exchanges
Extreme Sausage Sandwich	1	690	37	50	64	17	280	1265	0	25	2 1/2 carb, 3 med-fat meat, 7 fat
French Toast Sticks	1	560	89	18	30	4	10	490	2	8	6 carb, 4 fat
Hash Brown	1	150	13	10	60	3	0	230	2	1	1 carb, 2 fat
Sausage Biscuit	1	600	41	36	55	9	35	1200	2	13	3 carb, 1 med-fat meat, 6 fat
Sausage Croissant	1	605	42	41	61	13	240	725	1	18	3 carb, 1 med-fat meat, 7 fat
Sausage, Egg & Cheese Biscuit	1	970	50	68	63	21	280	1905	2	26	3 carb, 2 med-fat meat, 12 fat
Sourdough Breakfast Sandwich	1	445	37	26	52	8	215	845	2	16	2 1/2 carb, 1 med-fat meat, 4 fat
Supreme Croissant	1	475	41	27	52	9	220	815	1	16	3 carb, 1 med-fat meat, 4 fat
Ultimate Breakfast Sandwich	1	605	58	31	45	10	425	1630	2	26	4 carb, 2 med-fat meat, 4 fat

KFC

Salad & More

Item	Amount									Exchanges
Crispy BLT Salad	1	350	21	17	46	5	60	1170	4	27	1 1/2 carb, 3 med-fat meat

FAST FOODS

	Serving	Calories	Carb. (g)	Fat (g)	% Cal. Fat	Sat. Fat (g)	Chol. (mg)	Sod. (mg)	Fib. (g)	Prot. (g)	Servings/ Exchanges
Crispy Caesar Salad	1	370	20	19	46	7	65	1110	3	29	1 carb, 4 med-fat meat
Roasted BLT Salad	1	210	8	7	29	3	70	900	4	28	1/2 carb, 4 lean meat
Roasted Caesar Salad	1	220	6	9	36	5	75	850	3	29	1/2 carb, 4 lean meat
Tender Roast Filet Meal	1	360	41	7	17	2	85	2010	4	33	3 carb, 3 lean meat
Sandwiches											
KFC Snacker	1	320	31	16	47	3	25	700	2	14	2 carb, 1 med-fat meat, 2 fat
Honey BBQ KFC Snacker	1	220	32	4	16	1	35	490	2	15	2 carb, 1 med-fat meat
Honey BBQ Sandwich	1	300	41	6	17	2	55	920	1	22	3 carb, 2 lean meat
Triple Crunch Sandwich	1	650	49	34	47	7	75	1640	3	36	3 carb, 4 med-fat meat, 3 fat
Double Crunch Sandwich	1	530	42	28	48	6	55	1240	3	27	3 carb, 3 med-fat meat, 3 fat
Crispy Twister	1	670	55	38	51	7	60	1650	3	27	3 1/2 carb, 2 med-fat meat, 5 fat
Oven Roasted Twister	1	510	50	22	39	4	70	1400	4	29	3 carb, 3 med-fat meat, 1 fat
Tender Roast Sandwich	1	390	24	19	44	4	70	810	1	31	3 carb, 3 med-fat meat, 1 fat

Chicken

Original Chicken, Whole Wing	1	150	5	9	53	3	60	370	0	11	2 med-fat meat
Original Chicken, Breast	1	380	11	19	45	6	145	1150	0	40	1 carb, 5 med-fat meat
Original Chicken, Breast without Skin or Breading	1	140	0	3	18	1	95	410	0	29	4 very lean meat
Original Chicken, Drumstick	1	140	4	8	50	2	75	440	0	14	2 med-fat meat
Original Chicken, Thigh	1	360	12	25	64	7	165	1060	0	22	1 carb, 3 med-fat meat, 2 fat
Extra Crispy Chicken, Whole Wing	1	190	10	12	58	4	55	390	0	10	1/2 carb, 1 med-fat meat, 1 fat
Extra Crispy Chicken, Breast	1	460	19	28	54	8	135	1230	0	34	1 carb, 4 med-fat meat, 2 fat
Extra Crispy Chicken, Drumstick	1	160	5	10	56	3	70	420	0	12	2 med-fat meat
Extra Crispy Chicken, Thigh	1	370	12	26	62	7	120	710	0	21	1 carb, 3 med-fat meat, 2 fat

FAST FOODS

	Serving	Calories	Carb. (g)	Fat (g)	% Cal. Fat	Sat. Fat (g)	Chol. (mg)	Sod. (mg)	Fib. (g)	Prot. (g)	Servings/ Exchanges
Crispy Strips	3 piece	400	17	24	55	5	75	1250	0	29	1 carb, 4 med-fat meat, 1 fat
Popcorn Chicken											
Individual	1 order	380	23	21	50	5	60	1200	0	24	1 1/2 carb, 3 med-fat meat, 1 fat
Large	1 order	560	34	31	50	7	90	1790	1	36	2 carb, 4 med-fat meat, 2 fat
Pot Pie											
Chicken Pot Pie	1	770	70	40	47	15	115	1680	5	33	4 1/2 carb, 3 med-fat meat, 5 fat
Wings											
BBQ Wings Sauced	6	540	36	33	56	7	150	1130	1	25	2 1/2 carb, 3 med-fat meat, 4 fat
Hot Wings	6	450	23	29	58	6	145	1120	1	24	1 1/2 carb, 3 med-fat meat, 3 fat
Breads											
Biscuit	1	190	23	10	47	2	1.5	580	0	2	1 1/2 carb, 2 fat
Sides (Individual)											
Baked Beans	1	230	46	1	4	1	0	720	7	8	3 carb
Coleslaw	1	190	22	11	53	2	5	300	3	1	1 1/2 carb, 2 fat

	Serving										Exchanges
Corn on the Cob	3 inch	70	3	1.5	21	0.5	0	5	3	2	1 carb
Green Beans	1	50	7	1.5	30	0	5	570	2	2	1 vegetable
Macaroni & Cheese	1	400	45	18	40	5	15	1920	4	15	3 carb, 1 med-fat meat, 3 fat
Mashed Potatoes with Gravy	1	120	18	5	33	1	0	380	1	2	1 carb, 1 fat
Mashed Potatoes without Gravy	1	110	16	4	32	1	0	260	1	2	1 carb, 1 fat
Potato Salad	1	180	22	9	44	2	5	470	1	2	1 1/2 carb, 2 fat
Potato Wedges	1	240	30	12	46	3	0	830	3	4	2 carb, 2 fat
Seasoned Rice	1	150	32	1	7	0	0	640	2	4	2 carb
KRISPY KREME DONUTS											
Apple Fritter	1	380	46	21	50	5	5	290	2	4	3 carb, 4 fat
Caramel Kreme Crunch	1	350	43	19	49	5	5	170	<1	4	3 carb, 4 fat
Chocolate Iced Cake	1	270	36	14	47	3	20	320	<1	3	2 1/2 carb, 3 fat
Chocolate Iced Crème Filled	1	350	39	21	54	5	5	140	<1	3	2 1/2 carb, 4 fat

FAST FOODS

	Serving	Calories	Carb. (g)	Fat (g)	% Cal. Fat	Sat. Fat (g)	Chol. (mg)	Sod. (mg)	Fib. (g)	Prot. (g)	Servings/ Exchanges
Chocolate Iced Custard Filled	1	300	35	17	51	4	5	150	<1	3	2 carb, 3 fat
Chocolate Iced Glazed	1	250	33	12	43	3	5	100	<1	3	2 carb, 2 fat
Cinnamon Bun	1	260	28	16	55	4	5	125	<1	3	2 carb, 3 fat
Cinnamon Twist	1	230	33	9	35	2.5	5	85	<1	3	2 carb, 2 fat
Glazed Cinnamon	1	210	24	12	51	3	5	100	<1	2	1 1/2 carb, 2 fat
Glazed Crème Filled	1	340	39	20	53	5	5	140	<1	3	2 1/2 carb, 4 fat
Glazed Cruller	1	240	26	14	53	3.5	15	240	<1	2	2 carb, 3 fat
Glazed Lemon Filled	1	290	34	16	50	4	5	135	<1	3	2 carb, 3 fat
Glazed Strawberry Filled	1	290	35	16	50	4	5	135	<1	3	2 carb, 3 fat
Glazed Twist	1	210	28	9	39	2.5	5	80	<1	3	2 carb, 2 fat
Maple Iced	1	240	32	12	45	3	5	100	<1	2	2 carb, 2 fat
Maple Iced Cake	1	270	35	13	43	3	20	320	<1	3	2 carb, 3 fat
Original Glazed	1	200	22	12	54	3	5	95	<1	2	1 1/2 carb, 2 fat
Powdered Cake	1	280	37	14	45	3	20	320	<1	3	2 1/2 carb, 3 fat

Powdered Crème Filled	1	340	36	21	56	5	5	140	<1	3	2 1/2 carb, 4 fat
Sugar Coated	1	200	21	12	54	3	5	95	0	2	1 1/2 carb, 2 fat
Traditional Cake	1	230	25	13	51	3	20	320	<1	3	1 1/2 carb, 3 fat
Vanilla Iced Glazed	1	240	32	12	45	3	5	95	<1	2	2 carb, 2 fat

LONG JOHN SILVER'S

Fish and Seafood

Battered Fish	1 piece	230	16	13	52	4	30	700	0	11	1 carb, 1 med-fat meat, 2 fat
Baked Cod	1 piece	120	1	5	33	1	90	240	0	22	3 very lean meat
Battered Shrimp	1 piece	45	3	3	56	1	15	125	0	2	1 fat
Giant Shrimp	1 piece	80	5	5	56	2	20	250	0	2	1/2 carb, 1 fat
Crunchy Shrimp (basket)	21 pieces	340	32	19	50	5	105	720	2	12	2 carb, 1 med-fat meat, 3 fat
Breaded Clams	3 oz	240	22	13	50	2	10	1110	1	8	1 1/2 carb, 1 med-fat meat, 2 fat

Chicken

Chicken Plank	1 piece	140	9	8	50	3	20	400	0	8	1/2 carb, 1 med-fat meat, 1 fat

Sandwiches

Fish Sandwich	1	440	48	20	41	5	35	1120	3	17	3 carb, 1 med-fat meat, 3 fat

FAST FOODS

	Serving	Calories	Carb. (g)	Fat (g)	% Cal. Fat	Sat. Fat (g)	Chol. (mg)	Sod. (mg)	Fib. (g)	Prot. (g)	Servings/ Exchanges
Ultimate Fish Sandwich	1	500	48	25	46	8	50	1310	3	20	3 carb, 2 med-fat meat, 3 fat
Chicken Sandwich	1	360	41	15	36	4	25	810	3	13	3 carb, 1 med-fat meat, 2 fat
Salads											
Shrimp & Seafood Salad	1	260	22	12	42	5	85	820	4	18	1 1/2 carb, 2 med-fat meat
Chicken Club Salad	1	510	35	30	53	9	65	1550	5	28	2 carb, 3 med-fat meat, 3 fat
Dipping Sauces											
Cocktail Sauce	1 oz	25	6	0	0	0	0	250	0	0	1/2 carb
Tartar Sauce	1 oz	100	4	9	80	2	15	250	0	0	2 fat
Sides and Starters											
Regular Fries	3 oz	230	34	10	39	3	0	350	3	3	2 carb, 2 fat
Large Fries	5 oz	390	56	17	38	4	0	580	5	4	4 carb, 3 fat
Hushpuppies	1 pup	60	9	3	33	0.5	0	200	1	1	1/2 carb, 1 fat
Lobster Stuffed	1	170	16	9	47	2	30	390	1	6	1 carb, 2 fat
Crab Cake											

Slaw	4 oz	200	15	15	65	3	20	340	3	1	1 carb, 3 fat
Corn Cobbette	1	90	14	3	28	0.5	0	0	3	3	1 carb, 1 fat
Cheesesticks	3 sticks	140	12	8	50	2	10	320	1	4	1 carb, 2 fat
Rice	4 oz	180	34	4	19	1	0	540	3	3	2 carb, 1 fat
Crumblies	1 oz	170	14	12	65	3	0	420	1	1	1 carb, 2 fat
Clam Chowder	1 bowl	220	23	10	41	4	25	810	0	9	1 1/2 carb, 1 med-fat meat, 1 fat

Desserts

Chocolate Cream Pie	1	310	24	22	65	14	15	170	1	5	1 1/2 carb, 4 fat
Pecan Pie	1	370	55	15	38	3	40	190	2	4	3 1/2 carb, 3 fat
Pineapple Cream Pie	1	290	39	13	38	7	15	210	1	4	2 1/2 carb, 3 fat

McDONALD'S

Sandwiches

Hamburger	1	260	33	9	31	3.5	30	530	1	13	2 carb, 1 med-fat meat, 1 fat
Cheeseburger	1	310	35	12	35	6	40	740	1	15	2 carb, 1 med-fat meat, 1 fat
Double Cheeseburger	1	460	37	23	46	11	80	1140	1	25	2 1/2 carb, 2 med-fat meat, 3 fat
Quarter Pounder	1	420	40	18	38	7	70	730	3	24	2 1/2 carb, 2 med-fat meat, 2 fat

FAST FOODS

	Serving	Calories	Carb. (g)	Fat (g)	% Cal. Fat	Sat. Fat (g)	Chol. (mg)	Sod. (mg)	Fib. (g)	Prot. (g)	Servings/ Exchanges
Quarter Pounder with Cheese	1	510	43	25	43	12	95	1150	3	29	3 carb, 3 med-fat meat, 2 fat
Double Quarter Pounder with Cheese	1	730	46	40	49	19	160	1330	3	47	3 carb, 5 med-fat meat, 3 fat
Big Mac	1	560	46	30	48	10	80	1010	3	25	3 carb, 2 med-fat meat, 4 fat
Big N' Tasty	1	520	41	29	50	9	80	730	3	24	3 carb, 2 med-fat meat, 4 fat
Filet-O-Fish	1	400	42	18	40	4	40	640	1	14	3 carb, 1 med-fat meat, 3 fat
Chicken McGrill	1	400	38	16	35	3	70	1010	3	27	2 1/2 carb, 3 med-fat meat
Crispy Chicken	1	500	50	23	42	4	50	1090	3	24	3 carb, 2 med-fat meat, 3 fat
McChicken	1	420	41	22	48	4.5	45	760	1	15	3 carb, 1 med-fat meat, 3 fat
French Fries											
Small French Fries	1	230	30	11	43	2	0	140	3	2	2 carb, 2 fat
Medium French Fries	1	350	47	16	43	3	0	220	5	4	3 carb, 3 fat
Large French Fries	1	520	70	25	42	5	0	330	7	6	4 1/2 carb, 5 fat

Chicken McNuggets/Chicken Strips

Chicken McNuggets	4 pieces	170	10	10	53	2	25	450	0	10	1/2 carb, 1 med-fat meat, 1 fat
Chicken McNuggets	10 pieces	420	26	24	52	5	60	1120	0	25	2 carb, 3 med-fat meat, 2 fat
Chicken McNuggets	20 pieces	840	51	49	52	11	125	2240	0	50	3 1/2 carb, 6 med-fat meat, 4 fat
Chicken Selects Premium Breast Strips	3 pieces	380	28	20	47	3.5	55	930	0	23	2 carb, 2 med-fat meat, 2 fat
Chicken Selects Premium Breast Strips	10 pieces	1270	92	66	46	12	180	3100	0	77	6 carb, 8 med-fat meat, 5 fat

Salads

Bacon Ranch Salad	1	130	8	7	46	3.5	25	290	3	9	2 vegetable, 1 fat
Bacon Ranch Salad with Crispy Chicken	1	340	23	16	44	5	65	1030	3	27	1 1/2 carb, 3 med-fat meat
Bacon Ranch Salad with Grilled Chicken	1	240	11	9	33	4	85	940	3	31	2 vegetables, 4 lean meat
Caesar Salad	1	90	7	4	38	2.5	10	170	3	6	1 vegetable, 1 fat

FAST FOODS

	Serving	Calories	Carb. (g)	Fat (g)	% Cal. Fat	Sat. Fat (g)	Chol. (mg)	Sod. (mg)	Fib. (g)	Prot. (g)	Servings/ Exchanges
Caesar Salad with Crispy Chicken	1	300	22	14	40	4.5	50	910	3	24	1 1/2 carb, 3 med-fat meat
Caesar Salad with Grilled Chicken	1	200	10	6	25	3	70	830	3	28	2 vegetable, 3 lean meat
California Cobb Salad	1	150	7	9	53	4	85	400	3	11	1 vegetable, 1 med-fat meat, 1 fat
California Cobb Salad with Crispy Chicken	1	360	22	18	47	6	125	1140	3	29	1 1/2 carb, 3 med-fat meat, 1 fat
California Cobb Salad with Grilled Chicken	1	260	10	11	38	5	145	1060	3	32	2 vegetable, 4 lean meat
Side Salad	1	15	3	0	0	0	0	10	1	1	1 vegetable
Breakfast											
Egg McMuffin	1	290	30	11	34	4.5	235	850	2	17	2 strch, 2 med-fat meat
Sausage McMuffin	1	370	31	21	51	9	45	790	2	14	2 strch, 1 med-fat meat, 3 fat

Food											Exchanges
Sausage McMuffin with Egg	1	450	31	26	53	10	260	930	2	20	2 strch, 2 med-fat meat. 3 fat
English Muffin	1	150	27	2	10	1	0	260	2	5	2 strch
Bacon, Egg & Cheese Biscuit	1	440	36	24	50	8	245	1250	1	19	2 1/2 strch, 2 med-fat meat, 3 fat
Sausage Biscuit	1	410	34	26	59	8	30	990	1	10	2 strch, 1 med-fat meat, 4 fat
Sausage Biscuit with Egg	1	500	36	32	58	10	250	1080	1	18	2 1/2 strch, 2 med-fat meat, 4 fat
Biscuit	1	240	31	11	42	2.5	0	680	1	4	2 strch, 2 fat
Bacon, Egg & Cheese McGriddles	1	450	46	21	40	7	245	1260	1	20	3 strch, 2 med-fat meat, 2 fat
Sausage, Egg & Cheese McGriddles	1	560	48	32	50	11	260	1290	1	21	3 strch, 2 med-fat meat, 4 fat
Sausage McGriddles	1	420	44	22	48	7	30	990	1	11	3 strch, 4 fat
Big Breakfast	1	730	53	46	56	14	465	1460	3	27	3 1/2 strch, 3 med-fat meat, 6 fat

FAST FOODS

	Serving	Calories	Carb. (g)	Fat (g)	% Cal. Fat	Sat. Fat (g)	Chol. (mg)	Sod. (mg)	Fib. (g)	Prot. (g)	Servings/ Exchanges
Deluxe Breakfast	1	1220	136	60	44	17	480	1900	4	33	9 strch, 1 med-fat meat, 11 fat
Sausage Burrito	1	300	26	16	47	6	175	760	1	13	2 strch, 1 med-fat meat, 2 fat
Hotcakes & Sausage	1	770	104	33	39	9	50	930	2	15	7 carb, 7 fat
Hotcakes (2 pats margarine & syrup)	1	600	102	17	27	4	20	620	2	9	7 carb, 3 fat
Scrambled Eggs	2	180	5	11	56	4	435	180	0	15	2 med-fat meat
Warm Cinnamon Roll	1	420	57	18	38	4.5	60	400	2	8	4 carb, 3 fat
Desserts/Shakes											
Baked Apple Pie	1	250	34	11	40	3	0	150	2	2	2 carb, 2 fat
Apple Dippers with Low-Fat Caramel Dip	1	100	22	1	5	0.5	5	35	0	0	1 1/2 carb
Fruit 'n Yogurt Parfait (with Granola)	5.3 oz	160	31	2	13	1	5	85	<1	4	2 carb
Hot Caramel Sundae	6.4 oz	340	62	7	21	4.5	30	140	0	7	4 carb, 1 fat

Hot Fudge Sundae	6.4 oz	330	55	9	24	6	25	170	<1	8	4 carb, 2 fat
Strawberry Sundae	6.3 oz	280	51	6	18	3.5	25	85	0	6	3 1/2 carb, 1 fat
Kiddie Cone	1 oz	45	8	1	25	0.5	5	20	0	1	1/2 carb
M&M'S McFlurry	12.3 oz	620	96	20	29	12	55	190	<1	14	6 1/2 carb, 4 fat
Oreo McFlurry	11.9 oz	560	88	16	27	9	50	250	0	14	6 carb, 3 fat
McDonaldland Chocolate Chip Cookies	2 oz	270	39	11	37	6	35	170	1	3	2 1/2 carb, 2 fat
McDonaldland Cookies	2 oz	250	42	8	28	2	0	270	<1	4	3 carb, 2 fat
Vanilla Reduced-Fat Ice Cream Cone	3.2 oz	150	24	3.5	23	2	15	60	0	4	1 1/2 carb, 1 fat
Chocolate Triple Thick Shake (Small)	12 oz	440	76	10	20	6	40	190	<1	10	5 carb, 2 fat
Chocolate Triple Thick Shake (Medium)	16 oz	580	102	14	21	8	50	250	<1	13	7 carb, 3 fat
Chocolate Triple Thick Shake (Large)	21 oz	770	134	18	21	11	70	330	1	18	9 carb, 4 fat

FAST FOODS

	Serving	Calories	Carb. (g)	Fat (g)	% Cal. Fat	Sat. Fat (g)	Chol. (mg)	Sod. (mg)	Fib. (g)	Prot. (g)	Servings/ Exchanges
Vanilla Triple Thick Shake (Small)	12 oz	420	72	10	21	6	40	140	0	9	5 carb, 2 fat
Vanilla Triple Thick Shake (Medium)	16 oz	550	96	13	22	8	50	190	0	13	6 1/2 carb, 3 fat
Vanilla Triple Thick Shake (Large)	21 oz	740	128	18	22	11	70	250	0	17	8 1/2 carb, 4 fat
PANDA EXPRESS											
Chicken											
Black Pepper Chicken	5.5 oz	180	10	10	50	2	40	630	2	13	1/2 carb, 2 med-fat meat
Chicken with Mushrooms	5.5 oz	130	7	7	46	2	50	590	2	11	1/2 carb, 2 lean meat
Chicken with Potato	5.5 oz	220	17	11	45	2	55	910	1	12	1 carb, 1 med-fat meat, 1 fat
Chicken with String Beans	5.5 oz	170	12	8	41	1.5	30	560	3	11	1 carb, 1 med-fat meat, 1 fat
Mandarin Chicken	5.5 oz	250	8	9	32	3	125	960	2	34	1/2 carb, 4 lean meat
Orange Flavored Chicken	5.5 oz	480	50	21	40	5	80	820	2	21	3 carb, 2 med-fat meat, 2 fat

Spicy Chicken with Peanuts	5.5 oz	200	17	7	30	2	70	800	4	18	1 carb, 2 lean meat
Sweet & Sour Chicken	4 oz	310	28	14	42	3	50	330	2	18	2 carb, 2 med-fat meat, 1 fat
Beef											
Beef with Broccoli	5.5 oz	150	9	2	47	2	15	730	1	11	1/2 carb, 2 med-fat meat
Beef with String Beans	5.5 oz	170	11	9	47	2	20	640	2	12	1 carb, 1 med-fat meat, 1 fat
Pork											
BBQ Pork	4.5 oz	350	13	19	49	7	85	970	<1	32	1 carb, 4 med-fat meat
Sweet & Sour Pork	4 oz	410	17	30	66	7	55	350	3	19	1 carb, 2 med-fat meat, 4 fat
Vegetables											
Mixed Vegetables	5.5 oz	70	8	3	43	0.5	0	420	1	3	1 vegetable, 1 fat
Tofu											
String Beans with Fried Tofu	5.5 oz	180	11	11	56	2	0	650	3	10	1 carb, 1 med-fat meat, 1 fat
Rice & Noodles											
Steamed Rice	8 oz	330	74	0.5	2	0	0	20	2	7	5 carb

FAST FOODS

	Serving	Calories	Carb. (g)	Fat (g)	% Cal. Fat	Sat. Fat (g)	Chol. (mg)	Sod. (mg)	Fib. (g)	Prot. (g)	Servings/ Exchanges
Vegetable Chow Mein	8 oz	330	48	11	30	2	0	810	4	10	3 carb, 2 fat
Vegetable Fried Rice	8 oz	390	61	12	28	3	85	740	2	9	4 carb, 2 fat
Appetizers											
Chicken Egg Roll	1	190	21	8	37	2	25	450	3	8	1 1/2 carb, 1 med-fat meat, 1 fat
Fried Shrimp	6 pieces	260	26	12	42	3	65	730	<1	12	2 carb, 1 med-fat meat, 1 fat
Veggie Spring Roll	1	80	14	3	25	0	0	270	<1	2	1 carb, 1 fat
Sauces											
Hot Sauce	2 tsp	10	2	0.5	50	0	0	130	0	0	free
Mandarin Sauce	1.5 oz	70	16	0	0	0	0	670	0	<1	1 carb
Sweet & Sour Sauce	1.5 oz	60	15	0	0	0	0	120	0	<1	1 carb
PAPA JOHN'S											
Original Crust, Large 14 inch											
Cheese	1 slice	290	39	10	31	3	17	699	2	12	2 1/2 carb, 1 med-fat meat, 1 fat
Pepperoni	1 slice	343	39	15	39	5	27	913	2	14	2 1/2 carb, 1 med-fat meat, 2 fat

Sausage	1 slice	336	39	14	39	4	28	894	2	14	2 1/2 carb, 1 med-fat meat, 2 fat
All the Meats	1 slice	405	39	20	44	7	41	1114	2	18	2 1/2 carb, 2 med-fat meat, 2 fat
Garden Fresh	1 slice	287	40	9	29	2.5	14	685	3	12	2 1/2 carb, 1 med-fat meat, 1 fat
The Works	1 slice	370	40	16	39	5	34	1013	3	17	2 1/2 carb, 1 med-fat meat, 2 fat
Spinach Alfredo	1 slice	303	37	12	36	5	26	694	2	13	2 1/2 carb, 1 med-fat meat, 1 fat
Chicken Alfredo	1 slice	310	37	12	34	4	31	743	2	15	2 1/2 carb, 1 med-fat meat, 1 fat
BBQ Chicken & Bacon	1 slice	369	44	14	34	4	31	929	2	17	3 carb, 1 med-fat meat, 2 fat
Hawaiian BBQ Chicken	1 slice	376	46	14	34	4	31	1029	2	17	3 carb, 1 med-fat meat, 2 fat
Thin Crust, Large 14 inch											
Cheese	1 slice	238	23	13	48	3	17	490	1	10	1 1/2 carb, 1 med-fat meat, 2 fat
Pepperoni	1 slice	294	23	18	54	5	28	675	1.5	12	1 1/2 carb, 1 med-fat meat, 3 fat
Sausage	1 slice	303	24	18	54	5	31	724	1.5	13	1 1/2 carb, 1 med-fat meat, 3 fat
All the Meats	1 slice	371	24	24	57	7	44	945	1.5	17	1 1/2 carb, 2 med-fat meat, 3 fat
Garden Fresh	1 slice	228	24	11	45	3	14	447	2	9	1 1/2 carb, 1 med-fat meat, 1 fat
The Works	1 slice	315	25	18	53	5	32	809	2	14	1 1/2 carb, 1 med-fat meat, 3 fat
Spinach Alfredo	1 slice	251	22	15	52	5	26	470	1	10	1 1/2 carb, 1 med-fat meat, 2 fat

FAST FOODS

	Serving	Calories	Carb. (g)	Fat (g)	% Cal. Fat	Sat. Fat (g)	Chol. (mg)	Sod. (mg)	Fib. (g)	Prot. (g)	Servings/ Exchanges
Chicken Alfredo	1 slice	276	22	15	50	5	35	573	1	14	1 1/2 carb, 2 med-fat meat, 1 fat
BBQ Chicken & Bacon	1 slice	336	30	18	48	5	34	759	1	15	2 carb, 2 med-fat meat, 2 fat
Hawaiian BBQ Chicken	1 slice	324	31	17	46	5	31	805	1	14	2 carb, 1 med-fat meat, 2 fat
Side Items											
Cheese Sticks	1 order	180	20	8	40	3	13	380	1	8	1 carb, 1 med-fat meat, 1 fat
Bread Sticks	1 order	140	26	2	14	0	0	260	1	4	2 carb
Papa's Chicken Strips	1 order	83	5	4	49	1	13	178	<1	6	1 med-fat meat
Papa's Cinnapie	1	114	14	6	46	1	0	145	0	1	1 carb, 1 fat
Cheese Sauce	1	60	0	5	75	4	19	300	0	4	1 med-fat meat
Garlic Sauce	1	235	0	26	100	3	0	300	0	0	5 fat
Pizza Sauce	1	25	3	2	80	0	0	125	2	0	free
Ranch	1	140	2	14	93	3	15	280	0	0	3 fat
Honey Mustard	1	190	6	19	90	3	10	150	0	0	1/2 carb, 4 fat
BBQ Chicken & Bacon	1	48	10	0	0	0	0	310	0	0	1/2 carb

PIZZA HUT

Pan Pizza, Large 14 inch

Cheese	1 slice	270	27	13	44	5	25	470	1	11	2 carb, 1 med-fat meat, 2 fat
Pepperoni	1 slice	280	26	14	46	5	25	530	1	11	2 carb, 1 med-fat meat, 2 fat
Quartered Ham	1 slice	250	26	11	40	4	20	510	1	11	2 carb, 1 med-fat meat, 1 fat
Supreme	1 slice	300	27	16	47	6	25	600	2	12	2 carb, 1 med-fat meat, 2 fat
Chicken Supreme	1 slice	260	27	11	38	4	20	490	1	12	2 carb, 1 med-fat meat, 1 fat
Meat Lover's	1 slice	320	27	18	50	6	35	690	2	14	2 carb, 1 med-fat meat, 3 fat
Veggie Lover's	1 slice	250	28	11	40	4	15	440	2	9	2 carb, 2 fat
Pepperoni Lover's	1 slice	330	27	18	52	7	35	670	2	14	2 carb, 1 med-fat meat, 3 fat
Sausage Lover's	1 slice	300	27	17	50	6	30	590	2	12	2 carb, 1 med-fat meat, 2 fat

Thin 'N Crispy Pizza, Large 14 inch

Cheese	1 slice	190	20	8	37	5	25	460	1	9	1 carb, 1 med-fat meat, 1 fat
Pepperoni	1 slice	200	19	9	45	5	25	520	1	9	1 carb, 1 med-fat meat, 1 fat
Quartered Ham	1 slice	170	19	6	35	3	20	500	1	9	1 carb, 1 med-fat meat
Supreme	1 slice	220	21	11	45	5	25	600	2	11	1 1/2 carb, 1 med-fat meat, 1 fat

FAST FOODS

	Serving	Calories	Carb. (g)	Fat (g)	% Cal. Fat	Sat. Fat (g)	Chol. (mg)	Sod. (mg)	Fib. (g)	Prot. (g)	Servings/Exchanges
Chicken Supreme	1 slice	180	21	6	33	3	20	480	1	11	1 1/2 carb, 1 med-fat meat
Meat Lover's	1 slice	250	20	13	48	6	35	700	2	12	1 carb, 1 med-fat meat, 2 fat
Veggie Lover's	1 slice	170	21	7	35	3	15	450	2	8	1 carb, 1 med-fat meat
Pepperoni Lover's	1 slice	250	20	14	48	6	35	660	1	12	1 carb, 1 med-fat meat, 2 fat
Sausage Lover's	1 slice	230	20	12	43	5	30	580	1	10	1 carb, 1 med-fat meat, 1 fat
Hand-Tossed Style Pizzas, Large 14 inch											
Cheese	1 slice	220	27	8	32	5	25	480	1	11	2 carb, 1 med-fat meat, 1 fat
Pepperoni	1 slice	230	27	9	35	5	25	540	2	11	2 carb, 1 med-fat meat, 1 fat
Quartered Ham	1 slice	200	27	6	25	3	20	520	1	11	2 carb, 1 med-fat meat
Supreme	1 slice	250	28	10	36	5	25	620	2	13	2 carb, 1 med-fat meat, 1 fat
Chicken Supreme	1 slice	210	28	6	24	3	20	500	2	13	2 carb, 1 med-fat meat
Meat Lover's	1 slice	280	27	12	39	6	35	710	2	14	2 carb, 1 med-fat meat, 1 fat
Veggie Lover's	1 slice	200	28	6	25	3	15	460	2	9	2 carb, 1 fat
Pepperoni Lover's	1 slice	280	27	13	43	6	35	680	2	14	2 carb, 1 med-fat meat, 2 fat

Sausage Lover's	1 slice	260	27	11	38	5	30	600	2	12	2 carb, 1 med-fat meat, 1 fat

Stuffed Crust Pizzas, Large 14 inch

Cheese	1 slice	360	43	13	33	8	40	920	2	18	3 carb, 2 med-fat meat, 1 fat
Pepperoni	1 slice	370	42	15	35	8	45	970	3	18	3 carb, 2 med-fat meat, 1 fat
Quartered Ham	1 slice	340	42	11	29	6	40	960	2	18	3 carb, 2 med-fat meat
Supreme	1 slice	400	44	16	38	8	45	1070	3	20	3 carb, 2 med-fat meat, 1 fat
Chicken Supreme	1 slice	380	44	13	32	7	40	1020	3	20	3 carb, 2 med-fat meat, 1 fat
Meat Lover's	1 slice	450	43	21	42	10	55	1250	3	21	3 carb, 2 med-fat meat, 2 fat
Veggie Lover's	1 slice	360	45	14	33	7	35	980	3	16	3 carb, 1 med-fat meat, 2 fat
Pepperoni Lover's	1 slice	420	43	19	40	10	55	1120	3	21	3 carb, 2 med-fat meat, 2 fat
Sausage Lover's	1 slice	430	43	19	40	9	50	1130	3	19	3 carb, 2 med-fat meat, 2 fat

Fit 'N Delicious, Large 14 inch

Diced Chicken, Red Onion & Green Pepper	1 slice	160	22	4	22	2	15	420	2	9	1 1/2 carb, 1 med-fat meat
Diced Chicken, Mushroom & Jalapeño	1 slice	160	20	5	25	2	15	630	2	9	1 carb, 1 med-fat meat

FAST FOODS

	Serving	Calories	Carb. (g)	Fat (g)	% Cal. Fat	Sat. Fat (g)	Chol. (mg)	Sod. (mg)	Fib. (g)	Prot. (g)	Servings/ Exchanges
Ham, Red Onion & Mushroom	1 slice	150	21	4	27	2	15	440	2	8	1 1/2 carb, 1 med-fat meat
Ham, Pineapple & Diced Red Tomato	1 slice	150	22	4	23	2	15	440	1	7	1 1/2 carb, 1 fat
Green Pepper, Red Onion & Diced Tomato	1 slice	140	22	4	25	2	10	330	2	6	1 1/2 carb, 1 fat
Tomato, Mushroom & Jalapeño	1 slice	140	21	4	25	2	10	540	2	6	1 1/2 carb, 1 fat
P'Zone											
Pepperoni	1/2	610	69	22	33	11	55	1280	3	34	4 1/2 carb, 3 med-fat meat, 1 fat
Classic	1/2	610	71	21	31	11	50	1210	3	33	5 carb, 3 med-fat meat, 1 fat
Meat Lover's	1/2	680	70	28	37	14	65	1540	3	38	4 1/2 carb, 5 med-fat meat, 1 fat
Marinara Dipping Sauce	1	45	9	0	0	0	0	380	2	2	1/2 carb
Appetizers											
Bread Sticks	1	150	20	6	40	1	0	220	<1	4	1 carb, 1 fat

Cheese Breadsticks	1	200	21	10	45	4	15	340	<1	7	1 1/2 carb, 2 fat
Hot Wings	2	110	1	6	55	2	70	450	0	11	2 lean meat

Desserts

Cinnamon Sticks	2	170	27	5	26	1	0	170	<1	4	2 carb, 1 fat
White Icing Dipping Cup	2 oz	190	46	0	0	0	0	0	0	0	3 carb
Apple Dessert Pizza	1 slice	260	53	4	12	0.5	0	250	1	4	3 1/2 carb, 1 fat

RUBIOS

Baja Gourmet Seafood Burritos

Fish	1	740	70	40	49	8	50	1080	7	24	4 1/2 carb, 2 med-fat meat, 6 fat
Lobster	1	670	79	32	43	5	190	1410	8	16	5 carb, 6 fat
Mahi Mahi	1	700	56	38	49	11	60	1210	5	32	4 carb, 3 med-fat meat, 5 fat
Shrimp	1	630	75	25	37	7	165	1570	5	24	5 carb, 1 med-fat meat, 4 fat

Burritos

Baja Grill Carne Asada	1	680	58	32	43	13	100	2220	5	38	4 carb, 4 med-fat meat, 2 fat
Baja Grill Chicken	1	630	58	24	35	8	120	1800	5	46	4 carb, 5 med-fat meat
Cheesy Bean	1	820	88	36	40	19	105	1890	16	34	6 carb, 2 med-fat meat, 5 fat

FAST FOODS

	Serving	Calories	Carb. (g)	Fat (g)	% Cal. Fat	Sat. Fat (g)	Chol. (mg)	Sod. (mg)	Fib. (g)	Prot. (g)	Servings/Exchanges
Especial Carne Asada	1	940	117	37	35	10	65	2380	8	33	8 carb, 2 med-fat meat, 5 fat
Especial Chicken	1	890	117	29	29	6	85	2050	8	39	8 carb, 2 med-fat meat, 4 fat
HealthMex Chicken	1	530	77	10	18	1.5	70	1670	7	35	5 carb, 3 lean meat
HealthMex Veggie	1	520	98	8	14	1	0	1020	11	19	6 1/2 carb, 2 fat
Fish Tacos											
Especial	1	370	30	21	51	5	35	330	3	14	2 carb, 1 med-fat meat, 3 fat
Original	1	300	28	16	47	3	20	250	2	11	2 carb, 1 med-fat meat, 2 fat
Kid's Meals											
Baja Bites	5	230	19	8	35	1.5	40	1000	1	19	1 carb, 2 med-fat meat
Bean & Cheese Burrito	1	570	71	21	33	10	45	1190	9	21	5 carb, 1 med-fat meat, 3 fat
Cheese Quesadilla	1	360	32	18	47	10	50	680	1	17	2 carb, 2 med-fat meat, 2 fat
Original Fish Taco	1	300	27	16	47	3	20	120	2	11	2 carb, 1 med-fat meat, 2 fat
Taquitos	2	210	18	9	38	4.5	45	250	2	13	1 carb, 2 fat

Rubio's Favorites

Carne Asada Quesadilla	1	990	58	61	56	30	180	2290	4	53	4 carb, 6 med-fat meat, 6 fat
Cheese Quesadilla	1	830	56	52	57	27	125	1400	4	36	4 carb, 3 med-fat meat, 7 fat
Chicken Quesadilla	1	950	58	54	52	27	195	1960	4	59	4 carb, 7 med-fat meat, 4 fat
Chicken Taquitos	3	290	34	11	34	2	40	290	5	15	2 carb, 1 med-fat meat, 1 fat
Nacho Grande	1	1270	111	78	55	27	120	1800	20	37	7 carb, 2 med-fat meat, 14 fat
Nacho Grande Carne Asada	1	1420	113	87	55	31	175	2690	20	54	7 1/2 carb, 4 med-fat meat, 13 fat
Nacho Grande Chicken	1	1380	113	80	52	28	190	2360	20	59	7 1/2 carb, 5 med-fat meat, 11 fat

Sides

Black Beans	1	170	28	2	9	1	5	600	4	11	2 carb, 1 lean meat
Chips	1	430	56	22	47	1.5	0	480	7	5	4 carb, 4 fat
Churro	1	170	22	8	41	2	20	140	0	2	1 1/2 carb, 2 fat
Guacamole (small)	1	170	8	16	82	2.5	0	65	5	2	1/2 carb, 3 fat
Guacamole (large)	1	340	16	32	85	5	0	135	11	4	1 carb, 6 fat

FAST FOODS

	Serving	Calories	Carb. (g)	Fat (g)	% Cal. Fat	Sat. Fat (g)	Chol. (mg)	Sod. (mg)	Fib. (g)	Prot. (g)	Servings/ Exchanges
Pinto Beans	1	190	37	3	13	1.5	5	600	1	4	2 1/2 carb, 1 fat
Rice	1	160	33	1.5	9	0	0	290	1	2	2 carb
Salads & Bowls											
Grilled Chicken Chopped Salad	1	570	34	33	53	9	105	1490	7	36	2 carb, 4 med-fat meat, 3 fat
Grilled Grande Bowl Chicken	1	720	73	30	38	9	105	1710	8	41	5 carb, 4 med-fat meat, 2 fat
HealthMex Chicken Salad	1	250	31	2	8	0	70	990	6	27	2 carb, 3 very lean meat
Low Carb Chicken Salad	1	470	11	33	64	10	110	980	4	34	1 carb, 4 med-fat meat, 3 fat
Tacos											
Carne Asada	1	250	24	10	36	4.5	35	530	2	14	1 1/2 carb, 2 med-fat meat
Chicken	1	300	24	15	47	4	45	440	2	16	1 1/2 carb, 2 med-fat meat, 1 fat
HealthMex Chicken	1	170	23	2	12	0.5	30	400	2	14	1 1/2 carb, 1 lean meat
Mahi Mahi	1	310	24	16	45	4.5	30	230	2	18	1 1/2 carb, 2 med-fat meat, 1 fat

Street Burritos

	Serving										Exchanges
Carne Asada	1	330	34	13	33	4	45	1110	2	19	2 carb, 2 med-fat meat, 1 fat
Carnitas	1	300	35	11	33	3.5	40	900	2	17	2 carb, 2 med-fat meat
Chicken	1	300	34	7	20	1.5	55	640	2	24	2 carb, 3 lean meat

Street Tacos

Carnitas	1	110	11	5	41	1.5	20	270	1	8	1 carb, 1 med-fat meat
Carne Asada	1	130	10	6	38	2	20	380	1	8	1/2 carb, 1 med-fat meat
Chicken	1	110	10	3.5	27	0.5	30	240	1	11	1/2 carb, 1 lean meat

SUBWAY

6-Inch Sandwiches

Honey Mustard Ham	1	320	53	5	16	1.5	25	1420	4	18	3 1/2 carb, 1 med-fat meat
Oven Roasted Chicken Breast	1	330	47	5	15	1.5	45	1020	4	24	3 carb, 2 lean meat
Roast Beef	1	290	45	5	16	2	20	920	4	19	3 carb, 1 med-fat meat
Savory Turkey Breast	1	280	46	4.5	14	1.5	20	1020	4	18	3 carb, 1 med-fat meat

FAST FOODS

	Serving	Calories	Carb. (g)	Fat (g)	% Cal. Fat	Sat. Fat (g)	Chol. (mg)	Sod. (mg)	Fib. (g)	Prot. (g)	Servings/ Exchanges
Savory Turkey Breast & Ham	1	290	47	5	16	1.5	25	1230	4	20	3 carb, 2 lean meat
Subway Club	1	320	47	6	16	2	35	1310	4	24	3 carb, 2 lean meat
Sweet Onion Teriyaki	1	370	59	5	12	1.5	50	1220	4	26	4 carb, 2 lean meat
Veggie Delite	1	230	44	3	13	1	0	520	4	9	3 carb, 1 fat
6-Inch Hot Sandwiches											
Cheese Steak	1	250	47	10	25	4.5	35	1090	5	24	3 carb, 2 med-fat meat
Chicken & Bacon Ranch	1	530	47	25	43	10	90	1400	5	36	3 carb, 4 med-fat meat, 1 fat
Chipotle Southwest Cheese Steak	1	450	48	20	40	6	45	1310	6	24	3 carb, 2 med-fat meat, 2 fat
Italian BMT	1	450	47	21	42	8	55	1790	4	23	3 carb, 2 med-fat meat, 2 fat
Meatball Marinara	1	560	63	24	39	11	45	1610	7	24	4 carb, 2 med-fat meat, 3 fat
Turkey Breast, Ham & Bacon Melt	1	380	48	12	29	5	45	1610	4	25	3 carb, 2 med-fat meat

6-Inch Cold Sandwiches

Classic Tuna	1	530	45	31	53	7	45	1030	4	22	3 carb, 2 med-fat meat, 4 fat
Cold Cut Combo	1	410	47	17	37	7	60	1550	4	21	3 carb, 2 med-fat meat, 1 fat
Subway Seafood Sensation	1	450	51	22	44	6	25	1150	5	16	3 1/2 carb, 1 med-fat meat, 3 fat

Deli Style Sandwiches

Classic Tuna	1	350	35	18	49	5	30	750	3	14	2 carb, 1 med-fat meat, 3 fat
Ham	1	210	36	4	17	1.5	10	770	3	11	2 1/2 carb, 1 med-fat meat
Roast Beef	1	220	35	4.5	18	2	15	660	3	13	2 carb, 1 med-fat meat
Savory Turkey Breast	1	210	36	3.5	17	1.5	15	730	3	13	2 1/2 carb, 1 lean meat

Wraps

Chicken & Bacon Ranch with Cheese	1	440	18	27	55	10	90	1670	9	41	1 carb, 5 med-fat meat
Tuna, with cheese	1	440	16	32	66	6	45	1310	9	27	1 carb, 3 med-fat meat, 3 fat
Turkey Breast & Bacon Melt, with Chipotle Sauce	1	440	20	28	59	10	65	1870	9	34	1 carb, 4 med-fat meat, 2 fat

FAST FOODS

	Serving	Calories	Carb. (g)	Fat (g)	% Cal. Fat	Sat. Fat (g)	Chol. (mg)	Sod. (mg)	Fib. (g)	Prot. (g)	Servings/ Exchanges
Turkey Breast	1	190	18	6	26	1	20	1290	9	24	1 carb, 3 lean meat
Salads (Dressing & Croutons Not Included)											
Grilled Chicken & Baby Spinach	1	140	11	3	18	1	50	450	4	20	2 vegetable, 2 very lean meat
Subway Club	1	160	15	4	22	1.5	35	880	4	18	3 vegetable, 2 lean meat
Tuna, with Cheese	1	360	12	29	72	6	45	600	4	16	2 vegetable, 1 med-fat meat, 5 fat
Veggie Delite	1	60	12	1	17	0	0	90	4	3	2 vegetable
Breakfast Sandwiches on Deli Round											
Bacon & Egg	1	320	34	15	44	4.5	190	520	3	15	2 carb, 1 med-fat meat, 2 fat
Cheese & Egg	1	320	34	15	44	5	190	550	3	14	2 carb, 1 med-fat meat, 2 fat
Ham & Egg	1	310	35	13	35	3.5	190	720	3	16	2 carb, 1 med-fat meat, 2 fat
Steak & Egg	1	330	35	14	36	4	190	570	3	19	2 carb, 2 med-fat meat, 1 fat
Vegetable & Egg	1	290	36	12	38	3	180	410	3	12	2 1/2 carb, 1 med-fat meat, 1 fat

	Serving	Cal.									Exchanges
Western Egg	1	300	36	12	37	3.5	180	530	3	14	2 1/2 carb, 1 med-fat meat, 1 fat
Cookies											
Chocolate Chip	1	210	30	10	43	4	15	160	1	2	2 carb, 2 fat
M&M	1	210	30	10	43	3.5	15	105	1	2	2 carb, 2 fat
Oatmeal Raisin	1	200	30	8	35	2.5	15	170	2	3	2 carb, 2 fat
Peanut Butter	1	220	26	12	50	4	10	200	1	4	2 carb, 2 fat
Sugar	1	230	28	12	48	3.5	15	135	0	2	2 carb, 2 fat
White Chip Macadamia Nut	1	220	28	11	45	3.5	15	160	1	2	2 carb, 2 fat
Soup											
Brown & Wild Rice with Chicken	1 cup	190	17	11	53	4.5	20	990	2	6	1 carb, 2 fat
Chicken & Dumpling	1 cup	130	16	4.5	31	2.5	30	1030	1	7	1 carb, 1 med-fat meat
Chili Con Carne	1 cup	240	23	10	38	5	15	860	8	15	1 1/2 carb, 2 med-fat meat
Cream of Broccoli	1 cup	130	15	6	38	2	10	860	2	5	1 carb, 1 fat
Minestrone	1 cup	90	7	4	39	1	20	1180	1	7	1/2 carb, 1 med-fat meat

FAST FOODS

	Serving	Calories	Carb. (g)	Fat (g)	% Cal. Fat	Sat. Fat (g)	Chol. (mg)	Sod. (mg)	Fib. (g)	Prot. (g)	Servings/ Exchanges
New England Clam Chowder	1 cup	110	16	3.5	27	0.5	10	990	1	5	1 carb, 1 fat
Roasted Chicken Noodle	1 cup	60	7	1.5	25	0.5	10	940	1	6	1/2 carb, 1 very lean meat
Vegetable Beef	1 cup	90	15	1	11	0.5	5	1050	3	5	1 carb

TACO BELL
Fresco Style (Under 10 grams of fat)

	Serving	Calories	Carb. (g)	Fat (g)	% Cal. Fat	Sat. Fat (g)	Chol. (mg)	Sod. (mg)	Fib. (g)	Prot. (g)	Servings/ Exchanges
Crunchy Taco	1	150	14	7	47	3	20	360	2	7	1 carb, 1 med-fat meat
Soft Taco, Beef	1	190	22	8	37	3	20	630	2	9	1 1/2 carb, 1 med-fat meat, 1 fat
Ranchero Chicken Soft Taco	1	170	22	4	21	1	25	710	2	12	1 1/2 carb, 1 med-fat meat
Grilled Steak Soft Taco	1	170	21	5	26	2	15	560	2	11	1 1/2 carb, 1 med-fat meat
Gordita Baja, Beef	1	250	31	9	32	3	20	640	2	12	2 carb, 1 med-fat meat, 1 fat
Gordita Baja, Chicken	1	230	29	6	22	1	25	570	2	15	2 carb, 1 med-fat meat
Gordita Baja, Steak	1	230	29	7	26	2	15	570	3	13	2 carb, 1 med-fat meat

Bean Burrito	1	350	56	8	20	2	0	1220	9	13	4 carb, 2 fat
Burrito Supreme, Chicken	1	350	50	8	20	2	25	1270	6	19	3 carb, 2 med-fat meat
Burrito Supreme, Steak	1	350	50	9	23	3	15	1260	6	17	3 carb, 1 med-fat meat, 1 fat
Fiesta Burrito, Chicken	1	350	49	9	23	2	25	1100	4	16	3 carb, 1 med-fat meat, 1 fat
Tostada	1	200	30	6	25	1	0	670	8	8	2 carb, 1 fat
Enchirito, Beef	1	270	35	9	30	3	20	1300	5	12	2 carb, 1 med-fat meat, 1 fat
Enchirito, Chicken	1	250	34	5	20	2	25	1230	5	16	2 carb, 1 med-fat meat
Enchirito, Steak	1	250	34	7	24	2	15	1220	6	14	2 carb, 1 med-fat meat
Big Bell Value Menu											
Grande Soft Taco	1	450	44	21	42	8	45	1410	2	19	3 carb, 1 med-fat meat, 3 fat
Double Decker Taco	1	340	39	14	35	5	25	810	5	14	2 1/2 carb, 1 med-fat meat, 2 fat
Double Decker Taco Supreme	1	380	41	18	42	8	40	820	5	15	3 carb, 1 med-fat meat, 3 fat
Spicy Chicken Taco	1	180	21	7	33	2	20	580	2	10	1 1/2 carb, 1 med-fat meat
Spicy Chicken Burrito	1	430	50	19	40	5	30	1160	4	14	3 carb, 1 med-fat meat, 3 fat
1/2 lb. Bean Burrito Especial	1	600	82	21	32	5	15	1760	12	21	5 1/2 carb, 1 med-fat meat, 3 fat

FAST FOODS

	Serving	Calories	Carb. (g)	Fat (g)	% Cal. Fat	Sat. Fat (g)	Chol. (mg)	Sod. (mg)	Fib. (g)	Prot. (g)	Servings/Exchanges
1/2 lb. Bean Combo Burrito	1	470	52	19	36	7	45	1620	5	22	3 1/2 carb, 1 med-fat meat, 3 fat
Tacos											
Taco	1	170	13	10	53	4	25	350	<1	8	1 carb, 1 med-fat meat, 1 fat
Taco Supreme	1	220	14	14	55	7	35	360	1	9	1 carb, 1 med-fat meat, 2 fat
Soft Taco, Beef	1	190	22	8	37	3	20	630	2	9	1 1/2 carb, 1 med-fat meat, 1 fat
Soft Taco Supreme, Beef	1	260	23	14	50	7	35	640	1	11	1 1/2 carb, 1 med-fat meat, 2 fat
Ranchero Chicken Soft Taco	1	170	22	4	21	1	25	710	2	12	1 1/2 carb, 1 med-fat meat
Grilled Steak Soft Taco	1	170	21	5	26	2	15	560	2	11	1 1/2 carb, 1 med-fat meat
Gorditas											
Gordita Baja, Beef	1	250	31	9	32	3	20	640	2	12	2 carb, 1 med-fat meat, 1 fat
Gordita Baja, Chicken	1	230	29	6	22	1	25	570	2	15	2 carb, 1 med-fat meat
Gordita Baja, Steak	1	230	29	7	26	2	15	570	3	13	2 carb, 1 med-fat meat
Gordita Supreme, Beef	1	310	30	16	45	7	35	600	2	14	2 carb, 1 med-fat meat, 2 fat

Item											Exchanges
Gordita Supreme, Chicken	1	290	28	12	38	5	45	530	2	17	2 carb, 2 med-fat meat
Gordita Supreme, Steak	1	290	28	13	41	6	35	520	2	16	2 carb, 1 med-fat meat, 2 fat
Chalupas											
Chalupa Supreme, Beef	1	390	31	24	56	10	35	600	1	14	2 carb, 1 med-fat meat, 4 fat
Chalupa Supreme, Chicken	1	370	30	20	49	8	45	530	1	17	2 carb, 2 med-fat meat, 2 fat
Chalupa Supreme, Steak	1	370	29	22	51	8	35	520	2	15	2 carb, 1 med-fat meat, 3 fat
Chalupa Baja, Beef	1	430	32	27	58	8	30	760	2	12	2 carb, 1 med-fat meat, 4 fat
Chalupa Baja, Chicken	1	400	30	24	53	6	40	690	2	17	2 carb, 2 med-fat meat, 3 fat
Chalupa Nacho Cheese, Beef	1	380	33	22	53	7	20	740	1	12	2 carb, 1 med-fat meat, 3 fat
Chalupa Nacho Cheese, Chicken	1	350	31	18	46	5	25	670	1	16	2 carb, 1 med-fat meat, 3 fat
Burritos											
Bean Burrito	1	350	56	8	20	2	0	1220	9	13	4 carb, 2 fat
7-Layer Burrito	1	530	66	21	36	8	25	1350	10	18	4 1/2 carb, 1 med-fat meat, 3 fat
Chili Cheese Burrito	1	390	40	18	41	9	40	1080	3	16	2 1/2 carb, 1 med-fat meat, 3 fat

FAST FOODS

	Serving	Calories	Carb. (g)	Fat (g)	% Cal. Fat	Sat. Fat (g)	Chol. (mg)	Sod. (mg)	Fib. (g)	Prot. (g)	Servings/ Exchanges
Burrito Supreme, Chicken	1	350	50	8	20	2	25	1270	6	19	3 carb, 2 med-fat meat
Burrito Supreme, Steak	1	350	50	9	23	3	15	1260	6	17	3 carb, 1 med-fat meat, 1 fat
Fiesta Burrito, Chicken	1	350	49	9	23	2	25	1100	4	16	3 carb, 1 med-fat meat, 1 fat
Burrito Supreme, Beef	1	440	52	18	36	8	40	1330	5	17	3 1/2 carb, 1 med-fat meat, 3 fat
Fiesta Burrito, Beef	1	390	50	15	36	5	25	1160	3	14	3 carb, 1 med-fat meat, 2 fat
Grilled Stuft Burrito, Beef	1	720	79	33	42	11	55	2090	7	27	5 carb, 2 med-fat meat, 5 fat
Grilled Stuft Burrito, Chicken	1	680	76	26	34	7	70	1950	7	35	5 carb, 3 med-fat meat, 2 fat
Specialties											
Tostada	1	200	30	6	25	1	0	670	8	8	2 carb, 1 fat
Mexican Pizza	1	550	47	31	51	11	45	1040	5	21	3 carb, 2 med-fat meat, 4 fat
MexiMelt	1	290	23	16	48	8	40	880	2	15	1 1/2 carb, 2 med-fat meat, 1 fat
Fiesta Taco Salad	1	870	80	47	49	16	65	1780	12	31	5 carb, 2 med-fat meat, 7 fat
Fiesta Taco Salad without Shell	1	500	42	27	48	12	65	1520	10	24	3 carb, 1 med-fat meat, 4 fat

Expresso Taco Salad	1	630	58	33	48	13	65	1390	10	26	4 carb, 2 med-fat meat, 5 fat
Cheese Quesadilla	1	490	39	28	53	13	55	1150	3	19	2 1/2 carb, 2 med-fat meat, 4 fat
Chicken Quesadilla	1	540	40	30	50	13	80	1380	3	28	2 1/2 carb, 3 med-fat meat, 3 fat
Steak Quesadilla	1	540	40	31	52	14	70	1370	3	26	2 1/2 carb, 2 med-fat meat, 4 fat
Zesty Chicken Border Bowl	1	730	65	42	52	9	45	1640	12	23	4 carb, 2 med-fat meat, 6 fat

Nachos & Sides

Nachos	1 order	320	33	19	53	5	<5	530	2	5	2 carb, 4 fat
Nachos Supreme	1 order	450	42	26	51	9	35	810	5	13	3 carb, 1 med-fat meat, 4 fat
Nachos BellGrande	1 order	780	80	43	49	13	35	1300	11	20	5 carb, 1 med-fat meat, 8 fat
Pintos 'n Cheese	1 order	180	20	7	33	4	15	700	6	10	1 carb, 1 med-fat meat
Mexican Rice	1 order	210	23	10	43	4	15	740	3	6	1 1/2 carb, 2 fat
Cinnamon Twists	1 order	160	28	5	31	1	0	150	0	<1	2 carb, 1 fat

TACO JOHN'S

Burritos

Bean Burrito	6.6 oz	380	53	12	29	5	15	830	10	15	3 1/2 carb, 1 med-fat meat, 1 fat

FAST FOODS

	Serving	Calories	Carb. (g)	Fat (g)	% Cal. Fat	Sat. Fat (g)	Chol. (mg)	Sod. (mg)	Fib. (g)	Prot. (g)	Servings/ Exchanges
Beefy Burrito	6.6 oz	430	41	20	42	9	55	870	8	22	3 carb, 2 med-fat meat, 2 fat
Chicken & Potato Burrito	8.5 oz	460	54	19	37	7	35	1470	8	18	3 1/2 carb, 1 med-fat meat, 3 fat
Combination Burrito	6.6 oz	400	47	16	35	7	35	850	9	18	3 carb, 1 med-fat meat, 2 fat
Meat & Potato Burrito	8.5 oz	490	55	23	43	8	30	1190	9	15	3 1/2 carb, 1 med-fat meat, 4 fat
Super Burrito	8.9 oz	450	49	20	40	9	40	920	10	19	3 carb, 2 med-fat meat, 2 fat
Desserts											
Apple Grande	2.9 oz	240	36	9	33	3	5	220	0	5	2 1/2 carb, 2 fat
Choco Taco	4 oz	300	38	15	47	7	15	110	1	4	2 1/2 carb, 3 fat
Churros	1.9 oz	230	31	11	43	2	10	120	1	2	2 carb, 2 fat
Local Favorites											
Bean Tostada	3.5 oz	160	19	6	38	2	5	250	3	6	1 carb, 1 med-fat meat
Cheese Crisp	2 oz	210	11	14	62	7	35	260	1	10	1 carb, 1 med-fat meat, 2 fat
Chicken Fajita Burrito	6.4 oz	340	39	11	26	5	50	1120	7	22	2 1/2 carb, 2 med-fat meat
Chicken Testiva Burrito	9.2 oz	530	58	24	42	7	50	21	8	21	4 carb, 1 med-fat meat, 4 fat
Chili Enchilada	12.3 oz	740	71	38	46	12	75	1470	8	31	5 carb, 2 med-fat meat, 6 fat

El Grande Burrito	13.3 oz	720	67	36	46	17	90	1640	10	32	4 1/2 carb, 3 med-fat meat, 4 fat
El Grande Chicken Burrito	13.3 oz	660	64	28	38	13	100	2210	9	39	4 carb, 4 med-fat meat, 2 fat
El Grande Chicken Taco	7 oz	380	28	20	47	7	60	1010	2	22	2 carb, 2 med-fat meat, 2 fat
El Grande Taco	8.5 oz	510	32	32	55	11	75	820	4	24	2 carb, 3 med-fat meat, 3 fat
Mexi Rolls	7.5 oz	480	33	30	56	10	50	20	3	20	2 carb, 2 med-fat meat, 4 fat
Mexican Pizza	9.4 oz	500	46	25	44	12	60	1150	5	21	3 carb, 2 med-fat meat, 3 fat
Tostada	3.5 oz	180	14	10	50	4	25	270	3	9	1 carb, 1 med-fat meat, 1 fat
Sides											
Mexican Rice	6 oz	250	45	5	16	1	0	860	2	5	3 carb, 1 fat
Nachos	5 oz	380	38	23	55	6	10	970	<1	6	2 1/2 carb, 5 fat
Potato Oles	small order	440	48	26	52	6	0	1270	5	4	3 carb, 5 fat
Potato Oles	medium order	620	67	36	53	8	0	1780	6	5	4 1/2 carb, 7 fat
Potato Oles	large order	790	86	47	53	11	0	2290	8	7	6 carb, 9 fat
Potato Oles with Nacho Cheese	8 oz	550	52	35	58	10	10	2000	5	7	3 1/2 carb, 7 fat

FAST FOODS

	Serving	Calories	Carb. (g)	Fat (g)	% Cal. Fat	Sat. Fat (g)	Chol. (mg)	Sod. (mg)	Fib. (g)	Prot. (g)	Servings/ Exchanges
Refried Beans	9.5 oz	400	50	14	30	5	15	1110	11	18	3 carb, 1 med-fat meat, 2 fat
Side Salad without Dressing	3.5 oz	80	6	5	50	2	5	50	1	3	1 vegetable, 1 fat
Texas Style Chili	8.4 oz	270	26	12	41	6	35	1400	4	15	2 carb, 2 med-fat meat
Specialties											
Cheese Quesadilla	5.9 oz	480	39	28	52	15	50	960	6	20	2 1/2 carb, 2 med-fat meat, 4 fat
Chicken Festiva Salad without Dressing	10.7 oz	400	24	23	53	10	70	830	4	24	1 1/2 carb, 3 med-fat meat, 2 fat
Chicken Quesadilla	7.4 oz	540	41	29	48	15	75	1430	7	29	3 carb, 3 med-fat meat, 3 fat
Chicken Super Nachos	12.3 oz	780	62	45	53	15	90	2250	3	31	4 carb, 3 med-fat meat, 6 fat
Chicken Taco Salad without Dressing	12.8 oz	530	45	27	45	11	70	1330	5	27	3 carb, 3 med-fat meat, 2 fat
Potato Oles Brave	8.7 oz	580	55	36	55	11	20	1760	6	9	3 1/2 carb, 7 fat
Super Nachos	12.8 oz	830	73	51	54	17	60	1730	5	22	5 carb, 1 med-fat meat, 9 fat

Food	Amount	Cal.	Carb. (g)	Fat (g)	% Cal. Fat	Sat. Fat (g)	Chol. (mg)	Sod. (mg)	Fiber (g)	Pro. (g)	Exchanges/Choices
Super Potato Oles	16	980	82	62	57	22	60	2950	10	22	5 1/2 carb, 1 med-fat meat, 11 fat
Taco Salad without Dressing	12.8 oz	580	46	32	50	13	60	960	4	23	3 carb, 2 med-fat meat, 4 fat
Tacos											
Crispy Taco	3.3 oz	180	13	10	50	4	25	270	3	9	1 carb, 1 med-fat meat, 1 fat
Chicken Softshell Taco	4 oz	190	19	6	26	3	30	460	4	14	1 carb, 2 lean meat
Sierra Taco Beef	7 oz	430	38	23	47	8	45	980	4	17	2 1/2 carb, 1 med-fat meat, 4 fat
Sierra Taco Chicken	7 oz	390	37	17	38	5	50	1350	3	21	2 1/2 carb, 2 med-fat meat, 1 fat
Softshell Taco	4 oz	220	21	10	41	5	25	470	4	11	1 1/2 carb, 1 med-fat meat, 1 fat
Taco Bravo	6.5 oz	340	39	14	35	5	25	650	8	15	2 1/2 carb, 1 med-fat meat, 2 fat
Taco Burger	5 oz	280	28	12	39	5	35	600	3	14	2 carb, 1 med-fat meat, 1 fat
WENDY'S											
Sandwiches											
Big Bacon Classic	1	580	46	29	45	12	95	1390	3	35	3 carb, 4 med-fat meat, 2 fat
Cheeseburger, Kid's Meal	1	320	34	13	34	6	40	810	1	17	2 carb, 2 med-fat meat, 1 fat

FAST FOODS

	Serving	Calories	Carb. (g)	Fat (g)	% Cal. Fat	Sat. Fat (g)	Chol. (mg)	Sod. (mg)	Fib. (g)	Prot. (g)	Servings/ Exchanges
Classic Single with Everything	1	430	37	20	42	7	65	890	2	25	2 1/2 carb, 3 med-fat meat, 1 fat
Jr. Bacon Cheeseburger	1	380	34	18	45	7	55	810	2	20	2 carb, 2 med-fat meat, 2 fat
Jr. Cheeseburger	1	320	34	13	34	6	40	810	1	17	2 carb, 1 med-fat meat, 2 fat
Jr. Cheeseburger Deluxe	1	360	37	16	39	6	45	880	2	18	2 1/2 carb, 2 med-fat meat, 1 fat
Jr. Hamburger	1	280	34	9	29	3.5	30	600	1	15	2 carb, 1 med-fat meat, 1 fat
Hamburger Kid's Meal	1	270	33	9	30	3.5	30	600	1	15	2 carb, 1 med-fat meat, 1 fat
Homestyle Chicken Fillet Sandwich	1	540	57	22	35	4	55	1320	2	29	4 carb, 3 med-fat meat, 1 fat
Spicy Chicken Fillet Sandwich	1	510	57	19	33	3.5	55	1480	2	29	4 carb, 3 med-fat meat, 1 fat
Ultimate Chicken Grill Sandwich	1	360	44	7	17	1.5	75	1090	2	31	3 carb, 3 lean meat
French Fries											
Kid's Meal	3.2 oz	280	37	14	43	2.5	0	270	3	3	2 1/2 carb, 3 fat

Medium	5 oz	440	58	21	43	3.5	0	430	5	5	4 carb, 4 fat
Biggie	5.6 oz	490	65	24	43	4	0	480	6	5	4 carb, 5 fat
Great Biggie	6.7 oz	590	77	29	44	5	0	570	7	6	5 carb, 4 fat
Baked Potatoes											
Bacon & Cheese	1	560	69	25	39	7	40	850	8	16	4 1/2 carb, 5 fat
Broccoli & Cheese	1	440	69	15	30	3	10	540	9	10	4 1/2 carb, 3 fat
Plain	10 oz	270	61	0	0	0	0	25	7	7	4 carb
Sour Cream & Chives	1	340	62	6	18	3.5	10	40	7	8	4 carb, 1 fat
Homestyle Chicken Strips & Crispy Chicken Nuggets											
Homestyle Chicken Strips	3	410	33	18	39	3.5	60	1470	0	28	2 carb, 3 med-fat meat, 1 fat
Kid's Chicken Nugget Meal	4 piece	180	10	11	56	2.5	25	390	0	8	1/2 carb, 1 med-fat meat, 1 fat
Chicken Nugget Meal	5 piece	220	13	14	59	3	35	490	0	10	1 carb, 1 med-fat meat, 2 fat
Chicken Nugget Sauces											
Barbeque Sauce	1 pk Tbsp	40	11	0	0	0	0	160	0	1	1 carb
Deli Honey Mustard Sauce	1 pk Tbsp	170	6	16	82	2.5	15	210	0	1	1/2 carb, 3 fat
Heartland Ranch Sauce	1 pk Tbsp	200	1	21	95	3.5	20	280	0	1	4 fat

FAST FOODS

	Serving	Calories	Carb. (g)	Fat (g)	% Cal. Fat	Sat. Fat (g)	Chol. (mg)	Sod. (mg)	Fib. (g)	Prot. (g)	Servings/ Exchanges
Honey Mustard Nugget Sauce	1 pk Tbsp	130	6	12	77	2	10	220	0	5	1/2 carb, 2 fat
Spicy Southwest Chipotle Sauce	1 pk Tbsp	140	4	13	86	2	20	170	0	0	3 fat
Sweet & Sour Sauce	1 pk Tbsp	45	12	0	0	0	0	120	0	0	1 carb
Chili											
Small	8 oz	220	23	6	27	2.5	32	780	5	17	1 1/2 carb, 2 lean meat
Large	12 oz	330	35	9	24	3.5	55	1170	8	25	2 carb, 3 lean meat
Garden Sensations Salads and Fresh Fruit											
Chicken BLT Salad	1	330	10	18	49	9	103	840	4	35	2 vegetable, 4 med-fat meat
Fresh Fruit Bowl	1	130	33	0	0	0	0	35	3	2	2 fruit
Homestyle Chicken Strips Salad	1	440	33	22	45	8	70	1180	5	29	2 carb, 3 med-fat meat, 1 fat
Mandarin Chicken Salad	1	170	17	2	9	0.5	60	480	4	23	3 vegetable, 3 very lean meat

Spring Mix Salad	1	180	11	11	56	6	30	220	5	11	2 vegetable, 1 med-fat meat, 1 fat
Taco Supremo Salad	1	380	31	17	39	9	65	1000	9	27	2 carb, 3 med-fat meat
Side Salads											
Caesar Side Salad	1	70	3	4.5	57	2	15	150	2	6	1 vegetable, 1 fat
Fresh Fruit Cup	1	60	16	0	0	0	0	10	1	1	1 fruit
Mandarin Orange Cup	5 oz	80	20	0	0	0	0	15	1	1	1 fruit
Side Salad	1	35	7	0	0	0	0	20	3	2	1 vegetable
Salad Dressing											
Creamy Ranch Dressing	1 pk Tbsp	230	5	23	91	4	15	580	0	1	5 fat
Fat-Free French Style	1 pk Tbsp	80	19	0	0	0	0	210	0	0	1 carb
Honey Mustard Dressing	1 pk Tbsp	280	11	26	82	4	25	350	0	1	1 carb, 5 fat
House Vinaigrette Dressing	1 pk Tbsp	190	8	18	84	2.5	0	750	0	0	1/2 carb, 4 fat
Low-Fat Honey Mustard	1 pk Tbsp	110	21	3	23	0	0	340	0	0	1 1/2 carb, 1 fat
Oriental Sesame Dressing	1 pk Tbsp	190	21	11	53	1.5	0	490	0	1	1 1/2 carb, 2 fat
Reduced-Fat Creamy Ranch	1 pk Tbsp	100	6	8	70	1.5	15	550	1	1	1/2 carb, 2 fat

FAST FOODS

	Serving	Calories	Carb. (g)	Fat (g)	% Cal. Fat	Sat. Fat (g)	Chol. (mg)	Sod. (mg)	Fib. (g)	Prot. (g)	Servings/Exchanges
Salsa	1 each	30	6	0	0	0	0	440	0	1	1 vegetable
Sour Cream	1 pk Tbsp	60	2	5	75	3.5	20	20	0	1	1 fat
Salad Toppings											
Crispy Noodles	1 pk Tbsp	60	10	2	33	0	0	170	0	1	1 carb
Homestyle Garlic Croutons	1 pk Tbsp	70	9	3	36	0	0	125	0	2	1/2 carb, 1 fat
Honey Roasted Pecans	1 pk Tbsp	130	5	13	92	2	0	65	2	2	3 fat
Low-Fat Strawberry Flavored Yogurt	1	90	16	1	6	0	5	50	0	4	1 carb
Roasted Almonds	1 pk Tbsp	130	4	11	79	1	0	70	2	5	1 med-fat meat, 1 fat
Taco Chips	1 bag	210	29	9	38	1.5	0	240	2	3	2 carb, 2 fat
Frostys											
Junior	6 oz	160	28	4	22	2.5	15	75	0	4	2 carb, 1 fat
Medium	16 oz	430	74	11	23	7	45	200	0	10	5 carb, 2 fat
Small	12 oz	330	56	8	21	5	35	150	0	8	4 carb, 2 fat

FATS, OILS, BUTTER, MARGARINE, SALAD DRESSING, SOUR CREAM

	Serving	Calories	Carb. (g)	Fat (g)	% Cal. Fat	Sat. Fat (g)	Chol. (mg)	Sod. (mg)	Fib. (g)	Prot. (g)	Servings/Exchanges
Butter, Reduced-Fat	1 Tbsp	50	0	6	100	4	20	70	0	0	1 fat
Butter, Stick	1 tsp	36	0	4	100	3	11	41	0	0	1 fat
Butter, Whipped	2 tsp	40	0	5	100	3	13	50	0	0	1 fat
Chitterlings, Boiled	2 Tbsp	42	0	4	100	1	20	6	0	1	1 fat
Creamer, Nondairy, Liquid, Regular	1 Tbsp	18	2	1	50	1	0	5	0	0	free
Creamer, Nondairy Powder, Regular	1 tsp	22	2	1	41	1	0	7	0	<1	free
Dressing, Oil & Vinegar	2 Tbsp	144	<1	16	100	3	0	<1	0	0	3 fat
Dressing, Yogurt	1 Tbsp	11	1	<1	45	<1	2	59	<1	<1	free
Lard	1 tsp	36	0	4	100	2	4	0	0	0	1 fat
Margarine, Fat-Free/Nonfat	4 Tbsp	20	0	0	0	0	0	368	0	0	free

FATS, OILS, BUTTER, MARGARINE, SALAD DRESSING, SOUR CREAM

	Serving	Calories	Carb. (g)	Fat (g)	% Cal. Fat	Sat. Fat (g)	Chol. (mg)	Sod. (mg)	Fib. (g)	Prot. (g)	Servings/ Exchanges
Margarine, Reduced-Calorie	1 Tbsp	50	0	6	100	1	0	90	0	0	1 fat
Margarine, Squeeze	1 tsp	30	0	3	90	<1	0	37	0	0	1 fat
Margarine, Stick	1 tsp	34	0	4	100	<1	0	44	0	0	1 fat
Margarine, Tub	1 tsp	30	0	4	100	<1	0	33	0	0	1 fat
Mayonnaise	1 tsp	33	0	4	100	<1	3	26	0	0	1 fat
Mayonnaise, Fat-Free	1 Tbsp	10	2	0	0	0	NA	105	0	NA	free
Mayonnaise, Light/ Reduced-Fat	1 Tbsp	40	3	3	68	<1	6	120	0	0	1 fat
Oil, Canola	1 tsp	41	0	5	100	<1	0	0	0	0	1 fat
Oil, Cocoa Butter	1 tsp	40	0	5	100	3	0	0	0	0	1 fat
Oil, Coconut	1 tsp	39	0	5	100	4	0	0	0	0	1 fat
Oil, Cod Liver/Fish	1 tsp	41	0	5	100	1	0	26	0	0	1 fat
Oil, Corn	1 tsp	44	0	5	100	<1	0	0	0	0	1 fat

Food	Serving										Exchange
Oil, Cottonseed	1 tsp	40	0	5	100	1	0	0	0	0	1 fat
Oil, Olive	1 tsp	40	0	5	100	<1	0	0	0	0	1 fat
Oil, Palm	1 tsp	40	0	5	100	2	0	0	0	0	1 fat
Oil, Palm Kernel	1 tsp	39	0	5	100	4	0	0	0	0	1 fat
Oil, Peanut	1 tsp	40	0	5	100	<1	0	0	0	0	1 fat
Oil, Safflower	1 tsp	44	0	5	100	<1	0	0	0	0	1 fat
Oil, Sardine/Fish	1 tsp	41	0	5	100	1	0	32	0	0	1 fat
Oil, Sesame	1 tsp	40	0	5	100	<1	0	0	0	0	1 fat
Oil, Soybean	1 tsp	44	0	5	100	<1	0	0	0	0	1 fat
Salad Dressing, Fat-Free	1 Tbsp	20	5	0	0	0	0	145	0	0	free
Salad Dressing, Light/ Reduced-Calorie/ Reduced-Fat	2 Tbsp	80	5	6	68	1	NA	307	0	0	1 fat
Salad Dressing, Regular	1 Tbsp	64	2	6	84	NA	NA	150	NA	NA	1 fat
Salt Pork, Raw, Cured	1/2 oz	52	0	6	100	2	6	100	0	<1	1 fat
Shortening	1 tsp	35	0	4	100	1	0	0	0	0	1 fat

FATS, OILS, BUTTER, MARGARINE, SALAD DRESSING, SOUR CREAM

	Serving	Calories	Carb. (g)	Fat (g)	% Cal. Fat	Sat. Fat (g)	Chol. (mg)	Sod. (mg)	Fib. (g)	Prot. (g)	Servings/ Exchanges
Sour Cream, Fat-Free	1 Tbsp	15	3	0	0	0	0	20	0	<1	free
Sour Cream, Light	1 Tbsp	18	2	1	50	<1	5	15	0	<1	free
Sour Cream, Reduced-Fat	3 Tbsp	45	2	4	80	3	15	20	0	1	1 fat
Sour Cream, Regular	2 Tbsp	52	1	5	86	3	10	12	0	<1	1 fat
BUTTER, MARGARINE, AND SHORTENING											
Brands											
Benecol Spread											
Light	1 Tbsp	45	0	5	100	0.5	0	110	0	0	1 fat
Regular	1 Tbsp	70	0	8	100	1	0	110	0	0	2 fat
Blue Bonnet Margarine											
Light Stick	1 Tbsp	50	<1	5	100	1	0	80	0	0	1 fat
Light Tub	1 Tbsp	40	<1	4.5	100	1	0	90	0	0	1 fat
Regular Stick	1 Tbsp	80	0	9	100	2	0	110	0	0	2 fat
Regular Tub	1 Tbsp	60	0	7	100	1.5	0	120	0	0	1 fat

Food	Serving										
Brummel & Brown Margarine Spread with Yogurt											
Tub	1 Tbsp	45	0	5	100	1	0	90	0	0	1 fat
Butter Buds											
Butter Replacement, Dry	1 Tbsp	15	6	0	0	0	0	360	0	0	free
Canola Harvest Margarine											
Regular Soft Tub	1 Tbsp	100	0	11	100	1.5	0	110	0	0	2 fat
Premium Soft Tub	1 Tbsp	100	0	11	100	1.5	0	100	0	0	2 fat
Canoleo											
100% Canola Margarine	1 Tbsp	100	0	11	100	2	0	120	0	0	2 fat
Crisco											
Shortening, All Varieties	1 Tbsp	110	0	12	100	3	0	0	0	0	2 fat
Fleischmann's Margarine											
Light Stick	1 Tbsp	50	<1	5	100	1	0	NA	0	0	1 fat
Olive Oil Squeeze	1 Tbsp	70	0	8	100	1.5	0	95	0	0	2 fat
Original Light Tub	1 Tbsp	40	0	4.5	100	0	0	90	0	0	1 fat
Original Stick	1 Tbsp	100	0	11	100	2	0	115	0	0	2 fat

FATS, OILS, BUTTER, MARGARINE, SALAD DRESSING, SOUR CREAM

	Serving	Calories	Carb. (g)	Fat (g)	% Cal. Fat	Sat. Fat (g)	Chol. (mg)	Sod. (mg)	Fib. (g)	Prot. (g)	Servings/ Exchanges
Original Tub	1 Tbsp	80	0	9	100	1.5	0	90	0	0	2 fat
Tub with Olive Oil	1 Tbsp	70	0	8	100	1.5	0	95	0	0	2 fat
Unsalted Stick	1 Tbsp	100	0	11	100	2	0	0	0	0	2 fat
Unsalted Tub	1 Tbsp	80	0	9	100	1.5	0	0	0	0	2 fat
Gregg's											
Original Gold 'n Soft Tub	1 Tbsp	100	0	11	100	2	0	95	0	0	2 fat
I Can't Believe It's Not Butter											
Fat-Free Tub	1 Tbsp	5	0	0	0	0	0	90	0	0	free
Light Tub	1 Tbsp	50	0	5	100	1	0	85	0	0	1 fat
Regular Stick	1 Tbsp	90	0	10	100	2	0	95	0	0	2 fat
Regular Tub	1 Tbsp	80	0	9	100	2	0	90	0	0	2 fat
Regular Tub with Calcium Added	1 Tbsp	50	0	5	90	1	0	90	0	0	1 fat
Spray (All Flavors)	5 sprays	0	0	0	0	0	0	15	0	0	free

Food	Serving										
Whipped Squeeze	1 Tbsp	60	0	7	100	1	0	85	0	0	1 fat
Imperial											
Regular Stick	1 Tbsp	80	0	9	100	2	0	105	0	0	2 fat
Regular Tub	1 Tbsp	60	0	7	100	1.5	0	85	0	0	1 fat
Land O Lakes											
Butter and Vegetable Oil Blend Stick	1 Tbsp	90	0	10	100	2	0	95	0	0	2 fat
Butter and Vegetable Oil Blend Tub	1 Tbsp	30	0	8	100	1.5	0	75	0	0	2 fat
Country Morning Blend Margarine	1 Tbsp	100	0	11	100	2	0	90	0	0	2 fat
Garlic Flavored Butter Tub	1 Tbsp	100	0	11	100	5	20	95	0	0	2 fat
Honey Flavored Butter Tub	1 Tbsp	90	4	8	78	4	15	35	0	0	2 fat
Light Butter Stick	1 Tbsp	50	0	6	100	3.5	15	95	0	0	1 fat
Margarine Stick	1 Tbsp	100	0	11	100	2.5	0	115	0	0	2 fat
Margarine Tub	1 Tbsp	100	0	11	100	2	0	105	0	0	2 fat

FATS, OILS, BUTTER, MARGARINE, SALAD DRESSING, SOUR CREAM

	Serving	Calories	Carb. (g)	Fat (g)	% Cal. Fat	Sat. Fat (g)	Chol. (mg)	Sod. (mg)	Fib. (g)	Prot. (g)	Servings/ Exchanges
Salted Butter Stick	1 Tbsp	110	0	12	100	8	30	85	0	0	2 fat
Soft Baking Butter with Canola Oil Stick	1 Tbsp	100	0	11	100	5	20	90	0	0	2 fat
Spreadable Butter with Canola Oil Tub	1 Tbsp	100	0	11	100	4.5	20	90	0	0	2 fat
Ultra Creamy Butter Stick	1 Tbsp	110	0	12	100	8	30	85	0	0	2 fat
Unsalted Butter Stick	1 Tbsp	110	0	12	100	8	30	0	0	0	2 fat
Whipped Butter Tub	1 Tbsp	70	0	7	86	5	20	55	0	0	1 fat
Move Over Butter											
Whipped Margarine Tub	1 Tbsp	60	0	6	100	1	0	70	0	0	1 fat
Nucoa Margarine											
Regular Stick	1 Tbsp	100	0	11	100	2	0	160	0	0	2 fat
Parkay											
Fat-Free Spray	5 sprays	0	0	0	0	0	0	5	0	0	free

Regular Stick	1 Tbsp	90	0	10	100	2	0	105	0	0	2 fat
Regular Tub	1 Tbsp	80	0	8	100	1.5	0	100	0	0	2 fat
Tub with Calcium	1 Tbsp	45	0	5	100	1	0	115	0	0	1 fat
Squeeze	1 Tbsp	70	0	8	100	1.5	0	110	0	0	2 fat
Promise										
Fat-Free Tub	1 Tbsp	5	0	0	100	0	0	90	0	0	free
Light Tub	1 Tbsp	45	0	5	100	1	0	85	0	0	1 fat
Regular Tub	1 Tbsp	80	0	8	100	1.5	0	85	0	0	2 fat
Ultra Tub	1 Tbsp	35	0	3.5	100	1	0	90	0	0	1 fat
Shedd's Spread										
Country Crock Churn Style Tub	1 Tbsp	60	0	7	100	1.5	0	85	0	0	1 fat
Country Crock Easy Squeeze	1 Tbsp	60	0	7	100	1	0	85	0	0	1 fat
Country Crock Plus Calcium Tub	1 Tbsp	50	0	5	90	1	0	95	0	0	1 fat

FATS, OILS, BUTTER, MARGARINE, SALAD DRESSING, SOUR CREAM

	Serving	Calories	Carb. (g)	Fat (g)	% Cal. Fat	Sat. Fat (g)	Chol. (mg)	Sod. (mg)	Fib. (g)	Prot. (g)	Servings/ Exchanges
Country Crock Plus Yogurt Tub	1 Tbsp	40	0	4	100	1	0	80	0	0	1 fat
Country Crock Sticks	1 Tbsp	80	0	8	100	1.5	0	110	0	0	2 fat
Country Crock Tub	1 Tbsp	60	0	7	100	1.5	0	110	0	0	1 fat
Smart Balance											
Buttery Spread Tub	1 Tbsp	80	0	9	100	2.5	0	90	0	0	2 fat
Buttery Spread Tub with Omega Fatty Acids	1 Tbsp	80	0	9	100	2.5	0	90	0	0	2 fat
Light Buttery Spread Tub	1 Tbsp	45	0	5	100	1.5	0	90	0	0	1 fat
Smart Beat											
Smart Squeeze	1 Tbsp	5	0	0	0	0	0	100	0	0	free
Super Light Tub	1 Tbsp	20	0	2	100	0	0	105	0	0	free
Take Control											
Light Tub	1 Tbsp	45	0	5	100	0.5	<5	85	0	0	1 fat

Food	Serving										
Regular Tub	1 Tbsp	80	0	8	100	1	<5	85	0	0	2 fat

SALAD DRESSING

Brands

Bernstein's

Food	Serving										
Basil Parmesan	2 Tbsp	100	2	10	90	1	5	400	0	1	2 fat
Cheese & Garlic Italian	2 Tbsp	110	2	11	82	1	0	340	0	1	2 fat
Light Cheese Fantastico	2 Tbsp	25	2	1.5	40	1	0	340	0	1	free

Best Foods

Food	Serving										
Just 2 Good! Low-Fat Mayonnaise	1 Tbsp	25	2	2	80	0	0	120	0	0	free
Light Mayonnaise	1 Tbsp	45	1	4.5	89	0.5	<5	120	0	0	1 fat
Mayonnaise	1 Tbsp	90	0	10	100	1.5	5	85	0	0	2 fat

Cardini's

Food	Serving										
Balsamic Vinaigrette	2 Tbsp	140	4	14	86	2	0	240	0	0	3 fat
Caesar	2 Tbsp	160	1	17	94	2.5	30	240	0	1	3 fat
Caesar Light	2 Tbsp	80	5	7	75	1	30	250	0	1	1 fat

FATS, OILS, BUTTER, MARGARINE, SALAD DRESSING, SOUR CREAM

	Serving	Calories	Carb. (g)	Fat (g)	% Cal. Fat	Sat. Fat (g)	Chol. (mg)	Sod. (mg)	Fib. (g)	Prot. (g)	Servings/ Exchanges
Fat-Free Caesar	2 Tbsp	40	9	0	0	0	0	510	0	0	1/2 carb
Honey Mustard	2 Tbsp	140	5	13	86	2	0	220	0	0	3 fat
Italian	2 Tbsp	120	1	13	100	2	0	220	0	0	3 fat
Kalamata Olive	2 Tbsp	140	2	15	93	2.5	5	380	0	0	3 fat
Poppyseed	2 Tbsp	160	8	14	81	2	0	170	0	0	1/2 carb, 3 fat
Dorothy Lynch											
Fat-Free Dressing	2 Tbsp	60	14	0	0	0	0	160	0	0	1 carb
Homestyle Dressing	2 Tbsp	110	12	6	50	1	0	170	0	0	1 carb, 1 fat
Emeril's											
Bacon Vinaigrette	2 Tbsp	110	4	10	82	1	0	150	0	0	2 fat
Bleu Cheese	2 Tbsp	100	<1	11	100	1.5	<5	330	0	<1	2 fat
Caesar	2 Tbsp	130	2	14	100	1	10	190	0	0	3 fat
Romano	2 Tbsp	110	2	12	100	1	0	370	0	<1	2 fat

Girard's

Balsamic Basil	2 Tbsp	90	3	9	89	1.5	0	330	0	0	2 fat
Blue Cheese Vinaigrette	2 Tbsp	100	3	10	90	2	5	500	0	1	2 fat
Caesar	2 Tbsp	150	1	15	93	2.5	10	350	0	1	3 fat
Greek Feta Vinaigrette	2 Tbsp	110	1	11	91	2	0	320	0	0	2 fat
Light Caesar	2 Tbsp	90	5	8	78	1.5	10	360	0	1	2 fat
Raspberry	2 Tbsp	120	9	10	75	1.5	0	65	0	0	1/2 carb, 2 fat
Romano Cheese	2 Tbsp	130	2	13	92	2	0	500	0	1	3 fat
Shiitake Charconnay	2 Tbsp	100	4	9	80	1.5	0	210	0	0	2 fat
Spinach Salad	2 Tbsp	70	14	2	21	0	0	250	0	1	1 carb

Girard's Fat-Free

Balsamic Vinaigrette	2 Tbsp	25	6	0	0	0	0	400	0	0	1/2 carb
Raspberry	2 Tbsp	50	13	0	0	0	0	220	0	0	1 carb
Red Wine Vinaigrette	2 Tbsp	20	5	0	0	0	0	590	0	0	free

Hidden Valley

Coleslaw Dressing	2 Tbsp	150	5	15	93	2.5	10	170	0	0	3 fat

FATS, OILS, BUTTER, MARGARINE, SALAD DRESSING, SOUR CREAM

	Serving	Calories	Carb. (g)	Fat (g)	% Cal. Fat	Sat. Fat (g)	Chol. (mg)	Sod. (mg)	Fib. (g)	Prot. (g)	Servings/ Exchanges
Ranch	2 Tbsp	140	1	14	93	2.5	10	260	0	1	3 fat
Ranch Fat-Free	2 Tbsp	30	6	0	0	0	0	310	0	0	1/2 carb
Ranch Light	2 Tbsp	80	3	7	75	1	0	280	0	1	1 fat
Spicy Ranch	2 Tbsp	150	2	16	93	2	10	320	0	0	3 fat
White Cheddar	2 Tbsp	140	2	15	93	2	10	240	0	1	3 fat
Johnny's											
Great Caesar	2 Tbsp	170	1	18	94	1.5	5	260	0	1	4 fat
Great Caesar Lite	2 Tbsp	70	14	2	29	0	0	380	0	0	1 carb
Honey! You're Terrific	2 Tbsp	140	3	14	93	1	0	180	0	0	3 fat
Jamaica Mistake	2 Tbsp	140	7	12	79	1	0	380	0	0	1/2 carb, 2 fat
Ken's Steak House											
Buttermilk Ranch	2 Tbsp	180	1	20	100	3	5	280	0	0	4 fat
Country French	2 Tbsp	130	9	11	77	1.5	0	220	0	0	1/2 carb, 2 fat
Fat-Free Raspberry Pecan	2 Tbsp	45	10	0	0	0	0	250	0	0	1/2 carb

Lite Caesar	2 Tbsp	70	3	6	71	1	0	600	0	1	1 fat
Lite Olive Oil Vinaigrette	2 Tbsp	60	3	6	83	0.5	0	240	0	0	1 fat
Knott's Berry Farm											
Honey Dijon	2 Tbsp	130	4	12	92	1.5	<5	90	0	<1	2 fat
Honey Poppyseed	2 Tbsp	120	10	9	75	1.5	0	180	0	0	1/2 carb, 2 fat
Lowfat Raspberry Vinaigrette	2 Tbsp	50	8	2	30	0	0	105	0	0	1/2 carb
Oriental Chicken Salad	2 Tbsp	130	5	11	77	2	0	230	0	<1	2 fat
Sundried Tomato	2 Tbsp	100	3	10	90	1.5	0	200	0	<1	2 fat
Kraft											
Catalina	2 Tbsp	100	10	6	60	1	0	420	0	0	1/2 carb, 1 fat
Classic Caesar	2 Tbsp	110	<1	11	91	2	5	310	0	<1	2 fat
Ranch	2 Tbsp	110	2	11	91	1.5	5	310	0	0	2 fat
Roka Blue Cheese	2 Tbsp	120	1	13	100	2	<5	290	0	0	3 fat
Thousand Island	2 Tbsp	80	6	6	63	1	5	330	0	0	1/2 carb, 1 fat
Three Cheese Italian	2 Tbsp	130	<1	14	100	2.5	0	310	0	<1	3 fat

FATS, OILS, BUTTER, MARGARINE, SALAD DRESSING, SOUR CREAM

	Serving	Calories	Carb. (g)	Fat (g)	% Cal. Fat	Sat. Fat (g)	Chol. (mg)	Sod. (mg)	Fib. (g)	Prot. (g)	Servings/ Exchanges
Three Cheese Ranch	2 Tbsp	110	2	12	91	2	0	290	0	0	2 fat
Zesty Italian	2 Tbsp	80	3	8	88	1	0	310	0	0	2 fat
Kraft Carb Well											
Italian	2 Tbsp	70	0	8	100	1	0	300	0	0	2 fat
Light Buttermilk	2 Tbsp	60	0	6	83	1	5	430	0	<1	1 fat
Ranch	2 Tbsp	110	0	11	100	1.5	5	310	0	0	2 fat
Roka Blue Cheese	2 Tbsp	120	0	13	100	2	<5	260	0	0	3 fat
Kraft Free (Fat-Free)											
Caesar Italian	2 Tbsp	25	5	0	0	0	0	470	0	<1	free
Catalina	2 Tbsp	50	11	0	0	0	0	350	0	0	1 carb
Ranch	2 Tbsp	50	11	0	0	0	0	350	0	0	1 carb
Thousand Island	2 Tbsp	45	10	0	0	0	0	260	0	0	1/2 carb
Kraft Light Done Right (Reduced-Fat)											
Catalina	2 Tbsp	60	12	1	17	0	0	430	0	0	1 carb

Food	Serving										
House Italian	2 Tbsp	40	3	3	75	0.5	0	270	0	0	1 fat
Ranch	2 Tbsp	70	7	4.5	57	0.5	10	370	0	0	1/2 carb, 1 fat
Red Wine Vinaigrette	2 Tbsp	45	3	4	76	0	0	310	0	0	1 fat
Thousand Island	2 Tbsp	60	9	2	33	0	10	330	0	0	1/2 carb
Three Cheese Ranch	2 Tbsp	70	2	6	86	1	0	430	0	0	1 fat
Kraft Miracle Whip/Mayonnaise											
Fat-Free Mayonnaise	1 Tbsp	10	2	0	0	0	0	120	0	0	free
Fat-Free Miracle Whip	1 Tbsp	15	3	0	0	0	0	125	0	0	free
Light Miracle Whip	1 Tbsp	30	3	2	50	0	<5	140	0	0	1 fat
Mayonnaise	1 Tbsp	100	0	11	100	1.5	5	75	0	0	2 fat
Miracle Whip	1 Tbsp	45	2	4	78	0.5	<5	125	0	0	1 fat
Kraft Special Collection											
Caesar Italian with Oregano	2 Tbsp	100	2	10	90	1.5	0	470	0	<1	2 fat
Caesar Vinaigrette with Parmesan	2 Tbsp	60	1	5	75	1	<5	440	0	<1	1 fat

FATS, OILS, BUTTER, MARGARINE, SALAD DRESSING, SOUR CREAM

	Serving	Calories	Carb. (g)	Fat (g)	% Cal. Fat	Sat. Fat (g)	Chol. (mg)	Sod. (mg)	Fib. (g)	Prot. (g)	Servings/ Exchanges
Creamy Poppyseed	2 Tbsp	130	8	10	69	2	0	250	0	0	1/2 carb, 2 fat
Greek Vinaigrette	2 Tbsp	110	2	11	91	1.5	0	320	0	0	2 fat
Litehouse											
Big Bleu	2 Tbsp	160	1	17	100	2	15	230	0	1	3 fat
Coleslaw	2 Tbsp	90	7	7	78	0.5	5	95	0	0	1/2 carb, 1 fat
Lite Bleu Cheese	2 Tbsp	70	2	6	86	0.5	5	210	0	1	1 fat
Lite Ranch	2 Tbsp	60	2	6	83	0.5	5	200	0	1	1 fat
Original Bleu Cheese	2 Tbsp	150	1	16	100	1.5	15	210	0	1	3 fat
Poppyseed	2 Tbsp	130	6	12	85	1	10	210	0	0	1/2 carb, 2 fat
Ranch	2 Tbsp	120	2	12	92	1	10	180	0	1	2 fat
Litehouse Fat-Free											
Honey Dijon	2 Tbsp	35	8	0	0	0	0	120	0	0	1/2 carb
Sesame Ginger	2 Tbsp	35	8	0	0	0	0	230	0	0	1/2 carb

Litehouse One Carb Plus (Made with Canola Oil)

Bleu Cheese	2 Tbsp	150	1	16	100	1.5	15	210	0	1	3 fat
Caesar	2 Tbsp	140	1	14	93	1.5	15	200	0	1	3 fat
Italian	2 Tbsp	100	1	11	100	1	0	290	0	0	2 fat
Mediterranean	2 Tbsp	25	1	2	80	0	0	310	0	0	free
Ranch	2 Tbsp	120	1	13	100	1	10	230	0	1	3 fat

Litehouse Naturals

Balsamic Vinaigrette	2 Tbsp	80	4	7	75	0.5	0	150	0	0	1 fat
Caesar	2 Tbsp	150	1	17	100	1.5	10	120	0	1	3 fat
Chipotle Ranch	2 Tbsp	110	1	12	100	1	10	250	0	1	2 fat

Maple Grove Farms of Vermont

Balsamic Vinaigrette	2 Tbsp	50	6	3	60	0	0	40	0	0	1/2 carb, 1 fat
Fat-Free Balsamic Vinaigrette	2 Tbsp	5	1	0	0	0	0	160	0	0	free
Fat-Free Cranberry Balsamic Vinaigrette	2 Tbsp	30	7	0	0	0	0	180	0	0	1/2 carb

FATS, OILS, BUTTER, MARGARINE, SALAD DRESSING, SOUR CREAM

	Serving	Calories	Carb. (g)	Fat (g)	% Cal. Fat	Sat. Fat (g)	Chol. (mg)	Sod. (mg)	Fib. (g)	Prot. (g)	Servings/ Exchanges
Fat-Free Honey Dijon	2 Tbsp	40	10	0	0	0	0	200	<1	0	1 carb
Light Caesar	2 Tbsp	70	5	5	71	1	5	310	0	0	1 fat
Light Romano	2 Tbsp	40	1	3.5	75	0	0	260	0	<1	1 fat
Parmesan & Cracked Pepper	2 Tbsp	120	4	11	83	2	0	360	0	<1	2 fat
Marie's											
Balsamic Vinaigrette	2 Tbsp	50	3	4	80	0.5	0	220	0	0	1 fat
Caesar	2 Tbsp	170	1	19	100	3	15	150	0	1	4 fat
Chunky Blue Cheese	2 Tbsp	170	0	19	100	3.5	15	170	0	1	4 fat
Coleslaw	2 Tbsp	150	8	13	80	2	10	180	0	0	1/2 carb, 3 fat
Creamy Ranch	2 Tbsp	180	1	19	94	3	15	130	0	1	4 fat
Italian Vinaigrette	2 Tbsp	80	3	8	88	1	0	360	0	0	2 fat
Lite Chunky Blue Cheese	2 Tbsp	80	4	7	75	1.5	5	310	1	1	1 fat
Lite Creamy Ranch	2 Tbsp	90	8	7	67	1	5	260	0	1	1/2 carb, 1 fat

Poppyseed	2 Tbsp	150	8	13	80	2	10	180	0	0	1/2 carb, 3 fat
Raspberry Vinaigrette	2 Tbsp	40	8	0.5	13	0	0	60	0	0	1/2 carb
Red Wine Vinaigrette	2 Tbsp	60	5	4.5	67	0.5	0	200	0	0	1 fat
Spinach Salad	2 Tbsp	70	12	1.5	21	0	0	240	0	1	1 carb
Thousand Island	2 Tbsp	160	4	16	88	2.5	10	210	0	0	3 fat
Newman's Own											
Balsamic Vinaigrette	2 Tbsp	90	3	9	89	1	0	350	0	0	2 fat
Caesar	2 Tbsp	150	1	16	93	1.5	0	420	0	1	3 fat
Family Recipe Italian	2 Tbsp	120	1	13	100	1	0	400	0	1	3 fat
Olive Oil & Vinegar	2 Tbsp	150	1	16	100	2.5	0	150	0	0	3 fat
Ranch	2 Tbsp	140	2	15	93	2	10	270	0	0	3 fat
Newman's Own Lighten Up											
Balsamic Vinaigrette	2 Tbsp	45	2	4	89	0.5	0	470	0	0	1 fat
Caesar	2 Tbsp	70	3	6	71	1	5	520	0	1	1 fat
Honey Mustard	2 Tbsp	70	7	4	50	0.5	0	290	0	0	1 fat
Italian	2 Tbsp	60	0	6	83	1	0	260	0	0	1 fat

FATS, OILS, BUTTER, MARGARINE, SALAD DRESSING, SOUR CREAM

	Serving	Calories	Carb. (g)	Fat (g)	% Cal. Fat	Sat. Fat (g)	Chol. (mg)	Sod. (mg)	Fib. (g)	Prot. (g)	Servings/ Exchanges
Raspberry & Walnut	2 Tbsp	70	7	5	64	0.5	0	120	0	0	1/2 carb, 1 fat
Oriental Chef											
Creamy Lemon	2 Tbsp	60	6	5	67	0.5	10	490	0	0	1/2 carb, 1 fat
Delicate Sesame	2 Tbsp	60	6	4	67	0.5	0	530	0	0	1/2 carb, 1 fat
Honey & Orange	2 Tbsp	80	6	6	63	1	0	200	0	0	1/2 carb, 1 fat
Tangy Soy	2 Tbsp	80	4	8	88	1	0	510	0	0	2 fat
Paula's											
Classic Vinaigrette	2 Tbsp	140	1	15	96	1	0	130	0	0	3 fat
No-Fat Roasted Garlic	2 Tbsp	10	3	0	0	0	0	80	0	0	free
No-Oil Lemon & Dill	2 Tbsp	15	4	0	0	0	0	55	0	0	free
No-Oil Lime & Cilantro	2 Tbsp	15	4	0	0	0	0	40	0	0	free
No-Oil Orange & Basil	2 Tbsp	15	4	0	0	0	0	64	0	0	free
Wish Bone											
Berry Vinaigrette	2 Tbsp	50	2	5	90	0.5	0	135	0	0	1 fat

Chunky Blue Cheese	2 Tbsp	160	2	17	94	2.5	<5	260	0	<1	3 fat
Creamy Caesar	2 Tbsp	170	1	18	94	3	10	300	0	<1	4 fat
House Italian	2 Tbsp	100	3	10	90	1.5	5	260	0	0	2 fat
Italian	2 Tbsp	80	3	8	88	1	0	490	0	0	2 fat
Olive Oil Vinaigrette	2 Tbsp	60	4	5	75	0.5	0	250	0	0	1 fat
Ranch	2 Tbsp	160	1	17	94	2.5	10	200	0	<1	3 fat
Ranch Up	2 Tbsp	140	2	15	100	2.5	5	230	0	0	3 fat
Red Wine Vinaigrette	2 Tbsp	80	9	5	56	1	0	240	0	0	1/2 carb, 1 fat
Russian	2 Tbsp	110	14	6	45	1	0	360	0	0	1 carb, 1 fat
Thousand Island	2 Tbsp	130	6	12	85	2	10	330	0	0	1/2 carb, 2 fat
Western	2 Tbsp	160	12	12	69	1.5	0	230	0	0	1 carb, 2 fat
Wish Bone Carb Options											
Blue Cheese	2 Tbsp	150	0	16	93	2.5	10	230	0	0	3 fat
Italian	2 Tbsp	70	0	8	100	1	0	350	0	0	2 fat
Olive Oil Vinaigrette	2 Tbsp	50	0	6	100	0.5	0	230	0	0	1 fat
Ranch	2 Tbsp	150	0	16	93	2.5	10	200	0	0	3 fat

FATS, OILS, BUTTER, MARGARINE, SALAD DRESSING, SOUR CREAM

	Serving	Calories	Carb. (g)	Fat (g)	% Cal. Fat	Sat. Fat (g)	Chol. (mg)	Sod. (mg)	Fib. (g)	Prot. (g)	Servings/ Exchanges
Sweet & Spice French	2 Tbsp	100	1	11	100	1.5	0	220	<1	0	2 fat
Wish Bone Just 2 Good!											
Blue Cheese	2 Tbsp	45	6	2	44	0.5	0	310	0	<1	1/2 carb
Italian	2 Tbsp	35	4	2	57	0	0	490	0	0	free
Ranch	2 Tbsp	40	5	2	50	0	0	290	0	0	1/2 carb
Thousand Island	2 Tbsp	50	9	2	40	0	5	290	0	0	1/2 carb
Wish Bone Restaurant Style											
Blue Cheese	2 Tbsp	140	1	15	100	2.5	<5	310	0	0	3 fat
Caesar with Aged Romano	2 Tbsp	60	3	5	75	1	0	560	0	<1	1 fat
Creamy Lime Cilantro	2 Tbsp	160	3	16	88	2.5	0	300	0	0	3 fat
Raspberry Hazelnut Vinaigrette	2 Tbsp	80	9	5	56	0.5	0	260	0	0	1/2 carb, 1 fat

SOUR CREAM

Brands

Breakstone/Knudsen

Sour Cream	2 Tbsp	60	1	6	90	4	20	10	0	<1	1 fat
Sour Cream, Fat-Free	2 Tbsp	35	6	0	0	0	<5	25	0	2	1/2 carb
Sour Cream, Light	2 Tbsp	30	2	2	50	1	10	20	0	1	free

Daisy

Sour Cream	2 Tbsp	60	1	5	75	3.5	20	15	0	1	1 fat
Sour Cream, Light	2 Tbsp	40	2	3	63	2	10	25	0	2	1 fat
Sour Cream, No Fat	2 Tbsp	20	1	0	0	0	0	15	0	2	free

IMO

Sour Cream Substitute	2 Tbsp	60	2	5	83	5	0	35	0	1	1 fat

FROZEN PACKAGED FOOD, MEAT, CHICKEN, FISH, MEALS, PIZZA, SNACKS

FROZEN CHICKEN

Brands

Banquet

	Serving	Calories	Carb. (g)	Fat (g)	% Cal. Fat	Sat. Fat (g)	Chol. (mg)	Sod. (mg)	Fib. (g)	Prot. (g)	Servings/ Exchanges
Chicken Breast Nuggets	5 pieces	290	15	21	66	5	30	470	1	10	1 carb, 1 med-fat meat, 3 fat
Chicken Breast Patty	1	260	13	19	66	5	30	430	1	9	1 carb, 1 med-fat meat, 3 fat
Chicken Breast Strips	2	280	14	19	64	5	30	480	<1	11	1 carb, 1 med-fat meat, 3 fat
Chicken Breast Tenders	5 pieces	280	14	19	64	5	30	480	<1	11	1 carb, 1 med-fat meat, 3 fat
Chicken Nuggets	5 pieces	280	15	19	64	5	35	470	1	11	1 carb, 1 med-fat meat, 2 fat
Chicken Wings, Hot'n Spicy	3 oz	280	7	19	64	4	90	380	0	18	1/2 carb, 2 med-fat meat, 2 fat
Chicken, Original Fried	1 piece	380	13	25	61	7	80	1040	1	25	1 carb, 3 med-fat meat, 2 fat
Chicken, Popcorn	11 pieces	190	18	9	42	2	20	510	1	8	1 carb, 1 med-fat meat, 3 fat

Chicken, Skinless, Fried	1 piece	370	14	23	57	6	75	660	1	25	1 carb, 3 med-fat meat, 2 fat

Foster Farms

Breast Nuggets	4	160	9	9	50	2	25	360	1	13	1/2 carb, 2 med-fat meat
Buffalo Style Strips	3	190	15	8	37	2	30	1100	0	14	1 carb, 2 med-fat meat
Crispy Strips	3 oz	200	14	8	35	2	35	790	0	18	1 carb, 2 med-fat meat
Honey BBQ Glazed Wings	4	170	5	10	53	3	50	390	0	13	2 med-fat meat
Hot'N Spicy Wings	4	170	1	13	71	4	55	460	0	14	2 med-fat meat, 1 fat

Tyson

Breaded Chicken Breast Fillets	1 piece	240	20	9	33	2	30	680	0	19	1 carb, 2 med-fat meat
Buffalo Style Hot Wings	4 pieces	220	1	15	59	4	110	560	0	20	3 med-fat meat
Chicken Bites	13 pieces	270	15	18	59	4	40	400	1	13	1 carb, 2 med-fat meat, 2 fat
Chicken Breast Nuggets	5 pieces	280	21	16	54	4	50	430	0	13	1 1/2 carb, 2 med-fat meat, 1 fat
Chicken Breast Patties	1 patty	180	12	11	50	3	25	300	1	10	1 carb, 1 med-fat meat, 1 fat
Chicken Breast Strips	3 oz	120	1	4	25	1	60	500	0	21	3 very lean meat
Chicken Breast Tenderloins	1 piece	150	12	7	40	2	20	370	1	10	1 carb, 1 med-fat meat, 1 fat

FROZEN PACKAGED FOOD, MEAT, CHICKEN, FISH, MEALS, PIZZA, SNACKS

	Serving	Calories	Carb. (g)	Fat (g)	% Cal. Fat	Sat. Fat (g)	Chol. (mg)	Sod. (mg)	Fib. (g)	Prot. (g)	Servings/ Exchanges
Chicken Nuggets	5 pieces	280	16	18	57	4	45	490	0	14	1 carb, 2 med-fat meat, 2 fat
Crispy Chicken Strips	2 pieces	200	13	10	45	2	30	520	1	16	1 carb, 2 med-fat meat
Diced Chicken Strips	3 oz	90	0	1	6	0	45	250	0	20	3 very lean meat
Fajita Chicken Breast Strips	3 oz	110	3	2	18	1	60	450	0	19	3 very lean meat
Fun Shaped Chicken Nuggets	5 pieces	280	16	18	57	4	45	490	0	14	1 carb, 2 med-fat meat, 2 fat
Grilled Chicken Breast Strips	3 oz	110	2	3	23	1	50	480	0	19	3 very lean meat
Honey BBQ Wings	4 pieces	220	9	14	55	3	95	450	0	15	1/2 carb, 2 med-fat meat, 1 fat
Italian Style Chicken Meatballs	6 pieces	180	6	11	56	3	45	610	2	13	1/2 carb, 2 med-fat meat
Mesquite Breast Fillets	1 piece	130	1	7	46	2	45	540	0	17	2 lean meat
Popcorn Chicken Bites	6 pieces	250	22	12	40	2	30	760	2	14	1 1/2 carb, 1 med-fat meat, 1 fat

	Serving Size	Cal.	Carb. (g)	Fat (g)	% Cal. Fat	Sat. Fat (g)	Chol. (mg)	Sod. (mg)	Fiber (g)	Prot. (g)	Exchanges/Choices
Teriyaki Breast Fillets	1 piece	170	7	7	35	2	55	620	0	20	1/2 carb, 3 lean meat

FROZEN FISH

Brands

Captain's Choice

	Serving Size	Cal.	Carb. (g)	Fat (g)	% Cal. Fat	Sat. Fat (g)	Chol. (mg)	Sod. (mg)	Fiber (g)	Prot. (g)	Exchanges/Choices
Fish Portions	2 pieces	230	24	11	43	1	10	460	0	10	1 1/2 carb, 1 med-fat meat, 1 fat
Fish Sticks	6 sticks	210	19	11	48	1	5	290	0	10	1 carb, 1 med-fat meat, 1 fat
Grilled Garlic Butter Fish Fillets	1 fillet	100	1	3	27	0	70	310	0	17	2 very lean meat
Grilled Lemon Pepper Fillets	1 fillet	100	1	3	32	0	65	380	0	16	2 very lean meat

Fisher Boy

	Serving Size	Cal.	Carb. (g)	Fat (g)	% Cal. Fat	Sat. Fat (g)	Chol. (mg)	Sod. (mg)	Fiber (g)	Prot. (g)	Exchanges/Choices
Crispy Battered Fish Portions	1 piece	160	14	9	50	1	15	290	0	17	1 carb, 2 med-fat meat
Crunchy Breaded Fish Tenders	4 pieces	220	20	12	50	2	10	440	0	9	1 carb, 1 med-fat meat, 1 fat
Crunchy Fish Sticks	6 sticks	190	15	11	53	2	10	370	0	9	1 carb, 1 med-fat meat, 1 fat

FROZEN PACKAGED FOOD, MEAT, CHICKEN, FISH, MEALS, PIZZA, SNACKS

	Serving	Calories	Carb. (g)	Fat (g)	% Cal. Fat	Sat. Fat (g)	Chol. (mg)	Sod. (mg)	Fib. (g)	Prot. (g)	Servings/ Exchanges
Gorton's											
Batter Dipped Fish Portions	1 piece	160	12	10	56	2	20	400	0	6	1 carb, 1 med-fat meat, 1 fat
Caesar Parmesan Grilled Fillets	1 fillet	100	0	3	25	0	60	240	0	17	2 very lean meat
Cajun Blackened Grilled Fillets	1 fillet	100	1	3	25	0	60	330	0	17	2 very lean meat
Classic Char-Grilled Fillets	1 fillet	120	1	6	42	1	60	270	0	16	2 lean meat
Crunchy Golden Fish Fillets	2 fillets	250	20	15	56	4	25	600	0	9	1 carb, 1 med-fat meat, 2 fat
Crunchy Golden Fish Sticks	6 sticks	260	21	14	50	4	20	390	0	9	1 carb, 1 med-fat meat, 2 fat
Crunchy Lemon Herb Breaded Fish Fillets	2 fillets	220	21	11	45	3	30	600	0	10	1 carb, 1 med-fat meat, 1 fat

Garlic Butter Grilled Fillets	1 fillet	100	1	3	25	0	60	370	0	17	2 lean meat
Lemon Butter Grilled Fillets	1 fillet	120	1	6	42	1	60	380	0	16	2 lean meat
Lemon Pepper Grilled Fillets	1 fillet	100	1	3	25	0	60	370	0	17	2 very lean meat
Original Batter Tenders	3 1/2 pieces	250	20	14	52	4	30	530	0	11	1 carb, 2 high-fat meat
Traditional Seasoned Skillet Fillets	1 fillet	220	13	13	55	2	40	700	0	12	1 carb, 2 high-fat meat

Mrs. Paul's

Breaded Cod Fillets	1 fillet	240	16	14	50	2	35	330	0	14	1 carb, 2 high-fat meat
Breaded Flounder Fillets	1 fillet	160	10	8	50	1	25	210	0	10	1/2 carb, 1 high-fat meat
Cajun Grilled Fillets	1 fillet	130	0	6	38	1	65	240	0	18	3 lean meat
Lemon Pepper Grilled Fillets	1 fillet	130	0	6	38	1	65	210	0	18	3 lean meat

FROZEN PACKAGED FOOD, MEAT, CHICKEN, FISH, MEALS, PIZZA, SNACKS

	Serving	Calories	Carb. (g)	Fat (g)	% Cal. Fat	Sat. Fat (g)	Chol. (mg)	Sod. (mg)	Fib. (g)	Prot. (g)	Servings/ Exchanges
Van de Kamp's											
Crisp & Healthy Breaded Fish Sticks	6 sticks	170	24	2	15	0	25	420	0	10	1 1/2 carb, 1 lean meat
Crisp & Healthy Original Breaded Fish Fillets	2 fillets	170	25	3	15	0	25	400	0	11	1 1/2 carb, 1 lean meat
Crispy Golden Battered Fish Portions	1 piece	160	13	9	32	1	20	360	0	6	1 carb, 1 high-fat meat
Crunchy Golden Breaded Fish Fillets	2 fillets	260	17	17	62	3	25	380	0	10	1 carb, 1 high-fat meat, 2 fat
Crunchy Golden Breaded Fish Sticks	6 sticks	260	20	15	50	2	25	360	0	11	1 carb, 1 high-fat meat, 1 fat
Crunchy Golden Breaded Fish Strips	4 pieces	270	25	14	44	2	25	400	0	12	1 1/2 carb, 1 high-fat meat, 1 fat

	Serving										
Lemon Pepper Grilled Fillets	1 fillet	120	0	6	42	1	60	190	0	17	2 lean meat

FROZEN MEALS/ENTREES

Brands

Aunt Jemima Great Starts

Biscuit Sandwich, Sausage, Egg & Cheese	1	340	27	21	56	7	110	830	<1	12	2 carb, 1 med-fat meat, 2 fat
Croissant Sandwich, Sausage, Egg & Cheese	1	350	22	23	60	7	145	680	<1	13	1 1/2 carb, 1 med-fat meat, 4 fat
Scrambled Eggs & Bacon	1 pkg	320	16	22	63	8	300	740	<1	13	1 carb, 2 med-fat meat, 2 fat
Scrambled Eggs & Sausage	1 pkg	370	18	27	65	9	335	750	2	14	1 carb, 2 med-fat meat, 3 fat

Banquet

Barbeque Chicken	9.9 oz	310	37	11	32	3	50	1000	2	15	2 1/2 carb, 1 med-fat meat, 1 fat
Beef Enchilada	11 oz	380	57	13	32	4	15	1740	7	8	4 carb, 3 fat
Beef Pot Pie	7 oz	430	38	25	53	11	30	890	2	11	2 1/2 carb, 1 med-fat meat, 4 fat

FROZEN PACKAGED FOOD, MEAT, CHICKEN, FISH, MEALS, PIZZA, SNACKS

	Serving	Calories	Carb. (g)	Fat (g)	% Cal. Fat	Sat. Fat (g)	Chol. (mg)	Sod. (mg)	Fib. (g)	Prot. (g)	Servings/Exchanges
Chicken Fingers	7.1 oz	570	57	30	47	8	60	840	2	18	4 carb, 1 med-fat meat, 2 fat
Chicken Pot Pie	7 oz	400	37	23	53	9	35	950	2	10	2 1/2 carb, 1 med-fat meat, 4 fat
Country Fried Pork	10.3 oz	430	40	24	51	7	50	1220	5	13	2 1/2 carb, 1 med-fat meat, 4 fat
Lasagna with Meat Sauce	11 oz	340	46	10	26	4	20	1170	7	15	3 carb, 1 med-fat meat, 1 fat
Macaroni & Beef	11 oz	320	50	6	19	2.5	20	1200	7	16	3 carb, 1 med-fat meat
Pot Roast	9.4 oz	210	21	7	33	3	40	1150	5	15	1 1/2 carb, 2 lean meat
Sliced Beef	9 oz	250	17	10	36	3.5	55	1000	4	23	1 carb, 3 lean meat
Spaghetti & Meatballs	10.5 oz	440	43	20	41	8	40	1180	5	22	3 carb, 2 med-fat meat, 2 fat
Swedish Meatballs	10.3 oz	440	35	24	50	11	90	1100	4	19	2 carb, 2 med-fat meat, 3 fat
Banquet Hearty One											
Chicken Fried Beef Steak	16 oz	790	65	47	54	16	75	1770	8	26	4 carb, 2 med-fat meat, 7 fat
Fried Chicken	16 oz	930	69	53	52	13	175	2330	10	42	4 1/2 carb, 4 med-fat meat, 7 fat
Salisbury Steak	16 oz	630	44	40	57	15	65	2300	9	23	3 carb, 2 med-fat meat, 6 fat
Turkey	16 oz	520	48	22	38	6	80	2550	12	30	3 carb, 3 med-fat meat, 1 fat

Boston Market

Beef Sirloin & Noodles	14 oz	620	57	22	32	8	105	2270	3	28	4 carb, 2 med-fat meat, 2 fat
Chicken Pot Pie	1 cup	600	35	39	58	15	65	1110	2	15	2 carb, 1 med-fat meat, 7 fat
Glazed Rotisserie White Meat Chicken	10 oz	290	29	10	31	3	55	1220	2	20	2 carb, 2 med-fat meat
Lasagna with Meat Sauce	12.5 oz	470	43	20	38	9	70	1170	3	30	3 carb, 3 med-fat meat, 1 fat
Meatloaf	12 oz	530	38	33	55	13	105	1360	3	21	2 1/2 carb, 2 med-fat meat, 5 fat
Salisbury Steak	16 oz	770	48	43	49	18	110	2510	6	31	3 carb, 3 med-fat meat, 6 fat
Turkey Breast Medallions	11 oz	270	27	7	22	2	35	1230	1	23	2 lean meat

Green Giant Create-a-Meal

Stir-Fry Lo Mein	2 1/3 cup	320	33	7	19	2	60	920	3	30	2 carb, 3 lean meat
Stir-Fry Szechuan	1 3/4 cup	340	15	18	47	5	65	1050	4	30	1 carb, 4 med-fat meat
Teriyaki	1 3/4 cup	210	13	7	33	1	55	950	4	25	1 carb, 3 lean meat

Healthy Choice Flavor Adventures

Beef Merlot	10.1 oz	240	25	8	30	2	40	600	6	17	1 1/2 carb, 2 med-fat meat
Chicken Margherita	10.1 oz	340	42	8	21	1.5	50	600	6	25	3 carb, 2 med-fat meat

FROZEN PACKAGED FOOD, MEAT, CHICKEN, FISH, MEALS, PIZZA, SNACKS

	Serving	Calories	Carb. (g)	Fat (g)	% Cal. Fat	Sat. Fat (g)	Chol. (mg)	Sod. (mg)	Fib. (g)	Prot. (g)	Servings/ Exchanges
Chicken Tuscany	10.8 oz	340	39	9	24	3	40	600	4	24	2 1/2 carb, 2 med-fat meat
Creamy Herb Roasted Chicken	10.1 oz	240	29	5	19	1.5	60	580	5	18	2 carb, 2 lean meat
Grilled Basil Chicken	10.8 oz	330	37	9	25	3	40	600	5	23	2 1/2 carb, 2 med-fat meat
Grilled Chicken Caesar	10.1 oz	300	33	8	24	2.5	35	580	5	23	2 carb, 3 lean meat
Grilled Chicken Marinara	10.1 oz	270	35	4.5	15	1.5	35	580	5	22	2 carb, 2 lean meat
Grilled Steak in Roasted Garlic Sauce	10.1 oz	220	22	7	29	2.5	35	600	5	16	1 1/2 carb, 2 lean meat
Grilled Whiskey Steak	9.6 oz	280	38	6	19	2	40	600	6	17	2 1/2 carb, 1 med-fat meat
Oriental Style Beef	10.8 oz	310	33	9	26	2.5	35	580	5	22	2 carb, 3 lean meat
Princess Chicken	10.9 oz	310	41	7	20	2	60	580	5	19	3 carb, 1 med-fat meat
Roasted Chicken Chardonnay	10.8 oz	290	32	8	25	3	40	600	4	22	2 carb, 2 med-fat meat

Healthy Choice Meals

Beef Pot Roast	11.1 oz	320	39	9	25	3	45	550	6	19	2 1/2 carb, 2 med-fat meat
Beef Stroganoff	11.1 oz	320	39	9	25	3	65	580	6	20	2 1/2 carb, 2 med-fat meat
Beef Teriyaki	9.6 oz	310	44	7	20	2.5	40	600	5	16	3 carb, 1 med-fat meat
Beef Tips Portabella	11.4 oz	280	28	8	26	3	50	600	3	23	2 carb, 2 med-fat meat
Blackened Chicken	11.1 oz	300	36	6	18	2	35	600	5	20	2 1/2 carb, 2 lean meat
Boneless Beef Ribs with Classic BBQ Sauce	11.1 oz	360	47	9	23	3	55	580	8	22	3 carb, 2 med-fat meat
Breaded Chicken Breast Strips with Mac & Cheese	8 oz	290	35	5	16	2	40	600	3	24	2 carb, 3 very lean meat
Charbroiled Beef Patty	11.1 oz	310	37	9	26	3	40	600	6	18	2 1/2 carb, 2 med-fat meat
Cheddar Broccoli Potatoes	10.8 oz	270	41	7	23	3	20	600	7	11	3 carb, 1 fat
Cheesy Rice & Chicken	9.6 oz	250	27	5	18	2.5	50	600	4	23	2 carb, 2 lean meat
Chicken Breast & Vegetables	0.6 oz	260	30	7	24	2	45	550	6	18	2 carb, 2 lean meat

FROZEN PACKAGED FOOD, MEAT, CHICKEN, FISH, MEALS, PIZZA, SNACKS

	Serving	Calories	Carb. (g)	Fat (g)	% Cal. Fat	Sat. Fat (g)	Chol. (mg)	Sod. (mg)	Fib. (g)	Prot. (g)	Servings/ Exchanges
Chicken Broccoli Alfredo	11.6 oz	300	34	7	21	3	50	530	2	25	2 carb, 3 lean meat
Chicken Carbonara	9.1 oz	290	32	7	22	2.5	45	600	2	24	2 carb, 3 lean meat
Chicken Enchiladas	11.4 oz	360	59	7	18	3	30	580	8	13	4 carb, 1 fat
Chicken Fettuccini Alfredo	8.6 oz	290	32	7	22	2.5	45	570	3	24	2 carb, 3 lean meat
Chicken Parmigiana	11.1 oz	320	40	9	25	3	20	600	6	19	2 1/2 carb, 2 med-fat meat
Chicken Piccata	9.1 oz	260	36	5	17	2.5	40	600	2	16	2 1/2 carb, 1 med-fat meat
Chicken Teriyaki	11.1 oz	270	37	6	20	2	40	600	6	16	2 1/2 carb, 1 med-fat meat
Country Breaded Chicken	10.8 oz	370	55	9	22	3	45	600	5	17	3 1/2 carb, 1 med-fat meat, 1 fat
Country Glazed Chicken	8.6 oz	230	28	5	20	2	45	600	3	17	2 carb, 2 lean meat
Country Herb Chicken	11.5 oz	280	37	6	19	2.5	40	600	5	18	2 1/2 carb, 2 lean meat
Fettuccini Alfredo	9.4 oz	280	40	7	23	2.5	15	600	3	12	2 1/2 carb, 1 med-fat meat
Grilled Chicken Breast & Mashed Potatoes	8.6 oz	190	19	5	24	1.5	50	580	3	17	1 carb, 2 lean meat
Grilled Chicken Breast & Pasta	8.9 oz	250	25	7	25	2.5	40	560	4	20	1 1/2 carb, 2 lean meat

Item	Serving										Exchanges
Grilled Turkey Breast	10.1 oz	250	31	5	18	2	35	600	5	18	2 carb, 2 lean meat
Herb Baked Fish	11 oz	360	51	9	23	3	35	600	6	17	3 1/2 carb, 1 med-fat meat, 1 fat
Homestyle Chicken & Pasta	9.1 oz	250	28	6	22	2.5	40	570	5	21	2 carb, 2 lean meat
Honey Glazed Chicken	11.1 oz	320	46	6	17	2	40	580	6	18	3 carb, 1 med-fat meat
Lasagna Bake	9.1 oz	270	38	7	23	2.5	20	600	4	13	2 1/2 carb, 1 med-fat meat
Lemon Pepper Fish	10.8 oz	280	46	5	16	2	20	580	4	13	3 carb, 1 med-fat meat
Macaroni & Cheese	10.1 oz	290	44	7	22	2.5	15	600	5	12	3 carb, 1 med-fat meat
Mandarin Chicken	10.1 oz	250	36	3.5	13	0.5	40	520	4	18	2 1/2 carb, 2 lean meat
Manicotti	11.1 oz	280	44	5	16	3	45	600	4	14	3 carb, 1 med-fat meat
Mesquite Chicken BBQ	10.6 oz	300	44	5	15	2	45	480	5	18	3 carb, 1 med-fat meat
Oriental Style Chicken	8.6 oz	240	28	5	19	1.5	35	600	4	19	2 carb, 2 lean meat
Oven Roasted Beef	10.5 oz	280	33	7	23	2.5	60	600	5	22	2 carb, 2 lean meat
Rigatoni with Broccoli & Chicken	9.1 oz	270	29	7	23	2.5	40	600	5	22	2 carb, 2 lean meat
Roast Turkey Breast	8.6 oz	220	23	6	25	2	40	580	3	18	1 1/2 carb, 2 lean meat

FROZEN PACKAGED FOOD, MEAT, CHICKEN, FISH, MEALS, PIZZA, SNACKS

	Serving	Calories	Carb. (g)	Fat (g)	% Cal. Fat	Sat. Fat (g)	Chol. (mg)	Sod. (mg)	Fib. (g)	Prot. (g)	Servings/ Exchanges
Roasted Chicken Breast	11.1 oz	280	32	8	26	3	45	600	7	18	2 carb, 2 med-fat meat
Salisbury Steak	12.8 oz	360	45	9	23	3.5	45	580	5	23	3 carb, 2 med-fat meat
Salisbury Steak & Red Skin Mashed Potatoes	8.1 oz	200	20	6	27	2.5	40	600	4	15	1 carb, 2 lean meat
Sesame Chicken	9.1 oz	260	34	6	21	2	35	580	4	17	2 carb, 2 lean meat
Slow Roasted Turkey Breast & Mashed Potatoes	8.6 oz	210	17	7	30	1.5	45	600	4	18	1 carb, 2 lean meat
Spaghetti with Meat Sauce	11.6 oz	310	48	6	17	2.5	25	600	7	16	3 carb, 1 med-fat meat
Stuffed Pasta Shells	11.3 oz	290	40	6	19	3	20	470	5	17	2 1/2 carb, 1 med-fat meat
Sweet & Sour Chicken	11.1 oz	340	54	7	19	2	25	580	3	15	3 1/2 carb, 1 med-fat meat
Traditional Meatloaf	12.1 oz	300	36	9	27	3	40	600	6	18	2 1/2 carb, 2 med-fat meat
Traditional Turkey Breast	10.6 oz	330	50	5	14	2	35	600	16	21	3 carb, 2 lean meat

Tuna Casserole	9.6 oz	270	31	7	23	1.5	30	600	5	21	2 carb, 2 lean meat
Healthy Choice Mixed Grills											
Chicken with Honey BBQ Dipping Sauce	13.1 oz	380	53	7	17	1.5	25	580	8	24	3 1/2 carb, 2 lean meat
Chicken with Honey Mustard Dipping Sauce	13.6 oz	360	49	7	18	2	25	600	10	24	3 carb, 2 lean meat
Chicken with Roasted Garlic Red Peppers Dipping Sauce	13.1 oz	320	35	10	28	3	35	580	5	21	2 carb, 2 med-fat meat
Chicken with Teriyaki Dipping Sauce	14.1 oz	340	46	7	19	1.5	35	600	9	23	3 carb, 2 lean meat
Chicken with Tomato Garlic Dipping Sauce	13.1 oz	370	50	7	17	2	30	600	10	25	3 carb, 2 lean meat
Steak with BBQ Sauce	13.1 oz	420	59	8	17	3	45	600	7	26	4 carb, 2 med-fat meat
Steak with Teriyaki Dipping Sauce	13.1 oz	350	39	9	23	3	30	600	11	26	2 1/2 carb, 3 lean meat

FROZEN PACKAGED FOOD, MEAT, CHICKEN, FISH, MEALS, PIZZA, SNACKS

	Serving	Calories	Carb. (g)	Fat (g)	% Cal. Fat	Sat. Fat (g)	Chol. (mg)	Sod. (mg)	Fib. (g)	Prot. (g)	Servings/ Exchanges
Jimmy Dean											
Sausage Biscuit, Snack Size	2	390	24	29	67	10	35	620	1	9	1 1/2 carb, 1 med-fat meat, 5 fat
Sausage, Egg & Cheese Biscuit	1	400	27	26	60	9	115	820	1	14	2 carb, 1 med-fat meat, 4 fat
Lean Cuisine Café Classics											
Baked Chicken Florentine	8 oz	200	14	8	35	2	40	660	3	18	1 carb, 2 med-fat meat
Beef Portabello	9 oz	220	25	7	27	3	30	690	3	14	1 1/2 carb, 2 lean meat
Chicken Carbonara	9 oz	280	34	7	21	2	30	690	2	19	2 carb, 2 lean meat
Garlic Beef & Broccoli	9 oz	170	16	6	29	2	30	690	3	13	1 carb, 1 med-fat meat
Glazed Chicken	8.5 oz	230	25	5	20	1	45	510	1	21	1 1/2 carb, 2 lean meat
Grilled Chicken	9.4 oz	160	15	5	28	1	35	690	4	14	1 carb, 2 lean meat
Honey Dijon Grilled Chicken	8 oz	220	22	7	27	2.5	50	640	2	17	1 1/2 carb, 2 lean meat

Food	Serving										Exchanges
Honey Roasted Pork	9.5 oz	230	18	9	35	3.5	50	580	5	18	1 carb, 2 med-fat meat
Meatloaf	9.4 oz	270	30	8	26	3	45	540	3	19	2 carb, 2 med-fat meat
Roasted Garlic Chicken	8.9 oz	200	14	8	35	3	40	690	2	17	1 carb, 2 med-fat meat
Roasted Turkey & Vegetables	8 oz	150	12	5	30	1	25	650	3	15	1 carb, 2 lean meat
Salisbury Steak	9.5 oz	280	27	8	25	4	50	650	3	25	2 carb, 3 lean meat
Shrimp & Angel Hair Pasta	10 oz	240	35	5	19	1	50	640	2	14	2 carb, 1 med-fat meat
Steak Tips Portabello	7.5 oz	180	13	7	33	2	40	460	3	15	1 carb, 2 lean meat
Sweet & Sour Chicken	10 oz	290	51	2.5	9	0.5	25	690	1	16	3 1/2 carb, 1 lean meat
Teriyaki Chicken	10 oz	280	42	3.5	11	1.5	40	660	0	19	3 carb, 1 med-fat meat
Thai-Style Chicken	9 oz	250	35	4.5	16	2.5	30	660	1	18	2 carb, 2 lean meat
Three Cheese Chicken	8 oz	220	14	9	36	3	45	520	2	21	1 carb, 3 lean meat
Lean Cuisine Every-Day Favorites											
Angel Hair Pasta	10 oz	260	48	4	10	1.5	5	690	4	8	3 carb, 1 fat
Beef & Broccoli	8.5 oz	230	36	4	15	1.5	15	680	1	12	2 1/2 carb, 1 med-fat meat

FROZEN PACKAGED FOOD, MEAT, CHICKEN, FISH, MEALS, PIZZA, SNACKS

	Serving	Calories	Carb. (g)	Fat (g)	% Cal. Fat	Sat. Fat (g)	Chol. (mg)	Sod. (mg)	Fib. (g)	Prot. (g)	Servings/ Exchanges
Cheese Cannelloni	9.1 oz	240	31	4.5	17	2	20	640	3	18	2 carb, 2 lean meat
Cheese Ravioli	8.5 oz	250	38	6	20	3	35	620	3	10	2 1/2 carb, 1 med-fat meat
Chicken Chow Mein	9 oz	200	31	2.5	13	0.5	25	620	2	14	2 carb, 1 lean meat
Chicken Enchilada Suiza	9 oz	290	48	5	16	2	20	560	3	12	3 carb, 1 med-fat meat
Chicken Fettucini	9.3 oz	280	33	7	21	3	35	690	2	22	2 carb, 2 lean meat
Classic Five Cheese Lasagna	11.5 oz	310	44	7	19	4	25	660	4	17	3 carb, 1 med-fat meat
Fettucini Alfredo	9.3 oz	290	44	7	21	3.5	15	660	2	12	3 carb, 1 fat
Lasagna with Meat Sauce	10.5 oz	300	41	8	20	4	30	650	3	19	3 carb, 1 med-fat meat, 1 fat
Macaroni & Cheese	10 oz	300	43	7	20	4	20	650	1	16	3 carb, 1 med-fat meat
Mandarin Chicken	9 oz	270	46	3.5	11	1	30	690	2	14	3 carb, 1 med-fat meat
Penne Pasta with Tomato	10 oz	270	51	3	9	0.5	0	390	5	9	3 1/2 carb, 1 fat
Roasted Chicken with Lemon Pepper Fettuccine	8.1 oz	260	33	7	23	2	30	670	2	16	2 carb, 1 med-fat meat

Roasted Potatoes, Broccoli & Cheese Sauce	10.3 oz	240	37	5	19	3	15	660	4	11	2 1/2 carb, 1 med-fat meat
Santa Fe-Style Rice & Beans	10.4 oz	290	50	5	16	2	15	580	5	11	3 carb, 1 fat
Spaghetti	11.5 oz	240	35	5	19	1.5	20	690	3	14	2 carb, 1 med-fat meat
Swedish Meatballs	9.1 oz	290	36	7	21	3	55	640	2	21	2 1/2 carb, 2 lean meat

Lean Cuisine Dinnertime Selections

Chicken Fettuccine with Broccoli	13.6 oz	380	51	8	18	3.5	45	870	5	26	3 1/2 carb, 2 med-fat meat
Chicken Florentine	13.3 oz	330	44	6	15	2.5	40	840	6	25	3 carb, 2 lean meat
Glazed Chicken	13 oz	310	39	6	16	1	50	610	4	24	2 1/2 carb, 2 lean meat
Grilled Chicken & Penne Pasta	14 oz	340	46	6	15	2.5	35	680	5	25	3 carb, 2 lean meat
Jumbo Rigatoni	15.4 oz	390	50	10	23	3.5	30	790	6	24	3 carb, 2 med-fat meat
Roasted Turkey Breast	14 oz	340	50	7	18	1	30	840	6	20	3 carb, 2 lean meat

FROZEN PACKAGED FOOD, MEAT, CHICKEN, FISH, MEALS, PIZZA, SNACKS

	Serving	Calories	Carb. (g)	Fat (g)	% Cal. Fat	Sat. Fat (g)	Chol. (mg)	Sod. (mg)	Fib. (g)	Prot. (g)	Servings/ Exchanges
Salisbury Steak	15.5 oz	320	35	9	25	4.5	55	890	6	25	2 carb, 3 lean meat
Steak Tips Dijon	12 oz	310	44	7	19	3	35	820	5	18	3 carb, 1 med-fat meat
Lean Cuisine Spa Cuisine											
Chicken in Peanut Sauce	9 oz	280	32	7	21	1.5	25	690	2	21	2 carb, 2 lean meat
Chicken Mediterranean	10.5 oz	240	35	3.5	13	0.5	20	690	5	16	2 carb, 1 med-fat meat
Chicken Pecan	9 oz	260	34	6	19	2	30	570	4	18	2 carb, 2 lean meat
Lemon Chicken	9 oz	270	38	8	26	2	25	650	2	12	2 1/2 carb, 1 med-fat meat, 1 fat
Lemongrass Chicken	9.4 oz	240	29	6	21	3.5	30	660	4	17	2 carb, 2 lean meat
Pork with Cherry Sauce	8.3 oz	260	38	5	17	2	35	540	4	15	2 1/2 carb, 1 med-fat meat
Life Choice											
Beef Pot Roast	12 oz	280	12	9	32	4	80	940	3	36	1 carb, 5 lean meat
Chicken Parmesan	12.4 oz	300	13	10	30	5	85	960	2	38	1 carb, 5 lean meat
Hearty Meat Loaf	12.2 oz	360	16	16	42	7	85	830	6	38	1 carb, 5 lean meat
Homestyle Baked Chicken	12 oz	220	11	8	36	3	150	850	5	26	1 carb, 3 lean meat

Roasted Turkey Breast	12 oz	260	15	4.5	17	1.5	65	800	4	38	1 carb, 5 very lean meat
Slow Roasted Beef Tips	12 oz	260	12	8	31	4	75	910	4	35	1 carb, 4 lean meat
Marie Callender's											
Beef Pot Pie	10 oz	680	60	39	53	11	30	1200	4	20	4 carb, 1 med-fat meat, 7 fat
Beef Salisbury Steak & Gravy	14 oz	490	40	23	43	12	85	1570	7	29	2 1/2 carb, 3 med-fat meat, 2 fat
Beef Stroganoff	13 oz	410	39	16	37	7	140	1550	6	27	2 1/2 carb, 3 med-fat meat
Beef Tips in Mushroom Sauce	13.6 oz	360	35	12	31	4.5	70	1450	6	26	2 carb, 2 med-fat meat
Breaded Chicken Parmigiana	16 oz	670	60	34	46	9	60	970	8	31	4 carb, 3 med-fat meat, 4 fat
Cheesy Chicken Breast & Rice	14 oz	480	47	18	35	13	80	1500	5	31	3 carb, 3 med-fat meat, 1 fat
Chicken Pot Pie	10 oz	670	57	40	54	10	35	1000	4	19	4 carb, 1 med-fat meat, 7 fat
Chicken Teriyaki	14 oz	420	75	3	7	1	35	2220	5	23	5 carb, 1 med-fat meat
Chunky Chicken & Noodles	14 oz	630	53	35	51	14	100	1550	6	25	3 1/2 carb, 2 med-fat meat, 5 fat

FROZEN PACKAGED FOOD, MEAT, CHICKEN, FISH, MEALS, PIZZA, SNACKS

	Serving	Calories	Carb. (g)	Fat (g)	% Cal. Fat	Sat. Fat (g)	Chol. (mg)	Sod. (mg)	Fib. (g)	Prot. (g)	Servings/ Exchanges
Country Fried Beef Steak	15 oz	640	55	38	53	17	90	1980	8	18	3 1/2 carb, 1 med-fat meat, 7 fat
Country Fried Chicken & Gravy	16 oz	670	58	37	51	14	85	1830	8	24	4 carb, 2 med-fat meat, 5 fat
Country Fried Pork Chip	15 oz	590	50	33	51	12	80	1840	7	22	3 carb, 1 med-fat meat, 6 fat
Country Style Beef Stew	13 oz	440	52	16	34	6	55	1670	4	20	3 1/2 carb, 1 med-fat meat, 2 fat
Creamy Mushroom Chicken Pot Pie	10 oz	690	56	43	57	12	40	880	4	19	4 carb, 1 med-fat meat, 8 fat
Creamy Parmesan Chicken	1 cup	530	43	32	55	10	30	720	1	17	3 carb, 1 med-fat meat, 5 fat
Fettuccine Alfredo & Garlic Bread	14 oz	880	82	51	52	20	60	1270	6	23	5 1/2 carb, 1 med-fat meat, 9 fat
Fettuccine with Chicken & Broccoli	13 oz	630	43	37	54	15	90	900	6	30	3 carb, 3 med-fat meat, 4 fat
Golden Breaded Fish Fillet	12 oz	450	44	18	38	8	65	1450	5	26	3 carb, 2 med-fat meat, 2 fat
Grilled Chicken Alfredo Bake	13 oz	610	41	37	56	16	90	1000	6	26	3 carb, 2 med-fat meat, 5 fat

Food	Serving										
Herb Roasted Chicken	14 oz	530	20	35	60	12	215	1270	6	34	1 carb, 4 med-fat meat, 3 fat
Homestyle Chicken & Dumplings	14 oz	540	49	27	46	13	150	1550	6	24	3 carb, 2 med-fat meat, 3 fat
Honey Roasted Chicken Breast	14 oz	440	20	23	48	8	160	1060	7	37	1 carb, 5 med-fat meat
Honey Roasted Chicken Pot Pie	1 cup	520	47	29	52	7	25	880	3	16	3 carb, 1 med-fat meat, 5 fat
Lasagna Bake	14 oz	510	47	21	37	11	80	1590	8	31	3 carb, 3 med-fat meat, 1 fat
Macaroni & Cheese	1 cup	370	36	18	43	11	40	1130	3	16	2 1/2 carb, 2 med-fat meat, 2 fat
Meat Lasagna	1 cup	240	24	9	33	5	45	950	2	14	1 1/2 carb, 1 med-fat meat, 1 fat
Meatloaf & Gravy	14 oz	560	39	31	50	14	80	1510	6	31	2 1/2 carb, 3 med-fat meat, 3 fat
Old Fashioned Beef Pot Roast	15 oz	360	28	14	36	7	70	1490	4	30	2 carb, 3 med-fat meat
Slow Roasted Beef	14.5 oz	430	31	22	47	9	70	1530	9	26	2 carb, 3 med-fat meat, 1 fat
Southern Fried Chicken Tenderloins	13.5 oz	460	49	20	39	10	70	1460	9	20	3 carb, 2 med-fat meat, 2 fat

FROZEN PACKAGED FOOD, MEAT, CHICKEN, FISH, MEALS, PIZZA, SNACKS

	Serving	Calories	Carb. (g)	Fat (g)	% Cal. Fat	Sat. Fat (g)	Chol. (mg)	Sod. (mg)	Fib. (g)	Prot. (g)	Servings/ Exchanges
Spaghetti & Meat Sauce	17 oz	680	90	22	29	6	45	970	13	30	6 carb, 2 med-fat meat, 1 fat
Stuffed Pasta Medley	13 oz	450	58	15	31	8	75	1300	6	21	4 carb, 1 med-fat meat, 2 fat
Swedish Meatballs	14 oz	580	48	30	47	14	65	1140	7	28	3 carb, 3 med-fat meat, 3 fat
Sweet & Sour Chicken	14 oz	580	86	16	26	2.5	40	850	5	21	6 carb, 1 med-fat meat, 2 fat
Three Cheese Ravioli & Garlic Bread	16 oz	620	89	18	27	7	50	1480	10	25	6 carb, 1 med-fat meat, 3 fat
Turkey Breast with Stuffing	14 oz	380	38	13	32	4	60	1370	8	26	2 1/2 carb, 2 med-fat meat, 1 fat
Turkey Mushroom Chicken Pot Pie	1 cup	510	43	31	55	8	25	890	4	15	3 carb, 1 med-fat meat, 5 fat
Turkey Pot Pie	10 oz	660	58	39	53	10	30	1100	3	19	4 carb, 1 med-fat meat, 7 fat
Michael Angelo's											
Chicken Lasagna	1 cup	290	37	7	21	3	25	670	2	21	2 1/2 carb, 2 lean meat
Eggplant Parmesan	6 oz	280	23	19	61	3	40	330	4	5	1 1/2 carb, 4 fat

Lasagna	1 cup	290	25	10	31	8	50	490	4	24	2 carb, 3 lean meat
Vegetable Lasagna	1 cup	230	23	7	26	3	15	720	3	20	1 1/2 carb, 2 lean meat

Michelina's Budget Gourmet

Angel Hair Pasta	8 oz	240	41	4	15	1	5	490	3	9	3 carb, 1 fat
Chinese Style Vegetables & White Chicken	8 oz	300	52	7	20	1.5	5	690	3	7	3 1/2 carb, 1 fat
Escalloped Noodles & White Turkey	8 oz	280	36	13	39	5	65	600	2	11	2 1/2 carb, 1 med-fat meat, 2 fat
Fettuccine Alfredo with Four Cheeses	8 oz	310	42	10	29	4.5	65	590	2	12	3 carb, 2 fat
Italian Style Vegetables and White Chicken	8 oz	280	50	5	18	1.5	10	480	2	7	3 carb, 1 fat
Homestyle Macaroni & Cheese	8 oz	340	41	13	32	6	25	620	2	14	3 carb, 1 med-fat meat, 2 fat
Lasagna Alfredo with Broccoli	8 oz	290	36	11	34	5	25	720	2	11	2 1/2 carb, 1 med-fat meat, 1 fat

FROZEN PACKAGED FOOD, MEAT, CHICKEN, FISH, MEALS, PIZZA, SNACKS

	Serving	Calories	Carb. (g)	Fat (g)	% Cal. Fat	Sat. Fat (g)	Chol. (mg)	Sod. (mg)	Fib. (g)	Prot. (g)	Servings/ Exchanges
Lasagna with Meat Sauce	8 oz	240	37	7	25	2.5	15	520	2	10	2 1/2 carb, 1 fat
Macaroni & Cheese	8 oz	240	40	4.5	17	2.5	10	560	2	11	2 1/2 carb, 1 med-fat meat
Rigatoni in Cream Sauce	8 oz	260	41	4.5	15	1.5	15	440	2	12	3 carb, 1 fat
Spaghetti Marinara	8 oz	280	49	5	16	1	0	700	3	9	3 carb, 1 fat
Spicy Szechwan Style Vegetables & White Chicken	8 oz	300	47	7	20	1	5	740	3	10	3 carb, 1 fat
Stir Fry Rice & Vegetables	8 oz	450	61	19	38	3.5	10	780	3	7	4 carb, 4 fat
Wild Rice Pilaf with Vegetables	8 oz	390	60	13	28	13	10	760	2	7	4 carb, 3 fat
Ziti Parmesano	8 oz	230	36	7	26	2.5	10	430	2	9	2 1/2 carb, 1 fat
Michelina's Authentico											
Cheese Ravioli	8.1 oz	390	42	18	41	10	80	820	2	17	3 carb, 1 med-fat meat, 3 fat
Chicken Primavera	8.1 oz	250	37	6	20	3	30	750	3	13	2 1/2 carb, 1 med-fat meat

Food	Serving	Cal.									Exchanges
Fettucine Alfredo with Chicken & Broccoli	8.6 oz	300	37	11	30	6	40	600	2	14	2 1/2 carb, 1 med-fat meat, 1 fat
Four Cheese Lasagna	8.1 oz	230	43	7	21	3.5	25	550	3	13	3 carb, 1 med-fat meat
Fried Chicken	8.1 oz	310	27	18	52	6	40	960	2	11	2 carb, 1 med-fat meat, 3 fat
Glazed Chicken	8.1 oz	250	45	3.5	12	0.5	20	850	2	11	3 carb, 1 fat
Lasagna with Meat Sauce	9.1 oz	280	40	7	25	3	35	800	3	15	2 1/2 carb, 1 med-fat meat
Linguini with Clams	8.6 oz	290	50	3.5	12	0	10	560	2	11	3 carb, 1 fat
Macaroni & Cheese	8.1 oz	240	41	4	15	2.5	10	540	2	11	3 carb, 3 fat
Meatballs & Mashed Potatoes	8.6 oz	270	26	14	44	5	35	1150	3	11	2 carb, 1 med-fat meat, 2 fat
Meatloaf	8.1 oz	270	20	16	52	6	55	1380	2	11	1 carb, 1 med-fat meat, 2 fat
Noodles Stroganoff	8.1 oz	320	35	14	38	6	75	760	2	14	2 carb, 1 med-fat meat, 2 fat
Penne with Chicken	8.6 oz	330	48	9	24	3.5	40	610	2	16	3 carb, 1 med-fat meat, 1 fat
Peppersteak and Rice	8.1 oz	250	43	4	16	1.5	20	890	1	11	3 carb, 1 fat
Roast Turkey	8.1 oz	250	32	9	32	4	35	980	2	10	2 carb, 1 med-fat meat, 1 fat
Stuffed Cheese Rigatoni	8.6 oz	300	42	8	27	4.5	45	700	3	11	3 carb, 2 fat

FROZEN PACKAGED FOOD, MEAT, CHICKEN, FISH, MEALS, PIZZA, SNACKS

	Serving	Calories	Carb. (g)	Fat (g)	% Cal. Fat	Sat. Fat (g)	Chol. (mg)	Sod. (mg)	Fib. (g)	Prot. (g)	Servings/Exchanges
Teriyaki Chicken & Rice	8.6 oz	280	64	2.5	7	0.5	15	1160	1	11	4 carb, 1 fat
Michelina's Lean Gourmet											
Beef Peppersteak & Rice	8.1 oz	260	43	4.5	15	1.5	15	880	1	12	3 carb, 1 fat
Beef Stroganoff	8.1 oz	250	38	5	18	2	20	650	2	15	2 1/2 carb, 2 lean meat
Cheese Manicotti with Marinara Sauce	8.6 oz	290	48	5	16	2.5	25	780	3	12	3 carb, 1 fat
Cheese Stuffed Rigatoni	8.6 oz	260	37	7	27	3.5	35	700	3	10	2 1/2 carb, 1 med-fat meat
Chicken Alfredo Florentine	8.6 oz	270	38	6	19	3	40	610	2	15	2 1/2 carb, 1 med-fat meat
Fettucine Alfredo	9.1 oz	250	41	5	18	2.5	10	570	2	12	3 carb, 1 fat
Five Cheese Layered Lasagna	8.6 oz	220	36	5	20	2	10	760	5	10	2 1/2 carb, 1 fat
French Recipe Chicken	8.6 oz	180	23	4.5	22	1.5	30	830	4	10	1 1/2 carb, 1 med-fat meat
Glazed Chicken	8.1 oz	260	45	3.5	12	0.5	30	920	2	11	3 carb, 1 fat
Macaroni & Cheese	10.1 oz	300	51	5	15	3	15	670	3	14	3 1/2 carb, 1 med-fat meat

Meatloaf	3.1 oz	210	22	8	33	3	50	1170	2	13	1 1/2 carb, 1 med-fat meat, 1 fat
Roasted Sirloin Supreme	3.1 oz	230	30	5	22	2	45	920	2	13	2 carb, 1 med-fat meat
Salisbury Steak	8.5 oz	200	23	7	30	2.5	30	970	2	12	1 1/2 carb, 1 med-fat meat
Santa Fe Style Rice & Beans	9.1 oz	350	56	9	23	4.5	25	950	3	9	4 carb, 2 fat
Shrimp with Pasta & Vegetables	8.1 oz	260	37	6	23	3.5	55	590	2	12	2 1/2 carb, 1 med-fat meat
Spaghetti & Meat Sauce	9.1 oz	280	45	5	16	1.5	15	530	4	13	3 carb, 1 med-fat meat
Swedish Meatballs	9.1 oz	290	40	7	24	3.5	30	850	3	17	2 1/2 carb, 1 med-fat meat
Red Baron											
Scramblers, Bacon	1 piece	400	35	22	50	7	75	930	5	18	2 carb, 2 med-fat meat, 2 fat
Scramblers, Western	1 piece	390	36	21	49	7	45	790	2	15	2 1/2 carb, 1 med-fat meat, 3 fat
Stouffer's											
Baked Chicken Breast	8.9 oz	270	20	11	37	3.5	70	690	4	22	1 carb, 3 lean meat
Beef Pot Roast	8.9 oz	260	24	11	38	4	35	960	3	16	1 1/2 carb, 2 med-fat meat
Beef Stroganoff	9.8 oz	380	34	17	40	5	70	990	2	22	2 carb, 2 med-fat meat, 1 fat

FROZEN PACKAGED FOOD, MEAT, CHICKEN, FISH, MEALS, PIZZA, SNACKS

	Serving	Calories	Carb. (g)	Fat (g)	% Cal. Fat	Sat. Fat (g)	Chol. (mg)	Sod. (mg)	Fib. (g)	Prot. (g)	Servings/ Exchanges
Chicken a' la King	11.5 oz	370	45	12	30	4	50	780	2	20	3 carb, 2 med-fat meat
Chicken Tenderloins	10 oz	430	37	20	42	7	70	1230	3	26	2 1/2 carb, 3 med-fat meat, 1 fat
Corn Souffle	1/2 cup	170	21	7	35	1.5	55	480	1	5	1/2 carb, 1 fat
Creamed Chipped Beef	1/2 cup	140	9	8	50	4.5	40	610	0	9	1/2 carb, 1 med-fat meat, 1 fat
Escalloped Chicken & Noodles	10 oz	360	29	19	47	3.5	60	1020	4	17	2 carb, 2 med-fat meat, 2 fat
Fettuccine Alfredo	11.5 oz	530	52	28	47	16	105	970	4	17	3 1/2 carb, 1 med-fat meat, 5 fat
Fish Filet	9 oz	430	47	18	37	6	55	1040	2	20	3 carb, 2 med-fat meat, 2 fat
Five Cheese Lasagna	10.8 oz	370	39	14	35	7	35	960	4	21	2 1/2 carb, 2 med-fat meat, 1 fat
Fried Chicken Breast	8.9 oz	390	37	18	41	4.5	50	1040	2	19	2 1/2 carb, 2 med-fat meat, 2 fat
Grilled Chicken Portabello	9 oz	230	26	6	22	1	35	900	4	19	2 carb, 2 lean meat
Grilled Chicken Teriyaki	9.4 oz	300	45	3.5	1	1	40	880	3	21	3 carb, 2 lean meat
Grilled Herb Chicken	9 oz	250	33	4	14	1	35	590	3	20	2 carb, 2 lean meat
Grilled Lemon Pepper Chicken	9 oz	250	27	7	24	2	45	670	5	20	3 carb, 2 lean meat

Food	Serving										Exchanges
Lasagna with Meat Sauce	10.5 oz	360	37	11	28	6	35	800	3	28	2 1/2 carb, 3 lean meat
Macaroni & Beef	11.5 oz	360	39	13	33	5	40	1070	4	21	2 1/2 carb, 2 med-fat meat, 1 fat
Macaroni & Cheese	1 cup	320	32	15	44	7	25	950	2	14	2 carb, 1 med-fat meat, 1 fat
Meatloaf	9.9 oz	350	23	18	46	7	60	860	2	24	1 1/2 carb, 3 med-fat meat, 1 fat
Roast Turkey	9.6 oz	290	30	12	38	3.5	45	970	2	16	2 carb, 1 med-fat meat, 1 fat
Roasted Chicken	9.6 oz	460	34	24	48	6	80	990	5	26	2 carb, 3 med-fat meat, 2 fat
Salisbury Steak	9.6 oz	370	27	18	43	8	40	1120	1	25	2 carb, 3 med-fat meat, 1 fat
Spaghetti with Meat Sauce	12 oz	350	44	12	31	4	30	740	5	17	3 carb, 1 med-fat meat, 1 fat
Spaghetti with Meatballs	12.6 oz	460	58	16	30	5	40	880	4	21	4 carb, 1 med-fat meat, 2 fat
Spinach Souffle	1/2 cup	130	10	8	54	2	90	470	1	5	1/2 carb, 2 fat
Stuffed Pepper	10 oz	230	25	9	35	3.5	25	920	2	11	1 1/2 carb, 1 med-fat meat, 1 fat
Swedish Meatballs	11.5 oz	570	39	33	53	12	110	1150	2	28	2 1/2 carb, 3 med-fat meat, 4 fat
Tuna Noodle Casserole	10 oz	340	34	16	41	5	35	1140	2	16	2 carb, 1 med-fat meat, 1 fat
White Meat Chicken Pot Pie	10 oz	730	64	44	55	18	65	1180	4	20	4 carb, 1 med-fat meat, 8 fat

FROZEN PACKAGED FOOD, MEAT, CHICKEN, FISH, MEALS, PIZZA, SNACKS

	Serving	Calories	Carb. (g)	Fat (g)	% Cal. Fat	Sat. Fat (g)	Chol. (mg)	Sod. (mg)	Fib. (g)	Prot. (g)	Servings/ Exchanges
Stouffer's Skillet Sensations											
Chicken Alfredo	1 3/4 cup	240	25	9	33	3	25	630	2	15	1 1/2 carb, 1 med-fat meat, 1 fat
Garlic Chicken	1 2/3 cup	190	25	4	18	2	20	680	2	13	1 1/2 carb, 1 med-fat meat
Steak Teriyaki	1 2/3 cup	210	33	4	14	2	20	900	2	11	2 carb, 1 med-fat meat
Swanson											
Boneless White Meat Fried Chicken	11 oz	510	66	22	39	5	90	1250	5	20	4 1/2 carb, 1 med-fat meat, 3 fat
Breaded Fish Filet	10 oz	400	51	15	33	4	45	1300	3	16	3 1/2 carb, 1 med-fat meat, 2 fat
Chicken Strips	11 oz	610	75	28	41	6	45	940	5	20	5 carb, 1 med-fat meat, 5 fat
Classic Fried Chicken	11.5 oz	590	45	30	46	7	150	2030	4	35	3 carb, 4 med-fat meat, 2 fat
Meatloaf	11 oz	340	24	20	53	8	45	550	3	15	1 1/2 carb, 2 med-fat meat, 2 fat
Mexican Style Fiesta	13.3 oz	480	65	18	33	4	30	890	5	17	4 carb, 1 med-fat meat, 3 fat
Salisbury Steak	13 oz	380	24	20	47	7	80	920	3	25	1 1/2 carb, 3 med-fat meat, 1 fat
Turkey Breast & Stuffing	11.8 oz	350	43	11	26	2.5	35	1080	4	15	3 carb, 1 med-fat meat, 1 fat

Swanson Hungry-Man

Backyard Barbeque XXL	24 oz	1160	110	48	38	18	225	3290	4	66	7 carb, 5 med-fat meat, 5 fat
Beef Pot Roast	18.5 oz	430	47	16	33	5	55	1180	7	27	3 carb, 2 med-fat meat, 1 fat
Beer Battered Chicken & Cheese Fries	16 oz	660	64	26	35	10	125	1840	2	45	4 carb, 5 med-fat meat
Buffalo Style Chicken Strips	16 oz	870	106	28	29	6	105	2900	8	50	7 carb, 4 med-fat meat, 2 fat
Chopped Sirloin Beefsteak	16.3 oz	460	16	25	48	11	115	1480	3	37	1 carb, 5 med-fat meat
Classic Fried Chicken	16.5 oz	790	75	40	46	10	80	1940	6	33	5 carb, 3 med-fat meat, 5 fat
Country Fried Beef Steak	16 oz	630	64	29	41	10	70	1540	6	29	4 carb, 2 med-fat meat, 4 fat
Grilled BBQ Chicken	20 oz	870	116	28	30	8	110	1790	2	40	8 carb, 2 med-fat meat, 4 fat
Grilled Beef Steak Strips	20 oz	580	75	16	24	6	65	2370	6	34	5 carb, 3 med-fat meat
Meatloaf	16.5 oz	850	87	43	45	17	105	2500	6	34	6 carb, 2 med-fat meat, 7 fat
Mexican Style Fiesta	20 oz	780	96	33	37	9	45	1970	13	27	6 1/2 carb, 1 med-fat meat, 6 fat
Roasted Carved Turkey XXL	24 oz	1450	174	58	36	26	165	5410	13	47	12 carb, 2 med-fat meat, 10 fat

FROZEN PACKAGED FOOD, MEAT, CHICKEN, FISH, MEALS, PIZZA, SNACKS

	Serving	Calories	Carb. (g)	Fat (g)	% Cal. Fat	Sat. Fat (g)	Chol. (mg)	Sod. (mg)	Fib. (g)	Prot. (g)	Servings/Exchanges
Roasted Turkey Breast	18.7 oz	520	66	15	27	3.5	45	2620	5	29	4 1/2 carb, 2 med-fat meat, 1 fat
Roasted White Meat Chicken	16.5 oz	440	38	16	34	4	55	1560	5	36	2 1/2 carb, 4 med-fat meat
Salisbury Steak	16.3 oz	410	47	12	27	3	90	1020	3	28	3 carb, 2 med-fat meat
Southern Fried Chicken	12 oz	420	39	19	40	4	45	1240	3	21	2 1/2 carb, 2 med-fat meat, 2 fat
Uncle Ben's Bowls											
Chicken Fried Rice	12 oz	410	62	7	15	1.5	85	1270	2	23	4 carb, 2 lean meat
Roasted Chicken & Vegetables	12 oz	360	52	4.5	11	1	35	1040	3	24	3 1/2 carb, 2 lean meat
Spicy Beef & Broccoli	12 oz	360	61	5	13	1.5	25	1490	3	18	4 carb, 1 med-fat meat
Spicy Peanut Chicken	12 oz	400	49	11	25	2.5	60	1150	4	25	3 carb, 2 med-fat meat
Sweet & Sour Chicken	12 oz	360	68	2	6	0.5	30	540	2	17	4 1/2 carb, 1 lean meat
Teriyaki Chicken	12 oz	360	63	2.5	7	0.5	30	1290	2	20	4 carb, 1 lean meat
Thai Style Chicken	12 oz	370	54	7	16	2.5	60	1100	6	23	3 1/2 carb, 2 lean meat

Weight Watchers Smart Ones

Chicken Enchiladas Suiza	9 oz	340	38	10	26	4.5	40	800	3	12	2 1/2 carb, 1 med-fat meat, 1 fat
Chicken Marsala	9 oz	180	10	7	33	1.5	40	660	3	20	1/2 carb, 2 lean meat
Chicken Parmesan	11 oz	300	32	5	15	1	30	670	3	20	2 carb, 2 lean meat
Chicken Sante Fe	9 oz	140	11	2.5	14	0	30	800	4	20	1 carb, 2 lean meat
Creamy Chicken Tuscan	9 oz	180	8	8	38	3.5	50	690	3	18	1/2 carb, 2 med-fat meat
Creamy Parmesan Chicken	9 oz	210	12	8	33	4.5	65	800	3	24	1 carb, 3 lean meat
Fettucine Alfredo	9.3 oz	270	39	6	19	3.5	15	650	3	14	2 1/2 carb, 1 med-fat meat
Ravioli Florentine	8.5 oz	220	34	5	23	2	20	510	3	9	2 carb, 1 fat
Slow-Roasted Turkey Breast	10 oz	220	18	8	32	2.5	50	720	2	18	1 carb, 2 med-fat meat
Sweet & Sour Chicken	9 oz	150	10	3	17	0	30	800	3	20	1/2 carb, 3 very lean meat
Thai Style Chicken & Rice Noodles	9 oz	290	39	4	12	0.5	25	830	2	13	2 1/2 carb, 1 med-fat meat
Traditional Lasagna with Meat Sauce	10.5 oz	290	42	6	17	2.5	25	760	4	18	3 carb, 1 med-fat meat

FROZEN PACKAGED FOOD, MEAT, CHICKEN, FISH, MEALS, PIZZA, SNACKS

	Serving	Calories	Carb. (g)	Fat (g)	% Cal. Fat	Sat. Fat (g)	Chol. (mg)	Sod. (mg)	Fib. (g)	Prot. (g)	Servings/ Exchanges
Tuna Noodle Gratin	9.5 oz	260	39	6	19	2	30	730	3	13	2 1/2 carb, 1 med-fat meat
FROZEN PIZZA											
Brands											
DiGiorno											
Cheese Stuffed Crust Pepperoni	1/5 pizza	370	40	16	38	8	40	1030	3	19	2 1/2 carb, 2 med-fat meat, 1 fat
Cheese Stuffed Crust Supreme	1/6 pizza	350	35	16	43	7	35	950	3	18	2 carb, 2 med-fat meat, 1 fat
Deep Dish Supreme	1/6 pizza	320	33	15	44	6	30	810	2	14	2 carb, 1 med-fat meat, 2 fat
Deep Dish Three Meat	1/6 pizza	310	32	15	42	6	25	790	2	13	2 carb, 1 med-fat meat, 2 fat
Microwave Rising Crust Four Cheese	1/2 pizza	370	44	15	38	6	15	720	3	15	3 carb, 1 med-fat meat, 2 fat
Microwave Rising Crust Pepperoni	1/2 pizza	390	43	18	41	7	20	840	3	16	3 carb, 1 med-fat meat, 3 fat

Microwave Rising Crust Supreme	1/2 pizza	400	45	18	40	7	25	860	4	16	3 carb, 1 med-fat meat, 3 fat
Rising Crust Four Cheese	1/5 pizza	320	39	11	31	5	25	830	2	15	2 1/2 carb, 1 med-fat meat, 1 fat
Rising Crust Pepperoni	1/5 pizza	330	39	13	36	6	25	910	2	15	2 1/2 carb, 1 med-fat meat, 2 fat
Rising Crust Spinach, Mushroom, Garlic	1/6 pizza	290	40	9	28	4	20	770	3	14	2 1/2 carb, 1 med-fat meat, 1 fat
Rising Crust Three Meat	1/6 pizza	360	40	15	39	6	30	1000	2	17	2 1/2 carb, 1 med-fat meat, 2 fat
Thin Crispy Crust Four Cheese	1/5 pizza	300	34	11	33	5	25	660	3	15	2 carb, 1 med-fat meat, 1 fat
Thin Crispy Crust Four Meat	1/5 pizza	320	37	13	38	5	35	830	2	13	2 1/2 carb, 1 med-fat meat, 2 fat
Thin Crispy Crust Pepperoni	1/5 pizza	310	34	12	35	5	35	790	2	15	2 carb, 1 med-fat meat, 1 fat
Thin Crispy Crust Supreme	1/5 pizza	300	36	12	33	5	30	740	3	14	2 1/2 carb, 1 med-fat meat, 1 fat

FROZEN PACKAGED FOOD, MEAT, CHICKEN, FISH, MEALS, PIZZA, SNACKS

	Serving	Calories	Carb. (g)	Fat (g)	% Cal. Fat	Sat. Fat (g)	Chol. (mg)	Sod. (mg)	Fib. (g)	Prot. (g)	Servings/ Exchanges
Red Baron											
Carb Works Pepperoni	1 pizza	480	17	31	58	16	75	1510	4	36	1 carb, 5 med-fat meat, 1 fat
Classic 4-Cheese	1/4 pizza	400	37	20	45	8	30	720	2	18	2 1/2 carb, 2 med-fat meat, 2 fat
Classic 4-Meat	1/5 pizza	330	29	18	48	6	30	900	1	15	2 carb, 1 med-fat meat, 3 fat
Classic Mexican Style Supreme	1/5 pizza	360	33	19	47	9	35	690	2	14	2 carb, 1 med-fat meat, 3 fat
Classic Pepperoni	1/5 pizza	340	28	19	50	7	25	840	1	14	2 carb, 1 med-fat meat, 3 fat
Classic Supreme	1/5 pizza	340	29	19	50	7	25	790	2	14	2 carb, 1 med-fat meat, 3 fat
Deep Dish Mini Pizzas Cheese	4 pieces	410	46	19	41	6	20	800	2	17	3 carb, 1 med-fat meat, 3 fat
Deep Dish Mini Pizzas Pepperoni	4 pieces	450	46	23	47	8	30	990	2	17	3 carb, 1 med-fat meat, 4 fat
Deep Dish Pan Four-Cheese	1/3 pizza	370	39	17	41	7	20	620	2	14	2 1/2 carb, 1 med-fat meat, 2 fat

Deep Dish Pan Meat Trio	1/3 pizza	410	40	21	46	7	25	850	2	16	2 1/2 carb, 1 med-fat meat, 3 fat
Deep Dish Pan Pepperoni	1/3 pizza	410	40	21	46	7	25	850	2	15	2 1/2 carb, 1 med-fat meat, 3 fat
Deep Dish Singles Pepperoni	1	460	41	22	43	9	35	910	2	17	3 carb, 1 med-fat meat, 3 fat
Deep Dish Singles Supreme	1	470	40	20	38	9	40	960	2	18	2 1/2 carb, 2 med-fat meat, 2 fat
French Bread 5 Cheese & Garlic	1	420	39	23	48	9	30	830	2	15	2 1/2 carb, 1 med-fat meat, 4 fat
French Bread Pepperoni	1	360	42	15	36	6	30	1080	2	16	3 carb, 1 med-fat meat, 2 fat
Tombstone											
Brick Oven Style Cheese	1/3 pizza	350	38	15	37	7	35	690	3	17	2 1/2 carb, 1 med-fat meat, 2 fat
Brick Oven Style Supreme	1/4 pizza	320	29	16	44	7	40	700	3	15	2 carb, 1 med-fat meat, 2 fat
Original Pepperoni	1/4 pizza	380	36	19	45	8	40	860	3	16	2 1/2 carb, 1 med-fat meat, 3 fat
Original Pepperoni & Sausage	1/4 pizza	370	37	18	43	8	40	860	3	17	2 1/2 carb, 2 med-fat meat, 2 fat
Original Supreme	1/5 pizza	300	30	14	43	6	30	690	3	14	2 carb, 1 med-fat meat, 2 fat

FROZEN PACKAGED FOOD, MEAT, CHICKEN, FISH, MEALS, PIZZA, SNACKS

	Serving	Calories	Carb. (g)	Fat (g)	% Cal. Fat	Sat. Fat (g)	Chol. (mg)	Sod. (mg)	Fib. (g)	Prot. (g)	Servings/ Exchanges
Original Xtra Cheese	1/4 pizza	340	37	15	41	7	35	690	3	16	2 1/2 carb, 1 med-fat meat, 2 fat
Tony's											
Deep Dish Pepperoni	1 pizza	480	47	25	48	7	20	1150	2	17	3 carb, 1 med-fat meat, 4 fat
Original Cheese	1/3 pizza	370	40	17	41	6	20	780	2	16	2 1/2 carb, 1 med-fat meat, 2 fat
Original Meat Trio	1/4 pizza	330	31	17	48	5	15	860	1	13	2 carb, 1 med-fat meat, 2 fat
Original Pepperoni	1/3 pizza	420	40	22	48	6	15	1070	2	16	2 1/2 carb, 1 med-fat meat, 3 fat
Original Supreme	1/4 pizza	320	30	16	47	5	10	770	1	12	2 carb, 1 med-fat meat, 2 fat
Thin Crust Pepperoni	1/3 pizza	350	33	19	49	5	15	950	1	14	2 carb, 1 med-fat meat, 3 fat
Thin Crust Supreme	1/3 pizza	360	34	19	47	5	15	930	2	14	2 carb, 1 med-fat meat, 3 fat
Totino's											
Crisp Crust Party Pizza Canadian Style Bacon	1/2 pizza	330	34	16	42	3	10	850	1	13	2 carb, 1 med-fat meat, 2 fat
Crisp Crust Party Pizza Combination	1/2 pizza	390	35	22	51	5	15	850	2	13	2 carb, 1 med-fat meat, 3 fat

Crisp Crust Party Pizza Mexican Style	1/2 pizza	320	31	16	47	4	20	560	2	14	2 carb, 1 med-fat meat, 2 fat
Crisp Crust Party Pizza Pepperoni	1/2 pizza	380	34	22	53	6	15	870	1	12	2 carb, 1 med-fat meat, 3 fat
Crisp Crust Party Pizza Sausage	1/2 pizza	380	35	21	50	5	15	810	2	13	2 carb, 1 med-fat meat, 3 fat
Crisp Crust Party Pizza Supreme	1/2 pizza	380	35	21	50	5	15	840	2	13	2 carb, 1 med-fat meat, 3 fat
Crisp Crust Party Pizza Three Cheese	1/2 pizza	330	33	15	42	6	25	700	1	14	2 carb, 1 med-fat meat, 2 fat
Crisp Crust Party Pizza Three Meat	1/2 pizza	370	34	20	49	5	15	870	2	13	2 carb, 1 med-fat meat, 3 fat

FROZEN SNACKS

Brands

Bagel Bites

Cheese & Pepperoni	4	210	29	7	29	4	15	580	2	8	2 carb, 1 fat

FROZEN PACKAGED FOOD, MEAT, CHICKEN, FISH, MEALS, PIZZA, SNACKS

	Serving	Calories	Carb. (g)	Fat (g)	% Cal. Fat	Sat. Fat (g)	Chol. (mg)	Sod. (mg)	Fib. (g)	Prot. (g)	Servings/ Exchanges
Three Cheese	4	200	28	6	25	3	15	540	2	8	2 carb, 1 fat
Delimex											
Beef Taquitos	5	370	46	15	38	2	15	760	8	15	3 carb, 1 med-fat meat, 2 fat
Chicken Taquitos	5	370	47	14	35	3	30	480	8	15	3 carb, 1 med-fat meat, 2 fat
Hot Pockets											
Croissant Pockets Chicken Alfredo	1	320	35	15	44	5	20	690	3	11	2 carb, 1 med-fat meat, 2 fat
Croissant Pockets Five Cheese Pizza	1	390	37	20	46	8	20	880	3	14	2 1/2 carb, 1 med-fat meat, 3 fat
Croissant Pockets Ham & Cheddar	1	340	36	16	41	6	25	760	3	12	2 1/2 carb, 1 med-fat meat, 2 fat
Ham 'n Cheese	1	310	33	13	39	5	30	770	3	14	2 carb, 1 med-fat meat, 2 fat
Italian Style Meat Trio	1	350	39	16	40	6	30	890	3	13	2 1/2 carb, 1 med-fat meat, 2 fat
Lean Pockets Bacon, Egg & Cheese	1	150	21	5	27	1	40	280	2	7	1 1/2 carb, 1 med-fat meat

Food											
Lean Pockets Barbeque Sauce with Beef	1	290	47	7	21	2	20	850	3	11	3 carb, 1 fat
Lean Pockets Chicken, Cheddar & Broccoli	1	260	39	7	23	2	20	590	3	11	2 1/2 carb, 1 med-fat meat
Lean Pockets Chicken Fajita	1	260	38	7	23	3	25	730	3	11	2 1/2 carb, 1 med-fat meat
Lean Pockets Ham & Cheddar	1	280	40	7	21	4	25	700	3	14	2 1/2 carb, 1 med-fat meat
Lean Pockets Sausage. Egg & Cheese	1	140	19	5	29	2	45	310	2	7	1 carb, 1 med-fat meat
Pepperoni	1	360	41	17	42	6	25	730	3	11	3 carb, 1 med-fat meat, 2 fat
Philly Steak & Cheese	1	370	40	18	46	7	30	740	3	11	2 1/2 carb, 1 med-fat meat, 3 fat
Pot Pie Express Chicken	1	350	40	17	46	4	15	860	3	18	2 1/2 carb, 2 med-fat meat, 1 fat
Pot Pie Express Chicken with Broccoli	1	350	40	17	43	5	15	870	3	10	2 1/2 carb, 1 med-fat meat, 2 fat
Pot Pie Express Turkey	1	340	35	18	47	5	15	840	3	10	2 carb, 1 med-fat meat, 3 fat

FROZEN PACKAGED FOOD, MEAT, CHICKEN, FISH, MEALS, PIZZA, SNACKS

	Serving	Calories	Carb. (g)	Fat (g)	% Cal. Fat	Sat. Fat (g)	Chol. (mg)	Sod. (mg)	Fib. (g)	Prot. (g)	Servings/ Exchanges
Subs Ham 'N Cheese	1	360	49	10	25	4	25	920	4	18	3 carb, 1 med-fat meat, 1 fat
Subs Pepperoni Pizza	1	410	48	16	37	6	25	980	4	17	3 carb, 1 med-fat meat, 2 fat
Subs Philly Steak & Cheese	1	410	49	16	37	5	20	950	3	17	3 carb, 1 med-fat meat, 2 fat
Jose Ole Mexi-Minis											
Beef & Cheddar Mini Chimichangas	3	230	25	11	43	4	10	560	1	8	1 1/2 carb, 2 fat
Beef & Cheese Mini Tacos	4	200	18	11	50	4	20	430	3	7	1 carb, 1 med-fat meat, 1 fat
Chicken Taquitos	3	190	21	9	42	2	15	400	2	7	1 1/2 carb, 2 fat
Shredded Beef Taquitos	3	180	20	9	44	2	10	530	2	8	1 carb, 1 med-fat meat, 1 fat
Michelina's											
Hot Subs Chicken Alfredo with Broccoli	1	290	37	11	34	4	25	650	1	13	2 1/2 carb, 1 med-fat meat, 1 fat

Hot Subs Meatballs with Sauce	1	290	38	11	34	4	25	730	2	12	2 1/2 carb, 1 med-fat meat, 1 fat
Poppers										
Cheddar Cheese Jalapeño=	3	220	15	14	55	5	20	720	1	5	1 carb, 3 fat
Mozzarella Sticks	1	90	6	5	44	2	10	250	<1	3	1/2 carb, 1 fat
Totino's										
Pizza Rolls Cheese	6 rolls	200	26	7	30	3	10	420	1	9	1 1/2 carb, 1 fat
Pizza Rolls Supreme	6 rolls	210	25	10	43	3	10	360	1	7	1 1/2 carb, 2 fat
Sandwich Rolls Cheeseburger	6 rolls	210	24	9	38	3	10	450	1	8	1 1/2 carb, 2 fat

FROZEN DESSERTS, ICE CREAM, FROZEN YOGURT, FROZEN BARS, PUDDING, GELATIN

	Serving	Calories	Carb. (g)	Fat (g)	% Cal. Fat	Sat. Fat (g)	Chol. (mg)	Sod. (mg)	Fib. (g)	Prot. (g)	Servings/ Exchanges
Bread Pudding with Raisins	1/2 cup	212	31	7	30	3	83	291	1	7	2 carb, 1 fat
Fruit Juice Bar, Frozen, with Cream	1	87	19	1	10	<1	5	20	<1	1	1 carb
Fruit Juice Bar, Frozen, 100% Juice	1 3 oz	75	19	<1	0	0	0	3	0	1	1 carb
Frozen Yogurt, Fat-Free	1/3 cup	60	12	0	0	0	0	58	NA	3	1 carb
Frozen Yogurt, Low-Fat	1/3 cup	66	14	1	14	<1	3	26	<1	2	1 carb
Gelatin, Dessert	1/2 cup	80	19	0	0	0	0	57	0	2	1 carb
Gelatin Snacks, Grape	1	80	18	0	0	0	0	45	0	1	1 carb
Gelatin Snacks, Orange	1	80	18	0	0	0	0	45	0	1	1 carb
Ice Cream	1/2 cup	133	16	7	47	7	29	53	0	2	1 carb, 1 fat
Ice Cream, Fat-Free	1/2 cup	90	20	0	0	0	0	65	NA	4	1 carb

Food	Serving										
Ice Cream, Light	1/2 cup	100	14	4	36	3	25	35	1	3	1 carb, 1 fat
Ice Cream, No-Sugar-Added	1/2 cup	100	13	4	36	3	15	45	NA	3	1 carb, 1 fat
Ice Cream Bar, Creamsicle/Dreamsicle	1	92	18	2	20	1	7	43	0	2	1 carb
Ice Cream Bar, Drumstick	1	157	18	9	52	4	21	48	<1	3	1 carb, 2 fat
Ice Cream Bar, Fudgesicle	1	91	19	<1	0	<1	<1	55	<1	4	1 carb
Ice Cream Sandwich	1	144	22	6	38	3	20	36	<1	3	1 1/2 carb, 1 fat
Ice Pops/Popsicles, Double Stick	1	92	24	0	0	0	0	15	0	0	1 1/2 carb
Parfait, Lime	1/2 cup	120	21	3	23	3	0	105	0	3	1 1/2 carb, 1 fat
Pudding, Chocolate with Whole Milk, Homemade	1/2 cup	221	40	6	24	3	17	137	1	5	2 1/2 carb, 1 fat
Pudding, Regular	1/2 cup	144	27	3	19	2	9	201	NA	4	2 carb, 1 fat
Pudding, Rice with Raisins, Homemade	1/2 cup	217	40	4	17	3	17	85	<1	6	2 1/2 carb, 1 fat

FROZEN DESSERTS, ICE CREAM, FROZEN YOGURT, FROZEN BARS, PUDDING, GELATIN

	Serving	Calories	Carb. (g)	Fat (g)	% Cal. Fat	Sat. Fat (g)	Chol. (mg)	Sod. (mg)	Fib. (g)	Prot. (g)	Servings/ Exchanges
Pudding, Sugar-Free	1/2 cup	90	13	2	20	2	9	420	<1	4	1 carb
Pudding, Tapioca with 2% Milk	1/2 cup	147	28	2	12	2	9	172	0	4	2 carb
Pudding, Tapioca with Whole Milk, Homemade	1/2 cup	103	14	4	35	2	125	157	0	7	1 carb, 1 fat
Pudding, Vanilla with Whole Milk, Homemade	1/2 cup	130	20	4	28	3	16	113	0	4	1 carb, 1 fat
Pudding Pop, Chocolate	1	72	12	2	25	2	<1	78	<1	2	1 carb
Pudding Pop, Vanilla	1	75	13	2	24	2	<1	50	0	2	1 carb
Sherbet, Orange	1/2 cup	132	29	2	14	1	5	44	0	1	2 carb
Sorbet, Citrus Fruit	1/2 cup	92	23	0	0	0	0	8	<1	<1	1 1/2 carb
Sorbet, Non-Citrus Fruit	1/2 cup	70	17	<1	0	<1	0	46	0	1	1 carb
Sugar/Rolled Ice Cream Cone	1	40	8	<1	0	<1	0	32	<1	<1	1/2 carb

	Amount	Cal.	Carb. (g)	Fat (g)	% Fat Cal.	Sat. Fat (g)	Chol. (mg)	Sodium (mg)	Fiber (g)	Prot. (g)	Exchanges/Choices
Topping, Butterscotch	2 Tbsp	103	27	<1	0	<1	0	143	<1	<1	2 carb
Topping, Hot Fudge	2 Tbsp	147	25	6	37	2	5	28	<1	2	1 1/2 carb, 1 fat
Topping, Marshmallow Creme	2 Tbsp	118	30	<1	0	0	0	18	<1	<1	2 carb
Topping, Whipped	2 Tbsp	24	2	2	75	1	0	0	0	0	free
Topping, Whipped, Light	2 Tbsp	19	2	1	47	<1	0	0	0	0	free

ICE CREAM/FROZEN YOGURT

Brands

Ben & Jerry's

	Amount	Cal.	Carb. (g)	Fat (g)	% Fat Cal.	Sat. Fat (g)	Chol. (mg)	Sodium (mg)	Fiber (g)	Prot. (g)	Exchanges/Choices
Frozen Yogurt, Cherry Garcia	1/2 cup	170	32	3	16	2	20	65	<1	4	2 carb, 1 fat
Frozen Yogurt, Chocolate Fudge Brownie	1/2 cup	190	35	3	19	2	15	100	1	5	2 carb, 1 fat
Frozen Yogurt, Half Baked	1/2 cup	190	35	3	14	3	20	100	<1	5	2 carb, 1 fat
Ice Cream, Butter Pecan	1/2 cup	330	20	21	68	10	65	105	0	4	1 carb, 1 fat
Ice Cream, Cherry Garcia	1/2 cup	250	26	10	36	10	60	50	0	4	2 carb, 2 fat

FROZEN DESSERTS, ICE CREAM, FROZEN YOGURT, FROZEN BARS, PUDDING, GELATIN

	Serving	Calories	Carb. (g)	Fat (g)	% Cal. Fat	Sat. Fat (g)	Chol. (mg)	Sod. (mg)	Fib. (g)	Prot. (g)	Servings/ Exchanges
Ice Cream, Chocolate Chip Cookie Dough	1/2 cup	270	32	15	50	10	65	85	0	4	2 carb, 3 fat
Ice Cream, Chocolate Fudge Brownie	1/2 cup	260	32	13	45	9	35	80	2	5	2 carb, 3 fat
Ice Cream, Chubby Hubby	1/2 cup	330	31	15	41	11	55	150	1	7	2 carb, 3 fat
Ice Cream, Chunky Monkey	1/2 cup	300	30	18	54	10	55	45	1	5	2 carb, 3 fat
Ice Cream, Coffee Heath Bar Crunch	1/2 cup	290	32	18	56	65	115	29	0	4	2 carb, 4 fat
Ice Cream, Mint Chocolate Cookie	1/2 cup	260	26	16	55	9	65	100	0	4	2 carb, 3 fat
Ice Cream, Original Vanilla	1/2 cup	240	21	16	60	11	75	60	0	4	1 1/2 carb, 3 fat
Ice Cream, Peanut Butter Cup	1/2 cup	360	27	26	65	13	60	125	1	7	2 carb, 5 fat

Food	Serving										Exchanges
Ice Cream, Vanilla Caramel Fudge	1/2 cup	280	31	15	48	10	70	105	0	4	2 carb, 3 fat
Breyers											
Frozen Yogurt, Carb Smart, Vanilla	1/2 cup	90	14	5	44	3	15	40	4	3	1 carb, 1 fat
Ice Cream, 2% Light, Vanilla	1/2 cup	130	18	5	31	3	30	60	0	3	1 carb, 1 fat
Ice Cream, 98% Fat-Free Vanilla	1/2 cup	90	20	2	17	1	5	50	4	2	1 carb
Ice Cream, 98% Fat-Free No-Sugar-Added, Chocolate Fudge Brownie	1/2 cup	90	20	2	17	1	5	85	4	3	1 carb
Ice Cream, Carb Smart Vanilla	1/2 cup	130	9	9	62	6	40	5	3	5	1/2 carb, 2 fat
Ice Cream, Chocolate	1/2 cup	150	17	8	48	5	20	35	<1	3	1 carb, 2 fat

FROZEN DESSERTS, ICE CREAM, FROZEN YOGURT, FROZEN BARS, PUDDING, GELATIN

	Serving	Calories	Carb. (g)	Fat (g)	% Cal. Fat	Sat. Fat (g)	Chol. (mg)	Sod. (mg)	Fib. (g)	Prot. (g)	Servings/ Exchanges
Ice Cream, No-Sugar-Added, Chocolate Caramel	1/2 cup	100	18	4	35	3	10	60	3	3	1 carb, 1 fat
Ice Cream, No-Sugar-Added, Vanilla	1/2 cup	100	15	5	40	3	15	45	3	3	1 carb, 1 fat
Ice Cream, Strawberry	1/2 cup	120	15	6	45	4	15	30	0	2	1 carb, 1 fat
Ice Cream, Vanilla	1/2 cup	140	15	8	51	5	20	40	0	3	1 carb, 2 fat
Sherbet, Orange	1/2 cup	130	28	2	12	1	5	25	0	1	2 carb
Sherbet, Rainbow	1/2 cup	130	27	2	12	1	5	25	0	1	2 carb
Sorbet, Carb Smart, Chocolate	1/2 cup	70	9	5	64	4	0	30	2	2	1/2 carb, 1 fat
Häagen-Dazs											
Frozen Yogurt, Chocolate Fudge Brownie	1/2 cup	200	35	3	14	2	35	140	2	9	2 carb, 1 fat

Frozen Yogurt, Coffee	1/2 cup	200	31	5	23	3	65	50	0	8	2 carb, 1 fat
Frozen Yogurt, Vanilla	1/2 cup	200	31	5	23	3	65	55	0	9	2 carb, 1 fat
Frozen Yogurt, Vanilla Raspberry Swirl	1/2 cup	170	32	3	16	2	25	35	0	4	2 carb, 1 fat
Ice Cream, Chocolate	1/2 cup	270	22	18	60	11	115	60	1	5	1 1/2 carb, 4 fat
Ice Cream, Chocolate Chocolate Chip	1/2 cup	300	26	20	60	12	105	55	2	5	2 carb, 4 fat
Ice Cream, Light Coffee	1/2 cup	210	32	7	30	4	65	85	0	5	2 carb, 1 fat
Ice Cream, Light Vanilla Bean	1/2 cup	200	29	7	32	4	65	55	0	5	2 carb, 1 fat
Ice Cream, Vanilla	1/2 cup	270	21	18	59	11	120	70	0	5	1 1/2 carb, 4 fat
Healthy Choice											
Ice Cream, Brownie Bliss	1/2 cup	130	24	2	14	1	10	70	1	4	1 1/2 carb
Ice Cream, Chocolate Chocolate Chunk	1/2 cup	120	21	2	15	1	5	60	1	3	1 1/2 carb

FROZEN DESSERTS, ICE CREAM, FROZEN YOGURT, FROZEN BARS, PUDDING, GELATIN

	Serving	Calories	Carb. (g)	Fat (g)	% Cal. Fat	Sat. Fat (g)	Chol. (mg)	Sod. (mg)	Fib. (g)	Prot. (g)	Servings/ Exchanges
Ice Cream, Cookies & Cream	1/2 cup	120	21	2	15	1	5	90	<1	3	1 1/2 carb
Ice Cream, French Silk	1/2 cup	120	24	2	11	1	5	50	2	2	1 1/2 carb
Ice Cream, Praline & Caramel	1/2 cup	120	23	2	15	1	10	80	<1	2	1 1/2 carb
Ice Cream, Mint Chocolate Chip	1/2 cup	120	20	2	17	1	10	70	<1	3	1 carb
Ice Cream, No-Sugar-Added Vanilla	1/2 cup	100	17	2	20	1	10	55	1	3	1 carb
Ice Cream, Old Fashioned Butter Pecan	1/2 cup	100	18	2	20	1	10	65	2	2	1 carb
Ice Cream, Rocky Road	1/2 cup	130	25	2	14	1	5	60	<1	3	1 1/2 carb
Ice Cream, Vanilla	1/2 cup	110	19	2	16	1	5	60	<1	4	1 carb

Kraft

Cool Whip Free Whipped Topping	2 Tbsp	15	3	0	0	0	0	5	0	0	free
Cool Whip Lite Whipped Topping	2 Tbsp	20	3	1	50	1	0	0	0	0	free
Cool Whip Topping, Regular	2 Tbsp	25	2	2	60	2	0	0	0	0	free
Cool Whip Whipped Topping, Strawberry	2 Tbsp	25	2	2	60	2	0	0	0	0	free
Dream Whip Whipped Topping Mix	2 Tbsp	15	2	0	0	0	0	0	0	0	free
Marshmallow Creme	2 Tbsp	45	11	0	0	0	0	10	0	0	1 carb
Marshmallows, Jet Puffed	4	100	24	0	0	0	0	30	0	<1	1 1/2 carb
Marshmallows, Miniature	2/3 cup	100	24	0	0	0	0	30	0	<1	1 1/2 carb
Topping, Butterscotch	2 Tbsp	130	28	2	14	1	<5	150	0	<1	2 carb
Topping, Caramel	2 Tbsp	120	28	0	0	0	0	90	0	2	2 carb

FROZEN DESSERTS, ICE CREAM, FROZEN YOGURT, FROZEN BARS, PUDDING, GELATIN

	Serving	Calories	Carb. (g)	Fat (g)	% Cal. Fat	Sat. Fat (g)	Chol. (mg)	Sod. (mg)	Fib. (g)	Prot. (g)	Servings/ Exchanges
Topping, Chocolate	2 Tbsp	110	26	0	0	0	0	30	1	2	2 carb
Topping, Hot Fudge	2 Tbsp	140	24	5	32	2	0	100	<1	1	1 1/2 carb, 1 fat
Topping, Pineapple	2 Tbsp	110	28	0	0	0	0	15	0	0	2 carb
Topping, Strawberry	2 Tbsp	110	29	0	0	0	0	15	0	0	2 carb
FROZEN BARS											
Brands											
Atkins											
Endulge Vanilla Fudge Swirl Ice Cream Bars	2 oz bar	180	12	16	80	12	30	25	4	2	1 carb, 3 fat
Blue Bunny											
Banana Pops	1.8 oz pop	35	9	0	0	0	0	5	0	0	1/2 carb
Black Raspberry Ice Cream Bar	2.3 oz bar	230	20	16	62	11	25	45	1	2	1 carb, 3 fat
Chill'n Juice Pops	1.8 oz pop	40	10	0	0	0	0	5	0	0	1/2 carb

Food	Serving										
Citrus Snacks	1.8 oz bar	50	12	0	0	0	0	5	0	0	1 carb
Classic Sundae Cones	2.8 oz cone	270	32	14	47	9	25	105	1	4	2 carb, 3 fat
English Toffee Bars	1.3 oz bar	130	12	7	48	7	15	40	0	0	1 carb, 1 fat
Fudge Bars	2.6 oz bar	110	21	1.5	18	1	5	85	0	3	1 1/2 carb
Goin' Bananas	2.6 oz bar	110	21	1	8	0.5	5	80	0	3	1 1/2 carb
Health Smart No-Sugar-Added Fat-Free Creme Bars	2.1 oz bar	60–70	17	0	0	0	0	20–35	0	0–1	1 carb
Health Smart No-Sugar-Added Fat-Free Fudge/Vanilla Bars	2.2 oz bar	60	13–14	0	0	0	0	70–85	0	4	1 carb
Krunch Bars	1.6 oz bar	150	14	10	60	8	15	50	0	2	1 carb, 2 fat
Malt Cups	5.4 oz cup	220	35	7	29	5	30	105	0	4	2 carb, 1 fat
Mini Bomb Pops	2 pops (2.6 oz)	70	16	0	0	0	0	10	0	0	1 carb
Mississippi Mud Sandwich	2.2 oz bar	190	27	8	38	3.5	15	170	1	3	3 carb, 2 fat

FROZEN DESSERTS, ICE CREAM, FROZEN YOGURT, FROZEN BARS, PUDDING, GELATIN

	Serving	Calories	Carb. (g)	Fat (g)	% Cal. Fat	Sat. Fat (g)	Chol. (mg)	Sod. (mg)	Fib. (g)	Prot. (g)	Servings/ Exchanges
Nascar Speedway Sundae Bars	2.6 oz bar	300	25	20	60	12	30	80	<1	5	1 1/2 carb, 4 fat
Neapolitan Sandwich	2.2 oz bar	180	26	7	35	4	20	160	0	3	2 carb, 1 fat
Original Bomb Pop	1.7 oz pop	50	11	0	0	0	0	5	0	0	1 carb
Polar Pops	1.8 oz pop	40	10	0	0	0	0	5	0	0	1/2 carb
Root Beer Floats	1.9 oz bar	80	14	2	23	1.5	10	25	0	1	1 carb
Root Beer Pops	1.8 oz pop	40	10	0	0	0	0	10	0	0	1/2 carb
Slush Pops	1.7 oz pop	45	11	0	0	0	0	10	0	0	1 carb
Sour Power Bomb Pop	1.9 oz pop	50	12	0	0	0	0	5	0	0	1 carb
Star Bars	1.3 oz pop	110	11	7	57	6	5	30	0	1	1 carb, 1 fat
Sugar-Free Bomb Pop	1.8 oz pop	25	8	0	0	0	0	5	2	0	1/2 carb
Sundae Crunch Bars, All Varieties	2.1 oz bar	170	20–21	9	48	3.5	15	55–85	0	2	1 1/2 carb, 2 fat

Food	Serving										Exchanges
Sweet Freedom No-Sugar-Added Fudge Lites	2 bars (5.4 oz)	70	17	0.5	0	0	0	90	6	4	1 carb
Sweet Freedom No-Sugar-Added Ice Cream Lites	1.3 oz bar	90	10	5	5	5	5	30	2	2	2 1/2 carb, 1 far
Sweet Freedom No-Sugar-Added Vanilla Sundae Cone	2.9 oz cone	240	30	13	9	15	49	110	<1	5	2 carb, 3 fat
Sweet Freedom Sugar-Free Pops	1.8 oz pop	15	7	0	0	0	0	15	2	0	1/2 carb
Sweet Freedom White Chocolate Almond Lites	1.4 oz bar	100	10	7	5	5	63	30	2	2	1/2 carb, 1 fat
The Champ! Chocolate Lovers	3.4 oz cone	300	38	15	11	40	45	130	1	5	2 1/2 carb, 3 fat
Twin Pops	3.1 oz pop	70	18	0	0	0	0	10	0	0	1 carb
Vanilla Ice Cream Sandwich	2 oz bar	170	24	7	3.5	20	37	150	0	3	1 1/2 carb, 1 fat

FROZEN DESSERTS, ICE CREAM, FROZEN YOGURT, FROZEN BARS, PUDDING, GELATIN

	Serving	Calories	Carb. (g)	Fat (g)	% Cal. Fat	Sat. Fat (g)	Chol. (mg)	Sod. (mg)	Fib. (g)	Prot. (g)	Servings/ Exchanges
Vanilla Nutty Sundae Cones	2.8 oz cone	240	34	10	38	6	5	125	1	5	2 carb, 2 fat
Breyers											
All Natural Fruit Bars, All Varieties	1.75 oz bar	50	13–14	0	0	0	0	5	0	0	1 carb
Almond Ice Cream Bars	4 oz bar	270	20	19	63	12	20	85	<1	4	1 carb, 4 fat
Fruit Swirls	4 oz cup	160	19	9	51	5	20	30	<1	2	1 carb, 2 fat
Natural Strawberry Fruit Juice Bars	3.8 oz bar	120	30	0	0	0	0	10	<1	0	2 carb
No-Sugar-Added Fruit Bars	1.8 oz bar	25	5	0	0	0	0	0	0	0	free
Soft Frozen Lemonade Cup	12 oz cup	290	74	0	0	0	0	25	0	5	5 carb
Tropical Fruit Bars	2.8 oz bar	80	20	0	0	0	0	10	0	0	1 carb

Dole

Product	Serving										Exchanges/Choices
Fruit Juice Bars, All Varieties	1.8 oz bar	45	11–13	0	0	0	0	10	0		1 carb
No-Sugar-Added Fruit Juice Bars	1.8 oz bar	30	7	0	0	0	0	10	0		1/2 carb

Dove

Product	Serving										Exchanges/Choices
Dove Bars (Milk Chocolate with Vanilla)	2.6 oz bar	260	25	17	59	11	30	50	1	3	1 1/2 carb, 3 fat
Dove Bars (Milk Chocolate with Almonds)	2.6 oz bar	270	23	18	60	10	30	110	1	5	1 1/2 carb, 4 fat
Dove Bars (Miniatures)	5 pieces	320	32	20	56	13	45	40	2	4	2 carb, 4 fat

Dreyers

Product	Serving										Exchanges/Choices
Whole Fruit Bars, All Varieties	2.9 oz bar	80	20–21	0	0	0	0	0	0–1	0	1 1/2 carb
Whole Fruit No Added Sugar Bars	1.7 oz bar	30	8	0	0	0	0	0	1	0	1/2 carb

FROZEN DESSERTS, ICE CREAM, FROZEN YOGURT, FROZEN BARS, PUDDING, GELATIN

	Serving	Calories	Carb. (g)	Fat (g)	% Cal. Fat	Sat. Fat (g)	Chol. (mg)	Sod. (mg)	Fib. (g)	Prot. (g)	Servings/ Exchanges
Eskimo Pie											
Chocolate Éclair Bars	2.5 oz bar	220	26	12	49	5	15	45	<1	2	2 carb, 2 fat
King Size Ice Cream Bars	2.5 oz bar	220	21	15	61	11	25	50	0	3	1 1/2 carb, 3 fat
No-Sugar-Added Eskimo Pie	1.6 oz bar	120	13	8	60	6	10	40	0	3	1 carb, 2 fat
No-Sugar-Added Fudge Bars	1.8 oz bar	60	11	1	15	1	10	60	0	2	1 carb
No-Sugar-Added Vanilla Ice Cream Cones	2.5 oz cone	200	24	12	54	8	15	100	<1	5	1 1/2 carb, 2 fat
No-Sugar-Added Vanilla Ice Cream Sandwich	2.2 oz sandwich	160	27	4	23	2	10	135	<1	4	2 carb, 1 fat
Thin Mint Ice Cream Bars	2.6 oz bar	250	23	17	61	13	25	50	1	3	1 1/2 carb, 3 fat
Vanilla Milk Chocolate Bars	2.5 oz bar	220	21	15	64	11	25	50	0	3	1 1/2 carb, 3 fat

Good Humor

	Serving										Exchanges
Ice Cream Bars, All Varieties	3 oz bar	180–190	15	13	65	9	10–15	35–45	<1	2	1 carb, 3 fat
Chocolate Éclair Bars	3 oz bar	160	20	8	45	3	5	60	<1	2	1 carb, 2 fat
Cookies & Cream Bars	3 oz bar	190	21	12	57	6	10	120	<1	2	1 1/2 carb, 2 fat
Ice Cream Sandwiches	3 oz bar	160	25	6	34	2.5	10	140	<1	2	1 1/2 carb, 1 fat
Strawberry Shortcake Bars	3 oz bar	170	21	9	48	2.5	5	60	0	1	1 1/2 carb, 2 fat
Sundae Cones	4 oz cone	270	31	15	50	7	15	90	1	4	2 carb, 3 fat
Toasted Almond Bars	3 oz bar	180	22	10	50	2.5	5	35	<1	2	1 1/2 carb, 2 fat

Häagen-Dazs

	Serving										Exchanges
Chocolate & Dark Chocolate Ice Cream Bars	2.8 oz bar	290	23	20	62	12	70	35	2	4	1 1/2 carb, 4 fat
Sorbet & Yogurt Fat-Free Frozen Yogurt Bar	2.4 oz bar	90	21	0	0	0	0	15	<1	2	1 1/2 carb
Vanilla Caramel & Pecan Ice Cream Bars	3.1 oz bar	360	27	26	64	14	65	105	<1	4	2 carb, 5 fat

FROZEN DESSERTS, ICE CREAM, FROZEN YOGURT, FROZEN BARS, PUDDING, GELATIN

	Serving	Calories	Carb. (g)	Fat (g)	% Cal. Fat	Sat. Fat (g)	Chol. (mg)	Sod. (mg)	Fib. (g)	Prot. (g)	Servings/ Exchanges
Vanilla & Milk Chocolate Ice Cream Bars	2.7 oz bar	280	20	20	64	12	75	50	0	4	1 carb, 4 fat
Healthy Choice											
Caramel Swirl Sandwiches	2.1 oz bar	140	27	3	19	1	5	120	<1	2	2 carb, 1 fat
Fudge Bars	2.1 oz bar	80	13	1	11	0.5	5	60	0	3	1 carb
Sorbet & Cream Bars	2.1 oz bar	90	17	1	10	0.5	5	35	<1	1	1 carb
Strawberry & Cream Bars	2.1 oz bar	90	16	1	10	0.5	5	40	1	2	1 carb
Vanilla Ice Cream Sandwich	2 oz bar	130	24	3	21	1	5	150	<1	2	1 1/2 carb, 1 fat
Klondike											
Big Bear Ice Cream Cookie Sandwiches	4 oz bar	270	38	12	40	5	15	210	1	3	2 1/2 carb, 2 fat
Big Bear Vanilla Sandwiches	4.2 oz bar	190	28	7	33	4	15	170	0	3	2 carb, 1 fat

Cappuccino Bars	5 oz bar	280	24	19	61	14	20	70	0	3	1 1/2 carb, 4 fat
Caramel Crunch Bars	5 oz bar	270	26	17	56	13	25	80	0	3	2 carb, 3 fat
CarbSmart Fudge Bars	3.5 oz bar	100	9	7	63	4.5	20	45	1	2	1/2 carb, 1 fat
CarbSmart Ice Cream Sandwiches	2 oz bar	80	10	4.5	51	2.5	10	95	1	9	1/2 carb, 1 fat
CarbSmart Ice Cream Bars	3 oz bar	170	9	15	73	11	15	40	2	2	1/2 carb, 3 fat
Chocolate Bars	5 oz bar	280	23	19	61	14	20	55	<1	3	1 1/2 carb, 4 fat
Chocolate Cones	4.3 oz cone	280	29	16	50	7	15	75	1	5	2 carb, 3 fat
Dark Chocolate Bars	5 oz bar	280	24	19	61	13	20	55	<1	3	1 1/2 carb, 4 fat
Heath Bars	5 oz bar	300	26	20	60	14	20	100	0	3	2 carb, 4 fat
Hershey with Almond Bars	4 oz bar	250	20	18	64	11	20	80	<1	4	1 carb, 4 fat
Krunch Bars	5 oz bar	280	25	19	61	14	20	90	0	3	1 1/2 carb, 4 fat
Minis Snack Size Vanilla Ice Cream Bars	2 3-oz bars	170	15	11	59	8	15	45	0	2	3 carb, 2 fat
Neapolitan Bars	5 oz bar	280	24	19	61	14	20	65	<1	3	1 1/2 carb, 4 fat
Oreo Cookie Sandwich	4.2 oz bar	230	34	9	35	3.5	10	310	2	3	2 carb, 2 fat

FROZEN DESSERTS, ICE CREAM, FROZEN YOGURT, FROZEN BARS, PUDDING, GELATIN

	Serving	Calories	Carb. (g)	Fat (g)	% Cal. Fat	Sat. Fat (g)	Chol. (mg)	Sod. (mg)	Fib. (g)	Prot. (g)	Servings/ Exchanges
Original Vanilla Bars	5 oz bar	280	24	19	61	14	20	75	0	3	1 1/2 carb, 4 fat
Planters Caramel & Peanut Ice Cream Bars	4 oz bar	290	25	19	59	12	15	150	<1	4	1 1/2 carb, 4 fat
Slim-a-Bear 96% Fat-Free Cones	4 oz bar	160	32	3	18	1	5	110	3	4	2 carb, 1 fat
Slim-a-Bear 98% Fat-Free Mint/Vanilla Sandwiches	4 oz bar	130	28	1.5	12	0	5	120	3	4	2 carb
Slim-a-Bear No-Sugar-Added/Reduced-Fat Vanilla Bars	4 oz bar	170	21	9	47	7	5	65	4	4	1 1/2 carb, 2 fat
Slim-a-Bear No-Sugar-Added Vanilla Sandwich	3.8 oz bar	120	25	3	21	0.5	5	230	2	4	1 1/2 carb, 1 fat
Slim-a-Bear Premium Fudge Bar	3.5 oz bar	90	22	1.5	17	0.5	5	90	4	3	1 1/2 carb

Vanilla Cones	4.3 oz cone	280	29	16	50	7	15	85	<1	5	2 carb, 3 fat
York Peppermint Pattie Bars	5 oz bar	280	24	19	61	13	20	55	<1	3	1 1/2 carb, 4 fat
Luigi's											
Italian Ice, All Varieties	6 oz cup	120	31–32	0	0	0	0	10–15	<1	0	2 carb
Italian Ice (Chocolate)	6 oz cup	160	40	0	0	0	0	25	<1	0	2 1/2 carb
M&M/Mars											
Cookie Ice Cream Sandwich	2.2 oz bar	220	29	11	45	4.5	25	170	1	3	2 carb, 2 fat
Nestlé/Carnation											
Crunch Ice Cream Bar	2.1 oz bar	220	18	15	61	11	15	55	0	2	1 carb, 3 fat
Drumstick (Caramel)	3.3 oz cone	360	36	22	55	11	25	100	<1	5	2 1/2 carb, 4 fat
Drumstick (Cookies & Cream)	3.3 oz cone	350	40	19	49	13	25	140	<1	4	2 1/2 carb, 4 fat
Drumstick (Vanilla)	3.2 oz cone	340	33	21	56	11	20	90	<1	5	2 carb, 4 fat
Ice Cream Sandwich	2.1 oz bar	200	28	8	36	3.5	20	180	0	3	2 carb, 2 fat

FROZEN DESSERTS, ICE CREAM, FROZEN YOGURT, FROZEN BARS, PUDDING, GELATIN

	Serving	Calories	Carb. (g)	Fat (g)	% Cal. Fat	Sat. Fat (g)	Chol. (mg)	Sod. (mg)	Fib. (g)	Prot. (g)	Servings/ Exchanges
Ice Screamers Push-ups	2.1 oz bar	80	18	1	11	0.5	5	15	0	0	1 carb
Popsicle											
All Natural Ice Pops	1.8 oz pop	50	12	0	0	0	0	5	0	0	1 carb
Big Stick Cherry Pineapple Swirl Ice Pop	3.5 oz pop	50	12	0	0	0	0	5	0	0	1 carb
Creamsicle Bars	2.5 oz bar	100	18	2.5	25	1.5	5	30	0	1	1 carb, 1 fat
Creamsicle Pops	1.8 oz pop	70	12	2	26	1	5	20	0	1	1 carb
Fantastic Fruity Real Fruit Juice Pops	2 oz pop	50	13	0	0	0	0	5	0	0	1 carb
Fat-Free Fudgesicle	1.8 oz pop	60	14	0	0	0	0	50	<1	3	1 carb
Firecracker Ice Pops	1.6 oz pop	35	9	0	0	0	0	0	0	0	1/2 carb
Firecracker Super Heroes	1.6 oz pop	40	10	0	0	0	0	0	0	0	1/2 carb
Fudgesicle Bars	2.5 oz bar	90	16	1.5	15	1	5	65	<1	3	1 carb
Fudgesicle Pops	1.8 oz pop	60	11	1	15	0.5	5	45	<1	2	1 carb

Food	Serving										Exchanges/Choices
Great White Ice Pops	1.8 oz pop	45	11	0	0	0	0	0			1 carb
Ice Cream Scribblers Pops	2 (1.2 oz) pops	130	17	5	4	15	35	45	0	3	1 carb, 1 fat
Ice Pops	1.8 oz pop	45	11	0	0	0	0	0			1 carb
Intense Fruit Shots	1.7 oz pop	40	9	0.5	0	0	13	0	0		1/2 carb
Jell-O Pudding Pops	1.8 oz pop	90	16	3	3	0	33	40	<1	2	1 carb, 1 fat
Lick-A-Color Ice Pops	2 oz pop	50	13	0	0	0	0	0	0		1 carb
Mini Fruit Bars	1.2 oz bar	70	19	0	0	0	0	15	0	<1	1 carb
Mini Fudge Pops	2 (1.2 oz) pops	80	16	1.5	1.5	<5	19	60	<1	3	1 carb
Mini Ice Cream Pops	2 (1.4 oz) pops	190	18	13	9	15	63	35	0	2	1 carb, 3 fat
Mini Ice Cream Sandwiches	2 bars	100	15	3.5	1.5	5	30	95	0	0	1 carb, 1 fat
No-Sugar-Added Creamsicle Pops	1.8 oz pop	25	6	0	0	0	0	20	0	<1	1/2 carb

FROZEN DESSERTS, ICE CREAM, FROZEN YOGURT, FROZEN BARS, PUDDING, GELATIN

	Serving	Calories	Carb. (g)	Fat (g)	% Cal. Fat	Sat. Fat (g)	Chol. (mg)	Sod. (mg)	Fib. (g)	Prot. (g)	Servings/ Exchanges
No-Sugar-Added Fudgesicle Pops	2 pops	70	18	0.5	7	0.5	0	80	4	3	1 carb
Rainbow Floats	1.8 oz pop	60	11	1.5	23	1	5	15	0	1	1 carb
Rainbow Ice Pops	1.8 oz pop	45	11	0	0	0	0	0	0	0	1 carb
Rootbeer, Banana & Lemon Lime Ice Pops	1.8 oz pop	45	11	0	0	0	0	0	0	0	1 carb
Scribblers Juice Pops	2 (1.2 oz) pops	60	16	0	0	0	0	0	0	0	1 carb
Sherbet Cyclone Pops	1.8 oz pop	50	11	0.5	10	0	0	10	0	1	1 carb
SpongeBob SquarePants Pop Ups	2.8 oz pop	90	17	1.5	15	0.5	5	20	0	1	1 carb
Sprinklers Ice Cream Bars	2.1 oz bar	130	18	6	42	2.5	10	25	0	1	1 carb, 1 fat
Sugar-Free Creamsicle	2 (1.7 oz) pops	45	12	0.5	11	0.5	0	5	3	1	1 carb

	Serving Size	Cal.	Carb. (g)	Fat (g)	% Cal. Fat	Sat. Fat (g)	Chol. (mg)	Sod. (mg)	Fiber (g)	Prot. (g)	Exchanges/Choices
Sugar-Free Fudgesicle	2 (1.7 oz) pops	70	9	2	26	0	0	0	2	4	1 carb
Sugar-Free Ice Pops, All Varieties	1.8 oz pop	15	3	0	0	0	0	0	0	0	free
Tingle Twister Ice Pops	1.8 oz pop	45	11	0	0	0	0	0	0	0	1 carb
Wild Bunch! Ice Pops	2 (1.1 oz) pops	60	14	0	0	0	0	5	0	0	1 carb
Slim Fast											
Chocolate Fudge Bars	3.5 oz bar	110	22	1.5	29	1	10	80	<1	3	1 1/2 carb
Vanilla Ice Cream Sandwich	3.6 oz bar	130	27	1	7	0.5	<5	150	<1	3	2 carb
Snickers											
Snickers Almond Ice Cream Bars	2 2.8-oz bars	300	31	18	54	10	20	85	1	4	2 carb, 4 fat
Snickers Ice Cream Bars	1.7 oz bar	180	18	11	55	6	15	60	1	3	1 carb, 2 fat

FROZEN DESSERTS, ICE CREAM, FROZEN YOGURT, FROZEN BARS, PUDDING, GELATIN

	Serving	Calories	Carb. (g)	Fat (g)	% Cal. Fat	Sat. Fat (g)	Chol. (mg)	Sod. (mg)	Fib. (g)	Prot. (g)	Servings/ Exchanges
The Skinny Cow/Silhouette											
98% Fat-Free Chocolate Peanut Butter Cup	1 sandwich	140	27	2.5	32	1	0	145	2	5	2 carb, 1 fat
98% Fat-Free Ice Cream Sandwich, All Varieties	1 sandwich	130	23	2	14	1	0	145	2	5	1 1/2 carb
Fat-Free Fudge Bars	4 oz bar	100	22	0	0	0	<5	70	1	4	1 1/2 carb
Skinny Carb Bar	4 oz bar	150	13	11	66	6	30	65	5	4	1 carb, 2 fat
Weight Watchers											
Smart Ones Giant Fudge Bars	2.5 oz bar	80	20	0	0	0	<5	55	4	3	1 carb
Smart Ones Giant Sundae Cones	2.6 oz cone	130	29	2.5	17	1.5	<5	95	3	4	2 carb, 1 fat
Smart Ones Vanilla Low-Fat Ice Cream Sandwich	2.4 oz bar	130	28	1.5	10	0	0	140	3	3	2 carb

PUDDING/GELATIN

Brands											
Hunt's											
Pudding, Snack Pack, Chocolate	4 oz	140	22	5	32	2	0	140	0	2	1 1/2 carb, 1 fat
Pudding, Snack Pack, Fat-Free Chocolate	4 oz	90	20	0	0	0	0	140	0	2	1 carb
Pudding, Snack Pack, No-Sugar-Added Chocolate	4 oz	60	6	4	50	1	<1	115	0	1	1/2 carb, 1 fat
Pudding, Snack Pack, Vanilla	4 oz	130	21	5	31	2	0	140	0	1	1 1/2 carb, 1 fat
Jell-O											
Gelatin Dessert, Cherry	1/2 cup	80	19	0	0	0	0	100	0	2	1 carb
Gelatin Dessert, Cherry Sugar-Free	1/2 cup	10	0	0	0	0	0	70	0	1	free

FROZEN DESSERTS, ICE CREAM, FROZEN YOGURT, FROZEN BARS, PUDDING, GELATIN

	Serving	Calories	Carb. (g)	Fat (g)	% Cal. Fat	Sat. Fat (g)	Chol. (mg)	Sod. (mg)	Fib. (g)	Prot. (g)	Servings/ Exchanges
Gelatin Snacks, Cherry	1	70	17	0	0	0	0	40	0	1	1 carb
Gelatin Snacks, Sugar-Free, Strawberry	1	10	0	0	0	0	0	45	0	1	free
Handi-Snacks Pudding, Vanilla	1	110	20	4	33	1	0	130	0	<1	1 carb, 1 fat
Pudding Snacks, Chocolate	1	120	25	2	15	2	0	190	<1	2	1 1/2 carb
Pudding Snacks, Fat-Free, Chocolate	1	100	23	0	0	0	0	180	<1	2	1 1/2 carb
Pudding Snacks, Fat-Free, Chocolate Vanilla Swirl	1	100	23	0	0	0	0	210	<1	3	1 1/2 carb
Pudding Snacks, Tapioca	1	110	25	2	16	2	0	170	0	1	1 1/2 carb
Pudding Snacks, Vanilla	1	110	23	2	16	2	0	180	0	1	1 1/2 carb

Kraft

Handi-Snacks Gel Snacks, Cherry Tropical Punch	1	90	22	0	0	0	45	0	0	1 1/2 carb
Handi-Snacks Pudding, Chocolate	1	110	21	4	32	1	0	160	<1	1	1 1/2 carb, 1 fat
Handi-Snacks Pudding, Fat-Free Chocolate	1	80	21	0	0	0	135	<1	4	1 carb

FRUIT, FRUIT DRINKS, JUICES

FRUITS

	Serving	Calories	Carb. (g)	Fat (g)	% Cal. Fat	Sat. Fat (g)	Chol. (mg)	Sod. (mg)	Fib. (g)	Prot. (g)	Servings/ Exchanges
Apple, Unpeeled	1 large	125	32	<1	0	<1	0	0	6	<1	2 fruit
Apple, Unpeeled	1 small	63	16	<1	0	<1	0	0	3	<1	1 fruit
Apples, Dried	4 rings	63	17	<1	0	0	0	23	2	<1	1 fruit
Applesauce, Unsweetened	1/2 cup	52	14	<1	0	0	0	2	2	<1	1 fruit
Apricots, Canned, Extra Light Syrup	1/2 cup	60	15	<1	0	0	0	2	2	<1	1 fruit
Apricots, Canned, Juice Pack	1/2 cup	60	15	0	0	0	0	5	2	<1	1 fruit
Apricots, Dried	8 halves	66	17	<1	0	0	0	2	3	1	1 fruit
Apricots, Fresh	4	68	16	1	13	0	0	1	3	2	1 fruit
Banana	1 small	64	16	<1	0	<1	0	1	2	<1	1 fruit
Banana Chips	1/4 cup	120	14	8	60	7	0	1	2	<1	1 fruit, 2 fat

Blackberries, Fresh	3/4 cup	56	14	<1	0	0	0	0	5	<1	1 fruit
Blackberries, Frozen, Unsweetened	3/4 cup	73	18	<1	0	NA	0	2	6	1	1 fruit
Blueberries, Fresh	3/4 cup	61	15	<1	0	0	0	7	3	<1	1 fruit
Blueberries, Frozen, Unsweetened	3/4 cup	58	14	<1	0	NA	0	1	3	<1	1 fruit
Boysenberries, Frozen, Unsweetened	1 cup	66	16	0	0	0	0	1	7	1	1 fruit
Cantaloupe, Fresh	1 cup	56	13	<1	0	0	0	14	1	1	1 fruit
Cherries, Sweet, Canned, Juice Pack	1/2 cup	68	17	0	0	0	0	4	<1	1	1 fruit
Cherries, Sweet, Fresh	12	59	14	<1	0	<1	0	0	2	1	1 fruit
Cranberries	1 cup	47	12	<1	0	<1	0	<1	4	<1	1 fruit
Cranberry Sauce, Canned	1/4 cup	105	27	<1	0	<1	0	20	<1	<1	1 1/2 fruit
Currants, Red & White, Fresh	1 cup	63	15	0	0	0	0	1	5	2	1 fruit

FRUIT, FRUIT DRINKS, JUICES

	Serving	Calories	Carb. (g)	Fat (g)	% Cal. Fat	Sat. Fat (g)	Chol. (mg)	Sod. (mg)	Fib. (g)	Prot. (g)	Servings/ Exchanges
Currants, Zante, Dried	1/4 cup	102	27	0	0	0	0	3	2	1	2 fruit
Dates	3	68	18	<1	0	0	0	0	2	<1	1 fruit
Figs, Dried	1 1/2	71	18	<1	0	<1	0	3	3	<1	1 fruit
Figs, Fresh	1 1/2 large	71	18	<1	0	<1	0	1	3	<1	1 fruit
Fruit Cocktail, Canned, Extra Light Syrup	1/2 cup	55	14	<1	0	0	0	5	1	<1	1 fruit
Fruit Cocktail, Canned, Juice Pack	1/2 cup	57	15	0	0	0	0	5	1	<1	1 fruit
Grapefruit, Canned	1/2 cup	69	17	<1	0	0	0	13	<1	1	1 fruit
Grapefruit, Fresh	1/2 cup	51	13	<1	0	0	0	0	2	1	1 fruit
Grapes, Fresh, Seedless	17	60	15	<1	0	<1	0	2	<1	<1	1 fruit
Guava, Fresh	1	46	11	0	0	0	0	3	5	1	1 fruit
Honeydew Melon, Fresh	1 cup	59	16	<1	0	0	0	15	1	<1	1 fruit
Kiwi, Fresh	1	56	14	<1	0	0	0	5	3	<1	1 fruit

Kumquats, Fresh	2	27	6	0	0	0	4	2	1	1/2 fruit
Lemon, Fresh	1	24	8	0	0	0	2	2	1	1/2 fruit
Lime, Fresh	1	15	6	0	0	0	1	2	0	1/2 fruit
Mango, Fresh	1/2	68	18	<1	0	<1	2	2	<1	1 fruit
Melon Balls, Mixed, Frozen	1 cup	57	14	<1	0	<1	54	1	2	1 fruit
Mixed Fruit, Dried	1/4 cup	83	22	<1	0	<1	6	3	<1	1 1/2 fruit
Nectarine, Fresh	1	67	16	<1	0	<1	0	2	1	1 fruit
Orange, Fresh	1	62	15	<1	0	<1	0	3	1	1 fruit
Oranges, Mandarin, Canned, Juice Pack	3/4 cup	69	18	<1	0	<1	0	1	1	1 fruit
Papaya, Fresh	1/2 medium	59	15	<1	0	<1	4	3	<1	1 fruit
Peach, Fresh	1 medium	57	15	<1	0	0	0	3	<1	1 fruit
Peaches, Canned, Extra Light Syrup	1/2 cup	52	14	<1	0	0	6	1	<1	1 fruit
Peaches, Canned, Juice Pack	1/2 cup	55	14	0	0	0	5	1	<1	1 fruit

FRUIT, FRUIT DRINKS, JUICES

	Serving	Calories	Carb. (g)	Fat (g)	% Cal. Fat	Sat. Fat (g)	Chol. (mg)	Sod. (mg)	Fib. (g)	Prot. (g)	Servings/ Exchanges
Pear, Fresh	1/2 large	59	15	<1	0	0	0	0	2	<1	1 fruit
Pears, Canned	1/2 cup	62	16	<1	0	0	0	5	3	<1	1 fruit
Pears, Canned, Light Syrup	1/2 cup	58	15	<1	0	0	0	3	3	<1	1 fruit
Persimmons, Native, Fresh	2	64	17	0	0	0	0	1	NA	0	1 fruit
Pineapple, Canned, Juice Pack	1/2 cup	74	20	0	0	0	0	1	<1	<1	1 fruit
Pineapple, Fresh	1/2 cup	57	14	<1	0	0	0	1	1	<1	1 fruit
Plums, Canned, Juice Pack	1/2 cup	73	19	0	0	0	0	2	1	<1	1 fruit
Plums, Fresh	2 small	73	17	<1	0	<1	0	0	2	1	1 fruit
Pomegranate, Fresh	1	105	26	0	0	0	0	5	1	1	2 fruit
Prunes, Dried, Uncooked	3	60	16	<1	0	0	0	1	2	<1	1 fruit
Raisins, Dark, Seedless	2 Tbsp	54	14	<1	0	0	0	2	<1	<1	1 fruit
Raspberries, Black, Fresh	1 cup	60	14	<1	0	0	0	0	8	1	1 fruit
Rhubarb, Diced	2 cups	52	12	<1	0	<1	0	10	4	2	1 fruit

Food	Serving									Exchange
Star Fruit (Carambola)	1 medium	30	7	0	0	0	2	2	0	1/2 fruit
Strawberries, Fresh	1 1/2 cups	56	13	<1	0	0	2	4	1	1 fruit
Strawberries, Frozen, Unsweetened	1 1/2 cups	65	17	<1	0	0	4	4	<1	1 fruit
Tangerines, Fresh	2 small	74	19	<1	0	0	2	4	1	1 fruit
Watermelon, Fresh	1 1/2 cups	64	15	<1	0	NA	4	1	1	1 fruit
FRUIT JUICES										
Apple Juice/Cider, Canned/Bottled	1/2 cup	58	15	<1	0	0	4	<1	<1	1 fruit
Apricot Nectar, Canned	1/2 cup	71	18	<1	0	<1	4	<1	<1	1 fruit
Cranberry Juice Cocktail, Bottled	1/3 cup	48	12	<1	0		2	0	0	1 fruit
Cranberry Juice Cocktail, Reduced-Calorie	1 cup	50	11	0	0		7	0	0	1 fruit
Fruit Juice Blends, 100% Juice	1/3 cup	50	12	<1	0	0	10	<1	<1	1 fruit

FRUIT, FRUIT DRINKS, JUICES

	Serving	Calories	Carb. (g)	Fat (g)	% Cal. Fat	Sat. Fat (g)	Chol. (mg)	Sod. (mg)	Fib. (g)	Prot. (g)	Servings/ Exchanges
Grape Juice, Bottled	1/3 cup	51	13	<1	0	0	0	3	<1	<1	1 fruit
Grapefruit Juice, Canned	1/2 cup	47	11	<1	0	0	0	1	<1	<1	1 fruit
Orange Juice, Canned	1/2 cup	52	12	<1	0	<1	0	3	<1	<1	1 fruit
Orange Juice, Fresh	1/2 cup	56	13	<1	0	0	0	1	<1	<1	1 fruit
Orange Juice, Frozen, Reconstituted	1/2 cup	56	13	<1	0	0	0	1	<1	<1	1 fruit
Pineapple Juice, Canned	1/2 cup	70	17	<1	0	0	0	1	<1	<1	1 fruit
Prune Juice, Bottled	1/3 cup	60	15	0	0	0	0	3	<1	<1	1 fruit

FRUIT DRINKS, JUICES

Brands

Capri-Sun (Single Serving Pouch)

	Serving	Calories	Carb. (g)	Fat (g)	% Cal. Fat	Sat. Fat (g)	Chol. (mg)	Sod. (mg)	Fib. (g)	Prot. (g)	Servings/ Exchanges
Big Pouch, Fruit Punch Juice Drink Blend	11.1 oz	150–160	33–44	0	0	0	0	25	0	0	2–3 carb
Fruit Punch Juice Drink Blend, Assorted Flavors	6.75 oz	90–110	25–28	0	0	0	0	15	0	0	2 carb

Fruit Waves Fruit Punch Flavored Fruit Juice Blend	6.75 oz	100	23–25	0	●	0	25–30	0	1 1/2 fruit
Lemonade	6.75 oz	100	27	0	0	0	15	0	2 carb
Sports Drink, Assorted Flavors	6.75 oz	60	16	0	●	0	55	0	1 carb
Dole									
Berry Blend Fruit Juice	8 oz	140	35	0	0	0	15	0	2 fruit
Mango Lime Fiesta Fruit Juice Blend	8 oz	120	30	0	0	0	15	0	2 fruit
Orange Strawberry Banana Fruit Juice Blend	8 oz	120	28	0	0	0	10	0	2 fruit
Pineapple Juice	8 oz	130	30	0	0	0	10	0	2 fruit
Pineapple Juice, Single Serving	6 oz can	80	22	0	0	0	10	0	1 1/2 fruit

FRUIT, FRUIT DRINKS, JUICES

	Serving	Calories	Carb. (g)	Fat (g)	% Cal. Fat	Sat. Fat (g)	Chol. (mg)	Sod. (mg)	Fib. (g)	Prot. (g)	Servings/ Exchanges
Pine-Orange Banana Fruit Juice Blend	8 oz	130	30	0	0	0	0	10	0	0	2 fruit
Pine-Orange Strawberry Fruit Juice Blend	8 oz	120	29	0	0	0	0	10	0	0	2 fruit
Donald Duck											
Orange Juice Plus Calcium	8 oz	110	27	0	0	0	0	20	0	1	2 fruit
Orange Juice, Single Serving	5.5 oz can	80	20	0	0	0	0	10	0	0	1 fruit
Florida's Natural											
Apple Juice	8 oz	120	29	0	0	0	0	0	0	2	2 fruit
Orange Juice with Calcium & Vitamin D	8 oz	110	26	0	0	0	0	0	0	0	2 fruit
Original Orange Juice	8 oz	110	26	0	0	0	0	0	0	2	2 fruit
Ruby Red Grapefruit Juice	8 oz	90	22	0	0	0	0	0	0	0	1 1/2 carb

Hansen's

Food	Serving	Cal	Carb						Exchanges
Smoothie, Assorted Flavors, Single Serving	11.5 oz	170–180	42–44	0	•	0	35–50	0	3 carb

Hawaiian Punch

Food	Serving	Cal	Carb						Exchanges
Fruit Punch, Assorted Flavors	8 oz	120	29–30	0	•	0	115–120	0	2 carb

Hi-C

Food	Serving	Cal	Carb						Exchanges
Blast Fruit Drink, Assorted Flavors, Single Serving	6.75 oz pouch	100–110	26–29	0	•	0	15	0	2 carb
Punch, Assorted Flavors, Single Serving	6.75 oz pouch	90–100	25–28	0	•	0	15	0	2 carb

Hollywood

Food	Serving	Cal	Carb						Exchanges
Carrot Juice, Single Serving	12 oz can	150	31	0	•	0	460	1	4 vegetable

Kool-Aid (Single Serving)

Food	Serving	Cal	Carb						Exchanges
Bursts Soft Drink, Assorted Flavors	6.75 oz	100	24	0	•	0	30–35	0	1 1/2 carb

FRUIT, FRUIT DRINKS, JUICES

	Serving	Calories	Carb. (g)	Fat (g)	% Cal. Fat	Sat. Fat (g)	Chol. (mg)	Sod. (mg)	Fib. (g)	Prot. (g)	Servings/ Exchanges
Jammers Juice Drink, Assorted Flavors	6.75 oz	90	24	0	0	0	0	20–30	0	0	1 1/2 carb
Sugar-Free Jammers Juice Drink, Assorted Flavors	6.75 oz	10	2	0	0	0	0	25	0	0	free
Langer's											
Apple Juice	8 oz	120	28	0	0	0	0	0	0	0	2 fruit
Cranberry 100 Blend Juice	8 oz	140	35	0	0	0	0	15	0	0	2 fruit
Cranberry Grape 100 Blend	8 oz	150	38	0	0	0	0	15	0	0	2 1/2 fruit
Cranberry Juice Cocktail	8 oz	140	35	0	0	0	0	10	0	0	2 carb
Diet Low Carb Apple Juice Cocktail	8 oz	30	7	0	0	0	0	10	0	0	1/2 carb
Diet Low Carb Cranberry Juice Cocktail	8 oz	30	8	0	0	0	0	10	0	0	1/2 carb

Diet Low Carb Ruby Red Grapefruit Juice Cocktail	8 oz	30	8	0	■	0	10	0	1/2 carb
Harvest Apple Juice	8 oz	120	28	0		0	0	0	2 fruit
Ruby Red Grapefruit Juice Cocktail	8 oz	130	33	0		0	10	0	2 carb
Libby's									
Juicy Juice Blend, Assorted Flavors	8 oz	120–130	29–31	0	0	0	10–20	0	2 fruit
Kern's Aguas Frescas Limeade Juice Drink	8 oz	120	31	0	0	0	5	0	2 carb
Kern's Apricot Nectar, Single Serving	11.5 oz can	200	50	0	0	0	10	0	3 carb
Kern's Guava Nectar	8 oz	150	37	0	0	0	5	0	2 1/2 carb
Kern's Mango Nectar with Calcium & Vitamin C	8 oz	150	36	0	0	0	5	0	2 1/2 carb

FRUIT, FRUIT DRINKS, JUICES

	Serving	Calories	Carb. (g)	Fat (g)	% Cal. Fat	Sat. Fat (g)	Chol. (mg)	Sod. (mg)	Fib. (g)	Prot. (g)	Servings/ Exchanges
Kern's Mango Nectar, Single Serving	11.5 oz can	210	52	0	0	0	0	25	0	0	3 1/2 carb
Kern's Peach Nectar, Single Serving	11.5 oz can	200	46	0	0	0	0	10	0	0	3 carb
Kern's Strawberry Banana Nectar	8 oz	150	36	0	0	0	0	5	0	0	2 1/2 carb
Martinelli's											
Apple Juice	8 oz	140	35	0	0	0	0	0	0	0	2 fruit
Minute Maid											
Apple Juice, Single Serving	6.75 oz box	90	23	0	0	0	0	15	0	0	1 1/2 fruit
Berry Punch	8 oz	120	32	0	0	0	0	15	0	0	2 carb
Cherry Limeade	8 oz	120	34	0	0	0	0	15	0	0	2 carb
Coolers, Assorted Flavors, Single Serving	6.75 oz pouch	100	26–28	0	0	0	0	15	0	0	2 carb

Coolers, Pink Lemonade, Single Serving	6.75 oz pouch	90	25	0	0	0	0	15	0	0	1 1/2 carb
Country Style Orange Juice	3 oz	110	27	0	0	0	0	15	0	2	2 fruit
Fruit Punch	8 oz	120	31	0	0	0	0	15	0	0	2 carb
Fruit Punch Juice Blend, Single Serving	8 oz	100	24	0	0	0	0	15	0	0	1 1/2 fruit
Heart Wise Orange Juice	8 oz	110	27	0	0	■	0	20	0	2	2 fruit
Home Squeezed Orange Juice/Calcium & Vitamin D	8 oz	110	27	0	0	■	0	15	0	2	2 fruit
Kid's + Orange Juice	8 oz	110	27	0	0	0	0	20	0	2	2 fruit
Lemonade	8 oz	110	31	0	0	0	0	15	0	0	2 carb
Light Orange Juice with Calcium & Vitamin D	8 oz	50	13	0	0	0	0	15	0	0	1 carb
Light Orange Juice Beverage	8 oz	50	13	0	0	0	0	15	0	0	1 carb

FRUIT, FRUIT DRINKS, JUICES

	Serving	Calories	Carb. (g)	Fat (g)	% Cal. Fat	Sat. Fat (g)	Chol. (mg)	Sod. (mg)	Fib. (g)	Prot. (g)	Servings/ Exchanges
Limeade	8 oz	120	33	0	0	0	0	15	0	0	2 carb
Mixed Berry Juice, Single Serving	6.75 oz box	100	25	0	0	0	0	15	0	0	1 1/2 fruit
Orange Juice, Single Serving	6.75 oz box	100	23	0	0	0	0	15	0	0	1 1/2 fruit
Original Orange Juice	8 oz	110	27	0	0	0	0	15	0	2	2 fruit
Original Orange Juice, Single Serving	8 oz	110	27	0	0	0	0	20	0	2	2 fruit
Original Orange Juice with Calcium	8 oz	110	27	0	0	0	0	15	0	0	2 fruit
Mott's											
Clamato Tomato Juice Cocktail, Assorted Flavors	8 oz	60	11–13	0	0	0	0	820–960	1	1	1 carb

Naked

Anti Oxidant Berry Blast, Single Serving	8 oz	120	30	0		0	10	1	1	2 fruit
Anti Oxidant Mighty Mango, Single Serving	8 oz	120	30	0		0	15	0	1	2 fruit
Immunity Power-C, Single Serving	8 oz	120	29	0		0	15	3	1	2 fruit
Immunity Strawberry Banana-C, Single Serving	8 oz	120	28	0		0	5	3	2	2 fruit
Immunity Well-Being, Single Serving	8 oz	140	32	0		0	5	<1	1	2 fruit
Just Juice O-J, Single Serving	8 oz	110	25	0		0	0	0	2	1 1/2 fruit
Just Juice Tangerine Scream, Single Serving	8 oz	110	25	0		0	0	0	1	1 1/2 fruit

FRUIT, FRUIT DRINKS, JUICES

	Serving	Calories	Carb. (g)	Fat (g)	% Cal. Fat	Sat. Fat (g)	Chol. (mg)	Sod. (mg)	Fib. (g)	Prot. (g)	Servings/ Exchanges
Protein Zone, Single Serving	8 oz	210	27	3.5	15	1.5	20	135	<1	17	2 carb, 2 lean meat
Superfood Blue Machine Juice Blend, Single Serving	8 oz	170	41	1	5	1	0	10	8	1	3 fruit
Superfood Green Machine Juice Blend, Single Serving	8 oz	130	33	0	0	0	0	15	1	1	2 fruit
Superfood Red Machine, Single Serving	8 oz	160	32	3	17	0	0	15	4	2	2 fruit, 1 fat
Ocean Spray											
Cran-Apple Juice Drink	8 oz	160	40	0	0	0	0	35	0	0	2 1/2 carb
Cranberry Drink, Single Serving	8 oz bottle	130	32	0	0	0	0	35	0	0	2 carb

	Serving	Cal	Carb (g)				Sodium (mg)		Carb Choices
Cranberry Juice Blend	8 oz	140	35	0	0	0	35	0	2 fruit
Cranberry Juice Cocktail	8 oz	150	37	0	0	0	35	0	2 1/2 carb
Cranberry Juice Cocktail, Single Serving	12 oz bottle	200	50	0	0	0	50	0	3 carb
Cran-Grape Juice Drink	8 oz	160	40	0	0	0	35	0	2 1/2 carb
Cran-Raspberry Juice Drink	8 oz	140	34	0	0	0	35	0	2 carb
Diet Juice Drink with Tea, Assorted Flavors	8 oz	10	3	0	0	0	60	0	free
Grape Cranberry Drink, Single Serving	8 oz bottle	170	41	0	0	0	35	0	3 carb
Juice Drink with Tea, Assorted Flavors	8 oz	100	24–25	0	0	0	35	0	1 1/2 carb
Light Cran-Grape Juice Drink	8 oz	40	10	0	0	0	75	0	1/2 carb
Light Cranberry Juice Cocktail	8 oz	40	10	0	0	0	75	0	1/2 carb

FRUIT, FRUIT DRINKS, JUICES

	Serving	Calories	Carb. (g)	Fat (g)	% Cal. Fat	Sat. Fat (g)	Chol. (mg)	Sod. (mg)	Fib. (g)	Prot. (g)	Servings/ Exchanges
Light Ruby Grapefruit Juice Drink	8 oz	40	10	0	0	0	0	65	0	0	1/2 carb
Light White Cranberry Juice Drink	8 oz	40	10	0	0	0	0	75	0	0	1/2 carb
Pink Grapefruit Juice Drink	8 oz	40	28	0	0	0	0	35	0	0	2 fruit
White Cranberry Juice Drink, Single Serving	12 oz bottle	180	46	0	0	0	0	50	0	0	3 carb
White Grapefruit Juice	8 oz	100	24	0	0	0	0	35	0	0	1 1/2 fruit
Old Orchard											
Apple Cherry Juice Cocktail Blend	8 oz	120	29	0	0	0	0	15	0	0	2 carb
Apple Strawberry Juice Cocktail Blend	8 oz	120	29	0	0	0	0	15	0	0	2 carb
Healthy Balance Grape Juice Cocktail	8 oz	40	10	0	0	0	0	6	0	0	1/2 carb

Lo Carb Apple Cranberry Juice Cocktail Blend	8 oz	29	6	0	0	0	9	0		1/2 carb
Lo Carb Apple Juice Cocktail	8 oz	30	6	0	0	0	9	0		1/2 carb
SunnyD										
Lemonade	8 oz	130	31	0	0	0	190	0		2 carb
Sunny Delight, Assorted Flavors	8 oz	120–130	29–32	0	0	0	170–190	0		2 carb
Sunny Delight, Single Serving	11.3 oz	170	40	0	0	0	260	0		2 1/2 carb
Sunsweet										
Prune Juice	8 oz	170	43	0	0	0	35	3	1	3 fruit
Prune Juice +	8 oz	170	43	0	0	0	30	3	2	3 fruit
TreeSweet										
Grapefruit Juice	8 oz	90	21	0	0	0	10	0	0	1 1/2 fruit
Orange Juice	8 oz	120	28	0	0	0	10	0	0	2 fruit

FRUIT, FRUIT DRINKS, JUICES

	Serving	Calories	Carb. (g)	Fat (g)	% Cal. Fat	Sat. Fat (g)	Chol. (mg)	Sod. (mg)	Fib. (g)	Prot. (g)	Servings/ Exchanges
Tree Top											
Apple Cider	8 oz	120	29	0	0	0	0	25	0	0	2 fruit
Apple Juice	8 oz	120	29	0	0	0	0	25	0	0	2 fruit
Tropicana											
Grovestand Orange Juice with Calcium & Vitamin D	8 oz	110	26	0	0	0	0	0	0	2	2 fruit
Healthy Heart Orange Juice	8 oz	110	26	0	0	0	0	0	0	2	2 fruit
Immunity Defense Orange Juice	8 oz	110	26	0	0	0	0	0	0	0	2 fruit
Light 'n Healthy Juice Beverage	8 oz	55	13	0	0	0	0	10	0	<1	1 carb
Light 'n Healthy Juice Beverage, Single Serving	10 oz	65–70	16–17	0	0	0	0	10	0	0	1 carb

Low Acid Orange Juice	8 oz	110	26	0	0	0	0	2	2 fruit
Orange Juice with Calcium and Vitamin D	8 oz	110	26	0	0	0	0	0	2 fruit
Orange Strawberry Banana Juice Blend	8 oz	130	30	0	0	0	0	2	2 fruit
Orange Tangerine Juice with Calcium & Vitamin D	8 oz	110	25	0	0	0	0	0	1 1/2 fruit
Original Orange Juice	8 oz	110	26	0	0	0	0	2	2 fruit
Ruby Red Grapefruit Juice	8 oz	90	22	0	0	0	0	2	1 1/2 fruit
Twister Juice Beverage, Assorted Flavors	8 oz	120	29–30	0	0	0	10–30	0	2 carb
Twister Juice Beverage, Assorted Flavors, Single Serving	10 oz	150	36	0	0	0	15	0	2 1/2 carb

FRUIT, FRUIT DRINKS, JUICES

	Serving	Calories	Carb. (g)	Fat (g)	% Cal. Fat	Sat. Fat (g)	Chol. (mg)	Sod. (mg)	Fib. (g)	Prot. (g)	Servings/ Exchanges
Welch's											
Apple Juice, Single Serving	10 oz	140	36	0	0	0	0	25	0	0	2 1/2 fruit
Concord Grape Juice Cocktail	8 oz	150	36	0	0	0	0	10	0	0	2 1/2 carb
Fruit Punch Juice Drink, Single Serving	10 oz	160	39	0	0	0	0	20	0	0	2 1/2 carb
Grape Drink, Single Serving	10 oz	170	43	0	0	0	0	45	0	0	3 carb
Grape Juice	8 oz	170	42	0	0	0	0	20	0	0	3 fruit
Guava Pineapple Fruit Juice Cocktail	8 oz	140	36	0	0	0	0	5	0	0	2 1/2 carb
Light Grape Juice Cocktail	8 oz	70	18	0	0	0	0	80	0	0	1 carb
Light White Grape Juice Cocktail	8 oz	70	18	0	0	0	0	80	0	0	1 carb

Low Cal Flavored Juice Drink, Assorted Flavors, Single Serving	10 oz	15	3	0	0	C	0	10–20	0	free
Mountain Berry Juice Cocktail	8 oz	140	34	0	0	C	0	20	0	2 carb
Orange Pineapple Juice Drink, Single Serving	10 oz	160	39	0	0	0	0	60	0	2 1/2 carb
Passion Fruit Juice Cocktail	8 oz	150	38	0	0	0	0	5	0	2 1/2 carb
Strawberry Breeze Fruit Juice Cocktail	8 oz	130	33	0	0	0	0	5	0	2 carb
Strawberry Kiwi Juice Drink	10 oz	140	36	0	0	0	0	30	0	2 1/2 carb
White Grape Juice	8 oz	160	39	0	0	0	0	20	0	2 1/2 juice

GRAINS, PASTA, RICE

	Serving	Calories	Carb. (g)	Fat (g)	% Cal. Fat	Sat. Fat (g)	Chol. (mg)	Sod. (mg)	Fib. (g)	Prot. (g)	Servings/ Exchanges
Barley, Cooked	1/2 cup	135	30	1	7	<1	0	<1	7	4	2 strch
Barley, Pearled, Cooked	1/2 cup	97	22	<1	0	<1	0	3	3	2	1 1/2 strch
Brown Rice, Long-Grain, Cooked	1/2 cup	108	23	1	8	<1	0	5	2	3	1 1/2 strch
Brown Rice, Medium-Grain, Cooked	1/2 cup	110	23	<1	0	<1	0	<1	2	2	1 1/2 strch
Bulgur Wheat, Cooked	1/2 cup	76	17	<1	0	<1	0	5	4	3	1 strch
Couscous, Cooked	1/2 cup	88	18	<1	0	<1	0	4	1	3	1 strch
Noodles, Egg, Cooked	1/2 cup	107	20	1	8	<1	26	6	<1	4	1 strch
Grits, Yellow Corn, Cooked	1/2 cup	73	16	<1	0	<1	0	0	<1	2	1 strch
Lasagna, Cut, Cooked	1/2 cup	99	20	<1	0	<1	0	<1	<1	3	1 strch
Linguine, Cooked	1/2 cup	99	20	<1	0	<1	0	<1	2	3	1 strch
Macaroni, Cooked	1/2 cup	99	20	<1	0	<1	0	<1	<1	3	1 strch

Food	Serving									
Macaroni, Vegetable, Cooked	1/2 cup	86	18	<1	0	0	4	1	3	1 strch
Macaroni, Whole-Wheat, Cooked	1/2 cup	87	19	<1	0	0	2	2	4	1 strch
Millet, Cooked	1/2 cup	143	28	1	6	0	2	NA	4	2 strch
Noodles, Chow Mein	1/2 cup	119	13	7	53	0	99	<1	2	1 strch, 1 fat
Noodles, Ramen, Cooked	1 cup	156	29	2	12	38	1349	3	6	2 strch
Noodles, Rice, Cooked	1/2 cup	80	20	<1	0	0	5	<1	<1	1 strch
Noodles, Spinach Egg, Cooked	1/2 cup	106	20	1	8	27	10	2	4	1 strch
Pasta, Homemade without Egg, Cooked	2 oz	70	14	<1	0	0	42	<1	3	1 strch
Pasta/Noodles, Egg, Homemade, Cooked	2 oz	74	13	<1	0	23	47	2	3	1 strch
Pasta/Noodles, Fresh, Cooked	2 oz	74	14	<1	0	19	3	<1	3	1 strch

GRAINS, PASTA, RICE

	Serving	Calories	Carb. (g)	Fat (g)	% Cal. Fat	Sat. Fat (g)	Chol. (mg)	Sod. (mg)	Fib. (g)	Prot. (g)	Servings/ Exchanges
Pasta/Noodles, Spinach, Fresh, Cooked	2 oz	74	14	<1	0	<1	19	3	1	3	1 strch
Pasta/Spirals, Cooked	1/2 cup	95	19	<1	0	<1	0	<1	<1	3	1 strch
Pasta/Wagon Wheels, Cooked	1/2 cup	99	20	<1	0	<1	0	<1	<1	3	1 strch
Rice Pilaf	1 cup	268	46	7	24	1	0	754	1	5	3 strch, 1 fat
Rotini, Cooked	1/2 cup	99	20	<1	0	<1	0	<1	<1	3	2 strch
Shells, Jumbo, Cooked	2	65	13	<1	0	<1	0	<1	<1	2	1 strch
Shells, Small, Cooked	1/2 cup	81	17	<1	0	<1	0	<1	<1	3	1 strch
Shells, Whole-Wheat, Cooked	1/2 cup	87	19	<1	0	<1	0	2	2	4	1 strch
Spaghetti, Cooked	1/2 cup	99	20	<1	0	<1	0	<1	3	3	1 strch
Spaghetti, Spinach, Cooked	1/2 cup	91	91	<1	0	<1	<1	0	10	3	3
Spaghetti, Whole-Wheat, Cooked	1/2 cup	87	19	<1	0	<1	0	2	3	4	1 strch

Food	Serving	Cal.	Carb. (g)	Fat (g)	Sat. Fat (g)	Chol. (mg)	Sodium (mg)	Fiber (g)	Prot. (g)	Exchanges
Vermicelli, Cooked	1/2 cup	99	20	<1	0	0	<1	2	3	1 strch
Wheat Bran	1/2 cup	63	19	1	<1	0	<1	12	5	1 strch
Wheat Germ, Toasted	1 Tbsp	27	4	<1	0	0	<1	3	6	free
White Flour, All-Purpose	1 Tbsp	28	6	<1	0	~	<1	<1	<1	1/2 strch
White Hominy, Canned	1/2 cup	58	12	<1	0	0	168	2	1	1 strch
White Rice, Long-Grain, Cooked	1/2 cup	134	29	<1	0	0	1	2	<1	2 strch
White Rice, Long-Grain, Instant, Cooked	1/2 cup	81	18	<1	0	0	3	<1	2	1 strch
White Rice, Long-Grain, Parboiled, Cooked	1/2 cup	100	22	<1	0	0	3	<1	2	1/2 strch
White Rice, Medium-Grain, Cooked	1/2 cup	121	27	<1	0	0	0	<1	2	2 strch
White Rice, Short-Grain, Cooked	1/2 cup	121	27	<1	0	0	0	<1	2	2 strch
Wild Rice, Cooked	1/2 cup	83	18	<1	0	0	3	2	3	1 strch

GRAINS, PASTA, RICE

Brands	Serving	Calories	Carb. (g)	Fat (g)	% Cal. Fat	Sat. Fat (g)	Chol. (mg)	Sod. (mg)	Fib. (g)	Prot. (g)	Servings/ Exchanges
Alber's											
Cornmeal, Yellow	3 Tbsp	110	24	0	0	0	0	0	<1	2	1 1/2 strch
Di Giorno											
Angel Hair Pasta	2 oz	160	31	2	11	0	0	115	2	6	2 strch
Fettuccine Pasta	2.5 oz	200	38	2	9	0	0	140	2	8	2 1/2 strch
Herb Linguine Pasta	2.5 oz	200	38	2	9	0	0	140	2	8	2 1/2 strch
Red Bell Pepper Fettuccine Pasta	2.5 oz	200	38	2	9	0	0	140	2	8	2 1/2 strch
Spinach Fettuccine Pasta	2.5 oz	200	38	2	9	0	0	140	2	8	2 1/2 strch
Kraft											
Macaroni & Cheese	1 cup	380	49	16	37	4	10	910	1	9	3 strch, 3 fat
Macaroni & Cheese, 2% Light Deluxe	1 cup	290	50	5	16	2	15	850	2	13	3 strch, 1 med-fat meat

	Serving	Cal.						Sod.			Exchanges
Macaroni & Cheese, Deluxe Original	1 cup	320	46	9	25	3	20	820	2	12	3 strch, 2 fat
Macaroni & Cheese, Easy Mac, Original	1 pouch	240	40	6	25	3	5	570	<1	7	2 1/2 strch, 1 fat
Macaroni & Cheese, Thick 'n Creamy	1 cup	380	52	15	36	4	20	750	2	10	3 1/2 strch, 3 fat
Macaroni & Cheese, Three Cheese Blend	1 cup	380	44	16	37	4	10	770	2	9	3 strch, 2 fat
Velveeta Shells & Cheese, Original	1 cup	360	47	12	30	5	20	930	2	17	3 strch, 1 med-fat meat, 1 fat
La Choy											
Noodles, Chow Mein	1/2 cup	140	19	6	39	–	0	230	1	3	1 strch, 1 fat
Noodles, Rice	1/2 cup	130	21	4	28	–	0	350	<1	2	1 1/2 strch, 1 fat
Lipton											
Pasta Sides, Alfredo	2/3 cup	320	43	12	34	5	20	970	1	10	3 strch, 2 fat
Pasta Sides, Chicken	2/3 cup	260	43	7	24	–	<5	820	1	7	3 strch, 1 fat

GRAINS, PASTA, RICE

	Serving	Calories	Carb. (g)	Fat (g)	% Cal. Fat	Sat. Fat (g)	Chol. (mg)	Sod. (mg)	Fib. (g)	Prot. (g)	Servings/ Exchanges
Pasta Sides, Parmesan	2/3 cup	320	42	12	34	5	20	830	1	10	3 strch, 2 fat
Rice Cajun Side, Garlic Butter Rice	1 cup	300	48	8	23	3	10	790	1	7	3 strch, 2 fat
Rice Fiesta Side, Spanish Rice	1 cup	280	50	5	16	1	0	930	2	6	3 strch, 1 fat
Rice Sides, Chicken Broccoli	1 cup	280	48	6	18	0	<5	910	2	7	3 strch, 1 fat
Minute Rice											
Brown Rice, Whole-Grain, Instant, Cooked	2/3 cup	170	34	2	11	0	0	10	2	4	2 strch
Long Grain & Wild Rice, Seasoned	1 cup	230	50	<1	0	0	0	950	1	6	3 strch
Rice, Boil-in-Bag, Cooked	1 cup	190	42	0	0	0	0	10	<1	4	3 strch
White Rice, Instant, Cooked	3/4 cup	160	36	0	0	0	0	5	<1	3	2 1/2 strch

Pasta Roni

	Serving	Cal.	Carb. (g)	Fat (g)	% Cal. Fat	Sat. Fat (g)	Chol. (mg)	Sod. (mg)	Fiber (g)	Prot. (g)	Exchanges/Choices
Butter & Garlic	1 cup	260	40	8	27	5	5	760	2	8	2 1/2 strch, 2 fat
Fettuccine Alfredo	1 cup	460	48	25	50	10	10	1160	2	11	3 strch, 2 fat

Rice-A-Roni

	Serving	Cal.	Carb. (g)	Fat (g)	% Cal. Fat	Sat. Fat (g)	Chol. (mg)	Sod. (mg)	Fiber (g)	Prot. (g)	Exchanges/Choices
Beef, As Prepared	1 cup	310	52	9	26	3	3	1130	2	7	3 1/2 strch, 2 fat
Chicken, As Prepared	1 cup	310	51	9	26	3	3	1130	2	7	3 1/2 strch, 2 fat
Express, Hearty Beef	1 cup	270	50	6	19	<1	<1	1040	1	3	3 strch, 1 fat
Fried Rice, As Prepared	1 cup	320	50	11	31	3	3	1500	2	7	3 1/2 strch, 1 fat

Uncle Ben's

	Serving	Cal.	Carb. (g)	Fat (g)	% Cal. Fat	Sat. Fat (g)	Chol. (mg)	Sod. (mg)	Fiber (g)	Prot. (g)	Exchanges/Choices
Brown Rice, Instant Whole-Grain	1 cup	190	42	2	9	0	0	20	2	4	3 strch
Brown Rice, Original	2/3 cup	130	27	1	7	0	0	0	1	3	2 strch
Converted Rice	1 cup	170	38	0	0	0	0	0	1	4	2 1/2 strch
Converted Rice, Boil-in-Bag	1 cup	200	43	<1	0	0	0	0	<1	5	3 strch
Long-Grain Rice, Instant	1 cup	190	43	<1	0	0	0	15	1	3	3 strch

GRAINS, PASTA, RICE

	Serving	Calories	Carb. (g)	Fat (g)	% Cal. Fat	Sat. Fat (g)	Chol. (mg)	Sod. (mg)	Fib. (g)	Prot. (g)	Servings/ Exchanges
Pilaf, Country Inn	1 cup	200	43	<1	0	0	0	640	1	5	3 strch
Ready Rice, Rice Pilaf	1 cup	240	44	4	15	0	0	1110	1	5	3 strch, 1 fat
Spanish Rice	1 cup	200	45	<1	0	0	0	880	<1	4	3 strch
Wild Rice, Original Recipe	1 cup	190	41	<1	0	0	0	620	1	6	3 strch

LEGUMES (BEANS)

	Serving	Calories	Carb. (g)	Fat (g)	% Cal. Fat	Sat. Fat (g)	Chol. (mg)	Sod. (mg)	Fib. (g)	Prot. (g)	Servings/ Exchanges
Baby Lima Beans, Cooked	1/2 cup	115	21	<1	0	<1	0	3	7	7	1 1/2 strch
Baked Beans, Homemade	1/2 cup	190	27	7	33	3	6	532	7	7	2 strch, 1 fat
Baked Beans, Vegetarian Canned	1/2 cup	118	26	<1	0	<1	0	504	6	6	2 strch
Baked Beans with Beef, Canned	1/2 cup	161	23	5	27	2	29	632	7	9	1 1/2 strch, 1 med-fat meat
Black Beans, Cooked	1/2 cup	114	21	<1	0	<1	0	<1	8	8	1 1/2 strch, 1 very lean meat
Black Turtle Soup Beans, Cooked	1/2 cup	120	22	<1	0	<1	0	3	5	8	1 1/2 strch, 1 very lean meat
Black-Eyed Cowpeas with Pork	1/2 cup	100	20	2	18	<1	8	420	4	3	1 strch
Fava/Broadbeans, Canned	1/2 cup	91	16	<1	0	<1	0	580	5	7	1 strch, 1 very lean meat
French Beans, Cooked	1/2 cup	114	21	<1	0	<1	0	5	8	6	1 1/2 strch

LEGUMES (BEANS)

	Serving	Calories	Carb. (g)	Fat (g)	% Cal. Fat	Sat. Fat (g)	Chol. (mg)	Sod. (mg)	Fib. (g)	Prot. (g)	Servings/ Exchanges
Garbanzo Beans/ Chickpeas, Cooked	1/2 cup	135	23	2	13	<1	0	6	6	7	1 1/2 strch
Great Northern Beans, Cooked	1/2 cup	105	19	<1	0	<1	0	2	6	7	1 strch, 1 very lean meat
Hummus	1/2 cup	210	25	11	47	2	0	300	6	6	1 1/2 strch, 2 fat
Kidney Beans, California Red, Cooked	1/2 cup	109	20	<1	0	<1	0	4	8	8	1 strch, 1 very lean meat
Kidney Beans, Canned, Not Drained	1/2 cup	104	19	<1	0	<1	0	444	5	7	1 strch, 1 very lean meat
Kidney Beans, Red, Cooked	1/2 cup	112	20	<1	0	<1	0	2	7	8	1 strch, 1 very lean meat
Kidney Beans, Royal Red, Cooked	1/2 cup	108	19	<1	0	<1	0	4	8	8	1 strch, 1 very lean meat
Lentils, Cooked	1/2 cup	115	20	<1	0	<1	0	2	9	9	1 strch, 1 very lean meat
Navy Beans, Cooked	1/2 cup	129	24	<1	0	<1	0	1	6	8	1 1/2 strch, 1 very lean meat

Pink Beans, Cooked	1/2 cup	126	24	<1	0	0	2	5	8	1 1/2 strch, 1 very lean meat
Pinto Beans, Cooked	1/2 cup	117	22	<1	0	0	2	7	7	1 1/2 strch
Pork & Beans in Sweet Sauce, Canned	1/2 cup	140	27	2	13	9	425	7	7	2 strch
Pork & Beans in Tomato Sauce, Canned	1/2 cup	124	25	1	7	9	557	6	7	1 1/2 strch
Refried Beans/Frijoles, Canned	1/2 cup	118	20	2	15	10	377	7	7	1 strch, 1 lean meat
Split Peas, Ccoked	1/2 cup	116	21	<1	0	0	2	8	8	1 1/2 strch, 1 very lean meat
White Beans, Cooked	1/2 cup	124	23	<1	0	0	5	6	9	1 1/2 strch, 1 very lean meat
White Beans, Small Cooked	1/2 cup	127	23	<1	0	0	2	9	8	1 1/2 strch, 1 very lean meat
Yellow Beans, Cooked	1/2 cup	127	22	<1	0	0	4	9	8	1 1/2 strch, 1 very lean meat

Brands

B&M

Baked Beans, 99% Fat-Free Vegetarian	1/2 cup	170	31	1	5	0	220	7	8	2 strch

LEGUMES (BEANS)

	Serving	Calories	Carb. (g)	Fat (g)	% Cal. Fat	Sat. Fat (g)	Chol. (mg)	Sod. (mg)	Fib. (g)	Prot. (g)	Servings/ Exchanges
Baked Beans, Bacon & Onion with Brown Sugar	1/2 cup	190	36	2	9	<1	<5	450	8	8	2 1/2 strch
Baked Beans, Barbeque	1/2 cup	170	33	1	5	0	0	460	6	7	2 strch
Baked Beans, Original	1/2 cup	170	30	2	12	1	<5	380	6	7	2 strch
Baked Beans, Red Kidney	1/2 cup	170	32	2	11	<1	<5	440	6	7	2 strch
Baked Beans with Honey	1/2 cup	170	30	2	11	0	0	450	8	8	2 strch
Baked Beans with Pork	1/2 cup	180	33	2	10	<1	<5	430	7	8	2 strch
Baked Beans, Yellow Eye	1/2 cup	180	30	3	15	<1	<5	450	8	8	2 strch
Bush Beans											
Baked Beans, Barbequed	1/2 cup	160	32	1	6	0	0	510	6	6	2 strch
Baked Beans, Bold & Spicy	1/2 cup	120	24	1	8	0	0	560	5	6	1 1/2 strch
Baked Beans, Boston Recipe	1/2 cup	150	31	1	7	0	0	440	5	6	2 strch
Baked Beans, Homestyle	1/2 cup	150	29	2	10	0	5	480	8	6	2 strch

Baked Beans, Original	1/2 cup	140	29	1	7	0	0	550	5	6	2 strch
Baked Beans, Vegetarian	1/2 cup	130	29	0	0	0	0	550	5	6	2 strch
Black Beans	1/2 cup	100	20	1	5	0	0	460	7	7	1 strch, 1 very lean meat
Black Beans, Country Style	1/2 cup	160	33	1	6	0	0	680	5	6	2 strch
Chili Beans	1/2 cup	120	20	1	8	1	0	480	6	6	1 strch
Dark Red Kidney Beans	1/2 cup	130	21	1	8	0	0	260	7	8	1 strch, 1 very lean meat
Garbanzos Chick Peas	1/2 cup	130	22	2	15	1	0	500	9	6	1 1/2 strch
Pinto Beans	1/2 cup	110	19	0	0	0	0	390	6	6	1 strch
Campbell's											
Chili Beans in Zesty Sauce	1/2 cup	130	21	3	21	1	5	490	6	6	1 1/2 strch, 1 fat
New England-Style Baked Beans	1/2 cup	180	32	3	15	-	5	460	6	5	2 strch, 1 fat
Old-Fashioned Barbecue Beans	1/2 cup	170	29	3	16	<1	5	460	6	7	2 strch, 1 fat
Pork & Beans in Tomato Sauce	1/2 cup	140	27	1	6	<1	5	460	7	6	2 strch

LEGUMES (BEANS)

	Serving	Calories	Carb. (g)	Fat (g)	% Cal. Fat	Sat. Fat (g)	Chol. (mg)	Sod. (mg)	Fib. (g)	Prot. (g)	Servings/ Exchanges
Friends											
Baked Beans, Original	1/2 cup	170	32	1	5	0	<5	390	7	8	2 strch
Baked Beans, Red Kidney	1/2 cup	170	32	1	5	0	<5	510	6	7	2 strch
Green Giant											
Baked Beans	1/2 cup	160	31	2	11	1	5	580	7	6	2 strch
Barbecue Beans	1/2 cup	140	28	<1	0	0	0	460	5	6	2 strch
Beans, Honey Bacon	1/2 cup	160	34	<1	0	0	0	490	6	6	2 strch
Black Beans	1/2 cup	90	21	0	0	0	0	580	6	7	1 1/2 strch
Black-Eyed Peas	1/2 cup	90	18	1	10	0	0	300	4	7	1 strch, 1 very lean meat
Butter Beans, Frozen	1/2 cup	80	18	0	0	0	0	170	4	6	1 strch
Chili Beans in Spicy Sauce	1/2 cup	100	21	1	9	0	0	580	6	7	1 1/2 strch
Garbanzo Beans	1/2 cup	110	18	2	16	0	0	380	5	6	1 strch
Great Northern Beans	1/2 cup	80	18	1	11	0	0	290	5	6	1 strch
Italian Beans	1/2 cup	130	24	1	7	0	0	480	5	5	1 1/2 strch

Food	Serving										Exchanges
Kidney Beans, Dark Red	1/2 cup	90	20	1	10	C	0	330	5	7	1 strch, 1 very lean meat
Kidney Beans, Light Red	1/2 cup	90	20	1	10	C	0	330	5	7	1 strch, 1 very lean meat
Mexican Beans	1/2 cup	120	21	2	15	C	0	530	5	6	1 1/2 strch
Pinto Beans	1/2 cup	90	20	1	10	C	0	280	5	6	1 strch
Red Beans	1/2 cup	90	19	1	10	C	0	340	5	6	1 strch
Hunt's											
Chili Beans	1/2 cup	90	17	1	10	C	0	600	6	6	1 strch
Kidney Beans	1/2 cup	120	21	0	0	C	0	400	NA	7	1 1/2 strch
Navy Beans with Ham	9 oz	239	38	3	11	<1	10	735	10	16	2 1/2 strch, 1 lean meat
Red Beans, Small	1/2 cup	91	18	0	0	C	0	580	NA	6	1 strch
Old El Paso											
Black Beans	1/2 cup	110	17	1	8	C	0	400	7	7	1 strch, 1 very lean meat
Garbanzo Beans	1/2 cup	100	16	2	18	C	0	340	4	6	1 strch, 1 lean meat
Mexe Beans	1/2 cup	110	19	0	0	C	0	630	7	7	1 strch, 1 very lean meat
Pinto Beans	1/2 cup	100	19	<1	0	C	0	420	7	6	1 strch, 1 very lean meat
Refried Beans	1/2 cup	100	17	<1	0	C	0	570	6	6	1 strch, 1 lean meat

LEGUMES (BEANS)

	Serving	Calories	Carb. (g)	Fat (g)	% Cal. Fat	Sat. Fat (g)	Chol. (mg)	Sod. (mg)	Fib. (g)	Prot. (g)	Servings/ Exchanges
Refried Beans, Fat-Free	1/2 cup	100	18	0	0	0	0	480	6	6	1 strch, 1 very lean meat
Refried Beans, Fat-Free, Spicy	1/2 cup	100	18	0	0	0	0	720	6	6	1 strch, 1 fat
Refried Beans, Vegetarian	1/2 cup	100	17	1	9	0	0	490	6	6	1 strch, 1 very lean meat
Refried Beans & Cheese	1/2 cup	130	18	4	28	2	5	500	6	7	1 strch, 1 med-fat meat
Refried Beans with Green Chili	1/2 cup	100	17	<1	0	0	<5	720	6	6	1 strch, 1 very lean meat
Refried Beans with Sausage	1/2 cup	200	14	13	59	5	10	360	4	7	1 strch, 1 med-fat meat, 2 fat
Refried Black Beans	1/2 cup	110	18	2	16	0	0	340	6	7	1 strch, 1 lean meat
Pace											
Refried Beans, Salsa	1/2 cup	80	15	0	0	0	0	590	4	5	1 strch
Refried Beans, Spicy Jalapeño	1/2 cup	90	17	0	0	0	0	590	5	5	1 strch

Refried Beans, Traditional	1/2 cup	80	16	0	0	•	0	590	5	5	1 strch
Progresso											
Black Beans	1/2 cup	100	17	1	9	•	0	400	5	6	1 strch, 1 very lean meat
Cannellini Beans	1/2 cup	110	20	0	0	•	0	340	6	8	1 strch
Chickpeas	1/2 cup	120	20	3	23	•	0	280	5	5	1 strch, 1 fat
Fava Beans	1/2 cup	110	20	<1	0	•	0	250	5	6	1 strch, 1 very lean meat
Garbanzo Beans	1/2 cup	110	18	2	16	•	0	380	5	6	1 strch, 1 very lean meat
Kidney Beans, Red	1/2 cup	110	20	<1	0	•	0	280	8	7	1 strch, 1 very lean meat
Pinto Beans	1/2 cup	110	18	1	8	•	0	250	7	7	1 strch, 1 very lean meat
Ranch Style											
Black Beans	1/2 cup	100	19	1	9	•	0	420	5	6	1 strch
Original Texas Beans	1/2 cup	130	20	3	19	-	0	590	6	6	1 strch, 1 fat
Pinto Beans with Jalapeño Peppers	1/2 cup	110	21	1	9	•	0	750	6	5	1 1/2 strch
Ranch Style Beans, Original	1/2 cup	130	19	3	23	-	0	600	5	5	1 strch, 1 fat

LEGUMES (BEANS)

	Serving	Calories	Carb. (g)	Fat (g)	% Cal. Fat	Sat. Fat (g)	Chol. (mg)	Sod. (mg)	Fib. (g)	Prot. (g)	Servings/ Exchanges
Ranch Style Beans with Jalapeño Peppers	1/2 cup	130	21	3	19	1	0	740	6	6	1 1/2 strch, 1 fat
Rosarita											
Refried Beans, Low-Fat Black Beans	1/2 cup	90	18	1	10	0	0	560	5	6	1 strch
Refried Beans, No-Fat Traditional	1/2 cup	90	17	0	0	0	0	590	5	7	1 strch, 1 very lean meat
Refried Beans, Spicy Jalapeño	1/2 cup	100	18	2	18	1	0	630	6	6	1 strch
Refried Beans, Traditional	1/2 cup	100	18	2	18	1	0	510	5	6	1 strch
Refried Beans, Vegetarian	1/2 cup	100	18	2	18	0	0	520	5	6	1 strch
Refried Beans with Green Chilis & Lime, No-Fat	1/2 cup	90	18	0	0	0	0	570	5	6	1 strch

Taco Bell

Refried Beans	1/2 cup	100	18	0	0	●	0	540	5	6	1 strch

Van Camps

Baked Beans with Chicken	1 cup	360	62	2	6	●	20	1060	0	23	2 carb, 2 lean meat
Baked Beans with Ground Beef	1 cup	370	57	7	16	●	15	1060	0	19	4 carb, 1 med-fat meat
Baked Beans with Hot Dogs	1 cup	340	47	6	15	●	40	1140	0	23	3 carb, 2 lean meat
Pork and Beans	1/2 cup	110	23	1	9	●	0	420	6	6	1 1/2 strch

MEAT, POULTRY, FISH, SEAFOOD (FRESH, COOKED)

BEEF (TRIMMED)

Brisket

	Serving	Calories	Carb. (g)	Fat (g)	% Cal. Fat	Sat. Fat (g)	Chol. (mg)	Sod. (mg)	Fib. (g)	Prot. (g)	Servings/ Exchanges
Brisket, Flat Cut	3 oz	181	0	7	35	3	34	46	0	28	4 lean meat
Brisket, Whole	3 oz	247	0	17	62	6	79	55	0	23	3 med-fat meat
Chuck											
Arm Pot Roast	3 oz	238	0	14	53	6	85	53	0	25	3 med-fat meat
Blade Roast	3 oz	284	0	21	67	8	88	55	0	23	3 high-fat meat
Clod Roast	3 oz	176	0	9	46	3	59	60	0	22	3 lean meat
Mock Tender Steak	3 oz	136	0	5	33	2	54	60	0	22	3 lean meat
Top Blade Steak	3 oz	184	0	10	49	3	52	57	0	22	3 lean meat
Flank											
Flank	3 oz	160	0	7	39	3	38	48	0	24	3 lean meat

Ground Beef

75% lean ground beef	3 oz	236	0	16	61	6	76	66	0	22	3 med-fat meat
80% lean ground beef	3 oz	230	0	15	59	6	77	64	0	22	3 med-fat meat
85% lean ground beef	3 oz	213	0	13	55	5	77	61	0	22	3 med-fat meat
90% lean ground beef	3 oz	184	0	10	49	4	72	58	0	22	3 lean meat
95% lean ground beef	3 oz	145	0	6	37	3	65	55	0	22	3 lean meat

Plate

Inside Skirt Steak	3 oz	187	0	10	48	4	51	64	0	22	3 lean meat

Round

Bottom Round	3 oz	159	0	7	40	2	73	31	0	23	3 lean meat
Eye of Round	3 oz	145	0	5	31	2	59	53	0	24	3 lean meat
Tip Round	3 oz	162	0	7	39	2	69	54	0	24	3 lean meat
Top Round	3 oz	178	0	5	25	2	77	38	0	30	4 very lean meat

Ribs

Rib Eye	3 oz	210	0	13	56	5	94	48	0	23	3 med-fat meat
Short Ribs	3 oz	400	0	36	81	15	80	45	0	18	3 high-fat meat

MEAT, POULTRY, FISH, SEAFOOD (FRESH, COOKED)

	Serving	Calories	Carb. (g)	Fat (g)	% Cal. Fat	Sat. Fat (g)	Chol. (mg)	Sod. (mg)	Fib. (g)	Prot. (g)	Servings/ Exchanges
Shank											
Shank Crosscuts, Trimmed to 1/4 inch	3 oz	224	0	12	48	5	68	52	0	26	3 med-fat meat
Short Loin											
Porterhouse Steak	3 oz	235	0	16	61	6	57	55	0	20	3 med-fat meat
T-bone Steak	3 oz	210	0	14	60	5	51	57	0	21	3 med-fat meat
Tenderloin	3 oz	200	0	11	50	4	72	53	0	23	3 med-fat meat
Top Loin	3 oz	180	0	9	45	3	65	57	0	24	3 lean meat
Sirloin											
Bottom Sirloin Tri-Tip Roast	3 oz	177	0	9	46	3	71	45	0	22	3 lean meat
Top Sirloin	3 oz	183	0	8	39	3	76	55	0	25	3 lean meat
Variety Cuts											
Brain	3 oz	125	0	9	65	3	2635	92	0	10	1 high-fat meat

Food	Serving										Exchange
Liver	3 oz	162	0	4	22	1	337	67	0	25	3 very lean meat
Tongue	3 oz	236	0	19	72	7	112	55	0	16	2 high-fat meat
BUFFALO											
Buffalo	3 oz	120	0	2	15	<2	69	48	0	24	3 very-lean meat
LAMB											
Ground, broiled	3 oz	240	0	17	63	7	81	69	0	21	3 med-fat meat
Leg, sirloin, roast, lean	3 oz	174	0	8	40	3	78	60	0	24	3 lean meat
Loin, roast/chop, cooked	3 oz	183	0	8	44	3	81	72	0	26	4 lean meat
Rib, roasted	3 oz	198	0	11	52	3	75	69	0	22	3 med-fat meat
VEAL											
Breast	3 oz	226	0	14	56	6	96	55	0	23	3 med-fat meat
Ground Veal	3 oz	146	0	6	37	3	88	71	0	21	3 lean meat
Leg (Top Round)	3 oz	136	0	4	26	2	88	58	0	24	3 very lean meat
Loin	3 oz	184	0	10	49	4	88	79	0	21	3 lean meat
Rib	3 oz	194	0	12	56	5	94	78	0	20	3 med-fat meat
Shank	3 oz	152	0	5	28	2	105	79	0	27	4 very lean meat

MEAT, POULTRY, FISH, SEAFOOD (FRESH, COOKED)

	Serving	Calories	Carb. (g)	Fat (g)	% Cal. Fat	Sat. Fat (g)	Chol. (mg)	Sod. (mg)	Fib. (g)	Prot. (g)	Servings/ Exchanges
Shoulder	3 oz	156	0	7	40	3	96	82	0	22	3 lean meat
Sirloin	3 oz	172	0	9	47	4	87	71	0	21	3 lean meat
PORK											
Ground Pork	3 oz	252	0	18	64	7	80	62	0	22	3 high-fat meat
Leg (Ham)	3 oz	232	0	15	58	5	80	51	0	23	3 med-fat meat
Loin											
Back Ribs	3 oz	315	0	25	71	9	100	86	0	21	3 high-fat meat
Blade Chops	3 oz	272	0	21	69	8	73	60	0	19	3 high-fat meat
Center Loin Chops	3 oz	210	0	12	51	5	73	50	0	24	3 med-fat meat
Center Rib Roast	3 oz	214	0	13	55	5	69	41	0	23	3 med-fat meat
Country-Style Ribs	3 oz	279	0	22	71	8	78	44	0	20	3 high-fat meat
Sirloin Roast	3 oz	222	0	14	57	5	74	51	0	23	3 med-fat meat
Tenderloin	3 oz	147	0	5	31	2	67	47	0	24	3 very lean meat
Top Loin Roast	3 oz	192	0	10	47	4	66	37	0	24	3 lean meat

| Whole Loin | 3 oz | 211 | 0 | 12 | 51 | 5 | 70 | 50 | 0 | 23 | 3 med-fat meat |

Shoulder

Arm Picnic	3 oz	269	0	20	67	7	80	60	0	20	3 high-fat meat
Blade Boston Roast	3 oz	229	0	16	63	6	73	57	0	20	3 med-fat meat
Whole Shoulder	3 oz	248	0	18	65	7	77	58	0	20	3 med-fat meat

POULTRY

Chicken Back, No Skin, Roasted	3 oz	203	0	11	49	3	76	82	0	24	3 med-fat meat
Chicken Breast, No Skin, Roasted	3 oz	141	0	3	19	1	72	63	0	26	3 very lean meat
Chicken Capon	3 oz	195	0	10	46	3	73	42	0	25	3 lean meat
Chicken, Dark Meat with Skin, Roasted	3 oz	216	0	14	58	3.6	78	75	0	22	3 med-fat meat
Chicken, Dark Meat, No Skin, Roasted	3 oz	174	0	8	43	2	78	78	0	23	3 lean meat

MEAT, POULTRY, FISH, SEAFOOD (FRESH, COOKED)

	Serving	Calories	Carb. (g)	Fat (g)	% Cal. Fat	Sat. Fat (g)	Chol. (mg)	Sod. (mg)	Fib. (g)	Prot. (g)	Servings/ Exchanges
Chicken Drumstick, No Skin, Roasted	3 oz	146	0	5	31	1	79	81	0	24	3 very lean meat
Chicken Leg, No Skin, Roasted	3 oz	162	0	7	39	2	80	77	0	23	3 lean meat
Chicken, Light Meat with Skin, Roasted	3 oz	189	0	9	44	3	72	63	0	25	3 lean meat
Chicken Neck, No Skin, Simmered	3 oz	152	0	7	41	2	67	54	0	21	3 lean meat
Chicken Thigh, No Skin, Roasted	3 oz	178	0	9	46	3	81	75	0	22	3 lean meat
Chicken Wing, No Skin, Roasted	3 oz	173	0	7	36	2	72	78	0	26	4 lean meat
Chicken, with Skin, Roasted	3 oz	204	0	11	49	3	75	69	0	23	3 med-fat meat
Cornish Game Hen, Whole Bird, Cooked, No Skin	3 oz	114	0	3	24	1	90	54	0	20	3 very lean meat

Food	Serving										Exchange
Duck, Domestic, No Skin, Roasted	3 oz	171	0	10	51	3	75	54	0	20	3 lean meat
Geese, No Skin, Roasted	3 oz	201	0	11	48	3	81	66	0	25	3 med-fat meat
Ostrich, Cooked	3 oz	120	0	2	15	0	81	66	0	23	3 very lean meat
Pheasant, No Skin	3 oz	114	0	3	24	0	57	30	0	20	3 very lean meat
Turkey Back, No Skin, Roasted	3 oz	144	0	5	31	2	81	62	0	24	3 lean meat
Turkey Breast, Roasted	3 oz	114	0	1	8	0	69	45	0	26	3 very lean meat
Turkey Dark Meat, No Skin, Cooked	3 oz	159	0	6	34	3	72	66	0	24	3 lean meat
Turkey, Ground, Cooked	3 oz	201	0	11	49	3	87	90	0	23	3 med-fat meat
Turkey Leg, No Skin, Roasted	3 oz	135	0	3	20	1	101	69	0	25	3 very lean meat
Turkey Neck, No Skin, Roasted	3 oz	153	0	6	35	2	104	48	0	23	3 lean meat
Turkey Wing, No Skin, Roasted	3 oz	139	0	3	19	1	87	66	0	26	4 very lean meat

MEAT, POULTRY, FISH, SEAFOOD (FRESH, COOKED)

	Serving	Calories	Carb. (g)	Fat (g)	% Cal. Fat	Sat. Fat (g)	Chol. (mg)	Sod. (mg)	Fib. (g)	Prot. (g)	Servings/ Exchanges
FISH/SEAFOOD											
Bluefish, Baked	3 oz	130	0	5	27	1	65	65	0	22	3 very lean meat
Carfish, Baked	3 oz	129	0	7	49	2	54	68	0	16	2 lean meat
Catfish, Baked	3 oz	129	0	6	42	2	54	69	0	15	3 lean meat
Caviar, Black/Red, Granular	2 Tbsp	81	1	6	67	1	188	480	0	8	1 med-fat meat
Clams, Fresh, Steamed	1 oz	42	1	<1	12	<1	19	32	0	7	1 very lean meat
Cod, Baked	3 oz	89	0	1	10	0	47	66	0	19	3 very lean meat
Crab	3 oz	114	2	6	47	2	81	453	0	15	3 lean meat
Escargot/Snails	1 oz	51	1	<1	10	<1	28	34	0	9	1 very lean meat
Flounder/Sole, Baked	3 oz	99	0	1	14	0	58	89	0	21	3 very lean meat
Haddock, Baked	3 oz	95	0	1	7	0	63	74	0	21	3 very lean meat
Halibut, Baked	3 oz	119	0	2	19	0	35	59	0	23	3 very lean meat
Herring, Atlantic, Baked	3 oz	173	0	10	51	2	65	98	0	20	3 lean meat
Imitation Shellfish, from Surimi	1 oz	29	3	<1	0	<1	6	238	0	3	1 very lean meat

Food	Serving									Exchanges
Lobster, Fresh, Steamed	1 oz	28	<1	<1	0	20	108	0	6	1 very lean meat
Mackerel, Atlantic/Pacific, Baked	3 oz	223	15	54	4	64	71	0	20	3 med-fat meat
Mackerel, King, Baked	3 oz	114	2	18	0	58	173	0	22	3 very lean meat
Ocean Perch, Baked	3 oz	102	2	16	0	46	82	0	20	3 very lean meat
Octopus	1 oz	46	1	<1	<1	27	130	0	9	1 very lean meat
Orange Roughy, Baked	3 oz	76	1	9	0	22	69	0	16	2 very lean meat
Oyster, Medium	6	58	3	2	<1	44	177	0	6	1 lean meat
Pollock, Baked	3 oz	100	1	9	0	77	94	0	21	3 very lean meat
Rainbow Trout, Baked	3 oz	144	6	38	2	58	36	0	21	3 lean meat
Rockfish, Baked	3 oz	103	2	15	0	37	65	0	20	3 very lean meat
Sablefish, Baked	3 oz	212	17	72	3	54	61	0	15	2 high-fat meat
Salmon, Atlantic/Coho, Baked	3 oz	175	10	54	2	54	52	0	19	3 lean meat
Salmon, Chum/Pink, Baked	3 oz	130	4	25	0	81	54	0	22	3 very lean meat
Salmon, Sockeye, Baked	3 oz	184	9	46	2	75	55	0	23	3 lean meat

MEAT, POULTRY, FISH, SEAFOOD (FRESH, COOKED)

	Serving	Calories	Carb. (g)	Fat (g)	% Cal. Fat	Sat. Fat (g)	Chol. (mg)	Sod. (mg)	Fib. (g)	Prot. (g)	Servings/ Exchanges
Scallops, Fresh, Steamed	1 oz	32	0	<1	0	<1	15	78	0	7	1 very lean meat
Sea Bass, Baked	3 oz	105	0	2	19	0	45	74	0	20	3 very lean meat
Shark, Baked	3 oz	140	0	5	16	1	50	85	0	22	3 very lean meat
Shrimp, Fresh, Cooked in Water	1 oz	28	0	<1	0	<1	56	64	0	6	1 very lean meat
Swordfish, Baked	3 oz	130	0	4	30	1	43	98	0	22	3 very lean meat
Tilefish, Baked	3 oz	125	0	4	29	1	54	50	0	20	3 very lean meat
Trout	3 oz	162	0	6	33	2	63	57	0	24	3 very lean meat
Tuna, Yellowfin, Baked	3 oz	118	0	1	8	0	49	40	0	25	3 very lean meat
Whiting, Baked	3 oz	98	0	1	13	0	71	112	0	20	3 very lean meat
RABBIT											
Rabbit	3 oz	174	0	6	31	2	72	30	0	27	3 lean meat
VENISON											
Venison	3 oz	135	0	2	13	2	96	45	0	27	3 very lean meat

MEAT, POULTRY, FISH (PROCESSED/PREPARED)

	Serving	Calories	Carb. (g)	Fat (g)	% Cal. Fat	Sat. Fat (g)	Chol. (mg)	Sod. (mg)	Fib. (g)	Prot. (g)	Servings/ Exchanges
Beef											
Beef Jerky	1 oz	94	4	4	38	2	14	796	<1	9	1 med-fat meat
Chipped Beef, Dried	1 oz	47	0	1	19	<1	26	948	0	8	1 very lean meat
Hot Dog, Beef & Pork	1	144	1	13	81	5	22	504	0	5	1 high-fat meat, 1 fat
Meatball	1 oz	60	2	4	60	1	24	107	<1	5	1 med-fat meat
Meatloaf	1 oz	57	<1	4	63	3	26	186	0	5	1 med-fat meat
Pork											
Bacon	3 slices	105	0	9	77	3	15	288	0	5	1 high-fat meat
Bratwurst	1 oz	85	<1	7	74	3	17	158	0	4	1 high-fat meat
Canadian Bacon	1 oz	53	<1	2	34	<1	16	441	0	7	1 lean meat
Ham, Boiled, Lean	1 oz	46	<1	2	39	<1	15	362	0	5	1 lean meat
Ham, Cured	1 oz	45	0	2	40	<1	16	378	0	7	1 lean meat
Hot Dog, Fat-Free	1	30	3	<1	0	<1	11	286	0	4	1 very lean meat

MEAT, POULTRY, FISH (PROCESSED/PREPARED)

	Serving	Calories	Carb. (g)	Fat (g)	% Cal. Fat	Sat. Fat (g)	Chol. (mg)	Sod. (mg)	Fib. (g)	Prot. (g)	Servings/ Exchanges
Hot Dog, Low-Fat	1	50	<1	2	36	<1	15	450	0	6	1 lean meat
Knockwurst	1 oz	87	<1	8	83	3	16	286	0	3	1 high-fat meat
Pepperoni Sausage, Beef & Pork	1 oz	140	<1	13	84	5	22	578	0	6	1 high-fat meat, 1 fat
Pickle & Pimento Loaf	1 oz	74	2	6	73	2	10	394	0	3	1 high-fat meat
Salami, Beef & Pork	1 oz	71	<1	6	76	2	18	302	0	4	1 high-fat meat
Sausage, Hard, Fat-Free	1 oz	35	3	<1	0	<1	12	290	0	5	1 very lean meat
Sausage, Italian	1 oz	92	<1	7	68	3	22	263	0	6	1 high-fat meat
Sausage, Polish	1 oz	92	<1	8	78	3	20	248	0	4	1 high-fat meat
Sausage, Smoked	1 oz	96	<1	9	84	3	20	269	0	4	1 high-fat meat
Poultry											
Hot Dog, Chicken	1	116	3	9	70	3	45	617	0	6	1 high-fat meat
Hot Dog, Turkey	1	102	<1	8	71	2	48	642	0	6	1 high-fat meat
Turkey Kielbasa, Low-Fat	1 oz	45	2	3	60	1	16	300	0	4	1 lean meat
Turkey Pastrami, Low-Fat	1 oz	40	<1	2	45	<1	15	296	0	5	1 lean meat

Fish

Herring, Smoked	1 oz	62	0	4	58	<1	23	262	0	7	1 lean meat

LUNCH MEAT

Brands

Bar-S

Beef Bologna	1 slice	100	2	8	70	3	20	370	0	3	1 high-fat meat
Bologna	1 slice	100	2	9	80	3	35	370	0	3	1 high-fat meat
Chicken Bologna	1 slice	90	2	7	67	2	35	370	0	3	1 high-fat meat
Cooked Ham	1 slice	40	1	1	23	0	20	420	0	5	1 very lean meat
Cotto Salami	1 slice	90	2	8	78	3	40	390	0	4	1 high-fat meat
Extra Lean Cooked Ham	1 slice	40	1	1	25	0	20	420	0	5	1 very lean meat
Oven Roasted Turkey	1 slice	25	2	0	0	0	15	350	0	6	1 very lean meat
Thick Sliced Bologna	- slice	180	5	16	78	5	70	670	0	6	1 high-fat meat, 2 fat

Butterball Hearty Deli Sliced

Golden Oven Roasted Turkey Breast	- slice	30	1	<1	17	0	15	250	0	5	1 very lean meat

MEAT, POULTRY, FISH (PROCESSED/PREPARED)

	Serving	Calories	Carb. (g)	Fat (g)	% Cal. Fat	Sat. Fat (g)	Chol. (mg)	Sod. (mg)	Fib. (g)	Prot. (g)	Servings/ Exchanges
Honey Roasted & Smoked Turkey Breast	1 slice	30	1	<1	17	0	15	250	0	5	1 very lean meat
Smoked Turkey Breast	1 slice	30	1	<1	17	0	15	250	0	5	1 very lean meat
Butterball Premium Carved Slices											
Honey Roasted & Smoked Turkey Breast	2 slices	60	3	1	25	<1	20	420	0	9	1 very lean meat
Oven Roasted Chicken Breast	2 slices	60	3	1	25	<1	25	450	0	8	1 very lean meat
Oven Roasted Turkey Breast	2 slices	60	1	1	25	<1	20	410	0	9	1 very lean meat
Smoked Turkey Breast	2 slices	50	1	1	30	<1	15	420	0	9	1 very lean meat
Butterball Thin Sliced											
Honey Roasted & Smoked Turkey Breast	4 slices	50	3	0	0	0	25	480	0	9	1 very lean meat

	Serving Size	Calories	Fat (g)	Sat. Fat (g)	% Cal. Fat	Carb. (g)	Chol. (mg)	Sodium (mg)	Fiber (g)	Protein (g)	Exchanges/Choices
Oven Roasted Chicken Breast	4 slices	50	2	0		0	25	480	0	10	1 very lean meat
Oven Roasted Turkey Breast	4 slices	50	2	0		0	25	480	0	10	1 very lean meat
Smoked Turkey Breast	4 slices	45	2	0		0	25	480	0	9	1 very lean meat
Carl Budding											
Assorted Varieties Meats	12 slices	110–120	1–3	7	50	2–3	40–50	680–1020	0	12–14	2 lean meat
Farmer John											
Brown Sugar & Honey Ham	1 slice	50	3	1	20	0	15	440	0	7	1 very lean meat
Cooked Ham	2 slices	60	1	1	17	0	25	770	0	10	1 very lean meat
Healthy Choice											
Deli Thin Sliced Cold Cuts, Assorted Varieties	6 slices	60	1–4	1	25	0	25	470	0	9	1 very lean meat
Deli Traditions Hearty Deli Sliced, Assorted Varieties	1 slice	30–35	1–2	1	29	0	10–15	240	0	5	1 very lean meat

MEAT, POULTRY, FISH (PROCESSED/PREPARED)

	Serving	Calories	Carb. (g)	Fat (g)	% Cal. Fat	Sat. Fat (g)	Chol. (mg)	Sod. (mg)	Fib. (g)	Prot. (g)	Servings/ Exchanges
Regular Sliced	1 slice	30–35	1–2	0–1	0–33	0	5–15	240	0	5	1 very lean meat
Hebrew National											
Beef Salami	3 slices	150	0	13	80	6	35	420	0	8	1 high-fat meat, 1 fat
Fat-Free Oven Roasted Turkey	5 slices	50	1	0	0	0	20	430	0	11	1 very lean meat
Lean Beef Bologna	4 slices	90	1	5	50	2	20	440	0	8	1 med-fat meat
Lean Beef Salami	4 slices	90	1	5	56	3	25	480	0	9	1 med-fat meat
Pastrami	4 slices	90	1	4	39	1	35	500	0	13	2 lean meat
Hillshire Farm											
Deli Select Thin Sliced Cold Cuts, Assorted Varieties	6–7 slices	50–70	0–4	0–1	17	0	25	540–790	0	10–11	1 very lean meat
Ultra Thin Sliced Cold Cuts, Assorted Varieties	2 oz	60	0–2	0–3	25	0–1	25	340–620	0	9–11	1 very lean meat

Land O'Frost

Honey Ham	2 oz	80	2	3	38	1	30	660	0	10	1 lean meat
Oven Roasted Chicken Breast	2 oz	90	1	6	56	1	35	710	0	8	1 med-fat meat
Smoked Ham	2 oz	70	1	3	43	1	30	700	0	10	1 lean meat
Turkey Breast	2 oz	90	1	5	56	1	30	740	0	9	1 med-fat meat
Taste Escapes, Assorted Varieties	4–6 slices	70–80	2	3	38	1	30	630–720	0	9–11	1 lean meat
Thin Sliced, Assorted Varieties	2.5 oz	110–120	0–4	7	50	2–3	40–65	840–990	0	12–13	2 lean meat

Louis Rich

Smoked Chopped Turkey Ham	1 slice	45	1	2	44	1	20	350	0	5	1 lean meat
Turkey Bologna	1 slice	50	1	4	70	1	20	270	0	3	1 med-fat meat

Louis Rich Carving Board

Grilled Chicken Breast	2 slices	45	1	0	0	0	25	480	0	9	1 very lean meat

MEAT, POULTRY, FISH (PROCESSED/PREPARED)

	Serving	Calories	Carb. (g)	Fat (g)	% Cal. Fat	Sat. Fat (g)	Chol. (mg)	Sod. (mg)	Fib. (g)	Prot. (g)	Servings/ Exchanges
Oven Roasted Turkey Breast	3 slices	70	3	1	14	0	25	730	0	11	2 very lean meat
Oscar Mayer											
Baked Ham	3 slices	60	0	2	33	1	30	760	0	10	1 very lean meat
Beef Bologna	3 slices	90	1	8	78	3	20	310	0	3	1 high-fat meat
Boiled Ham	3 slices	60	0	2	33	1	30	820	0	10	1 lean meat
Bologna	1 slice	90	1	8	89	3	30	300	0	3	1 high-fat meat
Braunschweiger	2 oz	190	1	17	79	6	90	630	0	8	1 high-fat meat, 2 fat
Chopped Ham	1 slice	60	2	3	50	1	15	330	0	4	1 lean meat
Cooked Beef Salami	1 slice	70	1	6	86	3	20	320	0	4	1 med-fat meat
Cotto Beef Salami	1 slice	60	1	4	67	2	20	360	0	4	1 med-fat meat
Deli Style Brown Sugar Ham	4 slices	70	4	1	21	0	25	820	0	10	1 very lean meat
Deli Style Honey Turkey Breast	4 slices	60	2	1	17	0	25	600	0	10	1 very lean meat

Food	Serving										Exchanges
Deli Style Smoked Ham	4 slices	50	0	1	20	0	25	700	0	9	1 very lean meat
Fat-Free Bologna	1 slice	20	2	0	0	0	10	250	0	3	1 very lean meat
Ham & Cheese Loaf	1 slice	60	0	4	67	2	20	350	0	4	1 med-fat meat
Hard Salami	3 slices	100	1	8	70	3	25	510	0	7	1 high-fat meat
Honey Ham	3 slices	70	2	2	29	1	30	770	0	11	2 very lean meat
Light Beef Bologna	1 slice	60	2	4	58	1	15	310	0	3	1 med-fat meat
Liver Cheese	1 slice	120	1	10	75	3	80	420	0	6	1 high-fat meat
Olive Loaf	1 slice	70	2	6	79	2	20	360	0	3	1 med-fat meat
Oven Roasted White Turkey	1 slice	30	1	1	33	0	10	300	0	4	1 very lean meat
Pickle & Pimiento Loaf	1 slice	80	2	6	69	2	20	360	0	3	1 med-fat meat
Sandwich Spread	2 oz	130	9	9	62	4	25	460	0	4	1/2 carb, 1 high-fat meat
Sara Lee											
Brown Sugar Ham	2 slices	60	4	1	17	0	10	490	0	8	1 very lean meat
Honey Ham	2 slices	45	1	1	22	0	20	420	0	8	1 very lean meat

MEAT, POULTRY, FISH (PROCESSED/PREPARED)

	Serving	Calories	Carb. (g)	Fat (g)	% Cal. Fat	Sat. Fat (g)	Chol. (mg)	Sod. (mg)	Fib. (g)	Prot. (g)	Servings/ Exchanges
Honey Roasted Breast of Turkey	2 slices	50	1	0	0	0	20	450	0	10	1 very lean meat
Oven Roasted Breast of Chicken	3 slices	50	1	0	0	0	20	430	0	10	1 very lean meat
Slim Jim											
Beef Jerky, Big Jerk	0.25 oz	25	1	1	36	0	NA	220	0	3	1 very lean meat
Beef Jerky, Giant Jerk	0.63 oz	60	2	2	30	NA	NA	510	0	7	1 very lean meat
CANNED MEAT											
Fish/Seafood											
Anchovies in Oil, Canned, Drained	5	42	0	2	43	<1	17	734	0	8	1 lean meat
Clams, Canned, Drained Solids	1 oz	42	1	<1	12	<1	19	32	0	7	1 very lean meat

Food	Serving										Exchange
Clams, Smoked, Canned in Oil, Small	5	88	1	6	61	1	19	161	0	7	1 med-fat meat
Crab, Canned, Drained Solids	1 oz	28	0	<1	18	<1	26	95	0	6	1 very lean meat
Salmon, Canned in Water	1 oz	40	0	2	45	<1	11	139	0	6	1 lean meat
Sardines, Oil-Packed, Drained	2	50	0	3	54	<1	34	121	0	6	1 lean meat
Shrimp, Canned, Drained Solids	1 oz	34	<1	<1	0	<1	50	48	0	7	1 very lean meat
Squid, Pickled	1 oz	26	1	<1	0	<1	64	397	0	4	1 very lean meat
Tuna, Canned in Oil, Drained	1 oz	56	0	2	32	<1	5	100	0	8	1 lean meat
Tuna, Canned, Water-Packed, Solids Only	1 oz	33	0	<1	0	<1	9	96	0	7	1 very lean meat
Beef											
Liver Pate, Canned	2 Tbsp	52	2	3	52	1	66	100	0	4	1 lean meat
Pickled Beef Tripe	1 oz	18	0	<1	0	<1	19	13	0	3	1 very lean meat

MEAT, POULTRY, FISH (PROCESSED/PREPARED)

	Serving	Calories	Carb. (g)	Fat (g)	% Cal. Fat	Sat. Fat (g)	Chol. (mg)	Sod. (mg)	Fib. (g)	Prot. (g)	Servings/ Exchanges
Pork											
Ham, Canned	1 oz	48	<1	2	38	<1	12	304	0	6	1 lean meat
Sausage, Vienna, Canned	1 oz	79	<1	7	80	3	15	270	0	3	1 high-fat meat
Brands											
Bumble Bee											
Alaska Sockeye Red Salmon (in Water)	2 oz	110	0	7	55	1	40	270	0	13	2 med-fat meat
Skinless & Boneless Pink Salmon (in Water)	2 oz	50	0	1	20	0	20	150	0	11	2 very lean meat
Solid White Albacore Tuna (in Vegetable Oil)	2 oz	90	0	3	33	0	25	250	0	14	2 lean meat
Solid White Albacore Tuna (in Water)	2 oz	70	0	1	14	0	25	250	0	15	2 very lean meat

Chicken of the Sea

	Serving	Cal.									Exchanges
Chunk Light Tuna (in Water)	2 oz	60	0	<1	8	0	30	250	0	13	2 very lean meat
Chunk Light Tuna 50% Less Sodium (in Water)	2 oz	60	0	<1	8	0	30	120	0	13	2 very lean meat
Skinless, Boneless Pink Salmon (in Water)	2 oz	60	0	2	33	1	20	280	0	10	2 very lean meat
Solid White Albacore Tuna (in Water)	2 oz	70	0	1	14	0	25	250	0	15	2 very lean meat

Red Devil

	Serving	Cal.									Exchanges
Snackers, Chunky Chicken	⁻/4 cup	140	2	10	64	3	30	400	0	10	1 high-fat meat, 1 fat
Snackers, Deviled Ham	1/4 cup	140	3	11	71	4	30	410	0	7	1 high-fat meat, 1 fat

Season

	Serving	Cal.									Exchanges
Sardines, No-Salt-Added (in Water)	2 oz	160	1	9	50	4	75	80	0	19	3 lean meat

MEAT, POULTRY, FISH (PROCESSED/PREPARED)

	Serving	Calories	Carb. (g)	Fat (g)	% Cal. Fat	Sat. Fat (g)	Chol. (mg)	Sod. (mg)	Fib. (g)	Prot. (g)	Servings/ Exchanges
Starkist											
Chunk Light Tuna (in Vegetable Oil)	2 oz	110	0	6	45	1	30	250	0	13	2 lean meat
Chunk Light Tuna (in Water)	2 oz	60	0	<1	0	0	30	250	0	13	2 very lean meat
Low Sodium Chunk Light Tuna (in Water)	2 oz	60	0	<1	0	0	25	100	0	13	2 very lean meat
Solid White Albacore Tuna (in Water)	2 oz	80	0	3	31	1	35	250	0	12	1 very lean meat
Swanson											
Chicken Breast (in Water)	2 oz	50	1	1	20	<1	20	270	0	10	1 very lean meat
Underwood											
Chicken Spread, Chunky	1/4 cup	110	3	7	57	3	30	410	0	8	1 high-fat meat
Ham Spread, Deviled	1/4 cup	150	0	12	72	4	35	460	0	9	1 high-fat meat, 1 fat

Food	Serving										Exchanges
Ham Spread, Honey	1/4 cup	140	5	11	71	4	30	370	0	6	5 carbohydrate
Liverwurst Spread	1/4 cup	170	3	14	74	5	65	380	1	7	1 high-fat meat, 1 fat
Roast Beef Spread	1/4 cup	140	0	11	71	5	45	390	0	9	1 high-fat meat, 1 fat
Sardines in Mustard Sauce	3.8 oz can	180	2	12	60	3	105	820	1	17	2 med-fat meat
Sardines in Soy Oil, Drained	3.8 oz can	220	1	16	65	4	100	310	0	18	2 high-fat meat
Sardines in Tomato Sauce	3.8 oz can	180	4	11	55	3	115	960	1	16	2 med-fat meat
Tuna Spread, Lightly Seasoned	1/4 cup	50	2	1	18	0	30	480	0	9	1 very lean meat

MILK, YOGURT, SOY DRINKS

	Serving	Calories	Carb. (g)	Fat (g)	% Cal. Fat	Sat. Fat (g)	Chol. (mg)	Sod. (mg)	Fib. (g)	Prot. (g)	Servings/Exchanges
Buttermilk, Skim, Cultured	1 cup	99	12	2	18	1	9	257	0	8	1 skim milk
Carob Flavor Beverage Mix with Milk	1 cup	195	23	8	37	5	33	133	1	9	1 whole milk, 1 carb
Carob Flavor Beverage Mix, Powder	1 Tbsp	45	11	<1	0	<1	0	12	<1	<1	1 carb
Chocolate Drink, Syrup with Reduced-Fat Milk	1 cup	181	30	5	25	3	16	140	<1	8	1 reduced-fat milk, 1 carb
Chocolate Malted Milk Drink	1 cup	228	30	9	38	6	35	172	<1	9	1 whole milk, 1 carb
Cocoa/Hot Chocolate Mix with Water	1 pkt	102	22	1	9	<1	1	143	<1	3	1/2 skim milk, 1 carb
Cocoa/Hot Chocolate Mix with Whole Milk	1 cup	193	30	6	28	4	20	128	2	10	1 whole milk, 1 carb

Food	Serving										Exchanges
Cocoa Mix, Sugar-Free with Reduced-Fat Milk	1 cup	136	15	6	40	3	18	160	2	9	1 reduced-fat milk
Cocoa Mix, Sugar-Free with Water	1 cup	63	1	<1	0	<1	3	230	<1	5	1 skim milk
Cocoa, Sugar-Free, Mix with Water	1 pkt	48	9	<1	0	<1	1	168	<1	4	1/2 skim milk
Eggnog	1 cup	343	34	19	50	11	149	138	0	10	1 whole milk, 1 1/2 carb, 2 fat
Eggnog, 2% Reduced-Fat	1 cup	189	17	8	38	4	194	155	0	12	1 whole milk
Instant Breakfast Powder	1 pkt	131	25	<1	0	<1	4	142	<1	7	1 skim milk, 1 carb
Milk, 1%, Low-Fat	1 cup	102	12	3	26	2	10	123	0	8	1 skim milk
Milk, 1%, Low-Fat, Acidophilus	1 cup	102	12	3	26	2	10	123	0	8	1 skim milk
Milk, 1%, Low-Fat, Chocolate	1 cup	158	26	3	17	2	7	152	1	9	1 skim milk, 1 carb
Milk, 1%, Low-Fat, Protein-Fortified	1 cup	119	14	3	23	2	10	143	0	10	1 skim milk

MILK, YOGURT, SOY DRINKS

	Serving	Calories	Carb. (g)	Fat (g)	% Cal. Fat	Sat. Fat (g)	Chol. (mg)	Sod. (mg)	Fib. (g)	Prot. (g)	Servings/Exchanges
Milk, 2%, Reduced-Fat	1 cup	121	12	5	37	3	18	122	0	8	1 reduced-fat milk
Milk, 2%, Reduced-Fat, Chocolate	1 cup	179	26	5	25	3	17	151	1	9	1 reduced-fat milk, 1 carb
Milk, 2%, Reduced-Fat, Protein-Fortified	1 cup	137	14	5	33	3	19	145	0	10	1 reduced-fat milk
Milk, Evaporated Skim	1 cup	199	29	<1	0	0	9	293	0	19	2 skim milk
Milk, Evaporated Whole	1 cup	338	25	19	51	12	74	267	0	17	2 whole milk
Milk, Fat-Free	1 cup	86	12	<1	0	<1	4	126	0	8	1 skim milk
Milk, Fat-Free Chocolate	1 cup	144	27	1	6	<1	4	121	2	9	1 skim milk, 1 carb
Milk, Fat-Free, Lactose-Reduced	1 cup	86	12	<1	0	<1	4	126	0	9	1 skim milk
Milk, Fat-Free Powder with Water	1 cup	82	12	<1	0	<1	4	131	0	8	1 skim milk

Food	Serving										Exchanges
Milk, Fat-Free, Protein-Fortified	1 cup	100	14	<1	0	0	5	144	0	10	1 skim milk
Milk, Goat	1 cup	168	11	10	54	7	28	122	0	9	1 whole milk
Milk, Soy	1 cup	81	4	5	56	<1	0	29	3	7	1 reduced-fat milk
Milk, Sweetened Condensed, Canned	1 cup	982	166	27	25	17	104	389	0	24	3 whole milk, 9 carb
Milk, Whole	1 cup	150	11	8	48	5	33	120	0	8	1 whole milk
Milk, Whole, Chocolate	1 cup	209	26	9	39	5	31	149	2	8	1 whole milk, 1 carb
Yogurt, Low-Fat, Custard-Style, Fruit	1 cup	253	43	5	18	4	20	127	0	9	1 reduced-fat milk, 2 carb
Yogurt, Low-Fat, Fruit	1 cup	250	47	3	11	2	10	143	<1	11	1 1/2 skim milk, 2 carb
Yogurt, Low-Fat, Fruit & Nuts	1 cup	290	47	7	22	2	10	139	<1	11	1 1/2 low-fat milk, 2 carb
Yogurt, Low-Fat, Plain	1 cup	155	17	4	23	3	15	172	0	13	1 reduced-fat milk
Yogurt, Nonfat, Fruit with LoCal Sweetener	1 cup	122	19	<1	0	<1	3	139	1	12	1 skim milk, 1/2 carb

MILK, YOGURT, SOY DRINKS

	Serving	Calories	Carb. (g)	Fat (g)	% Cal. Fat	Sat. Fat (g)	Chol. (mg)	Sod. (mg)	Fib. (g)	Prot. (g)	Servings/ Exchanges
Yogurt, Nonfat, Plain	1 cup	137	19	<1	0	<1	4	187	0	15	1 1/2 skim milk
Yogurt, Whole-Milk, Plain	1 cup	150	11	8	48	5	31	114	0	9	1 whole milk
Brands											
8th Continent											
Soymilk, Light	8 oz	60	5	1	17	0	0	190	0	7	1 skim milk
Soymilk, Original	8 oz	80	8	3	31	<1	0	160	0	7	1 skim milk
Soymilk, Vanilla	8 oz	100	11	3	25	<1	0	170	0	7	1 skim milk
Breyers											
Yogurt, Crème Savers Lowfat, Strawberry Crème	8 oz	240	45	3	11	2	25	240	0	7	1 skim milk, 2 carb
Yogurt, Crème Savers Smoothie, Strawberry & Crème	10 oz	190	32	3	14	2	20	280	0	8	1 skim milk, 1 carb

Food	Serving										Exchanges
Yogurt, Fruit-on-the-Bottom, Strawberry	8 oz	240	46	2	8	1	20	130	0	9	1 skim milk, 2 carb
Yogurt, Light Classic Nonfat Strawberry	4 oz	60	11	0	0	0	5	50	0	4	1 skim milk
Yogurt, Smooth & Creamy Strawberry	4 oz	115	23	1	8	<1	10	50	0	4	1/2 skim milk, 1 carb
Carnation											
Milk, Evaporated	2 Tbsp	40	3	2	45	2	10	30	0	2	2 whole milk
Milk, Evaporated, Fat-Free	2 Tbsp	25	4	0	0	0	0	40	0	2	free
Milk, Evaporated, Low-Fat	2 Tbsp	25	3	<1	0	0	5	35	0	2	free
Milk, Sweetened Condensed	2 Tbsp	130	22	3	21	2	10	45	0	3	1 1/2 carb, 1 fat
Colombo											
Yogurt, Classic Fruit on the Bottom	8 oz	230	47	2	9	2	15	90	0	7	1 skim milk, 2 carb
Yogurt, Fat-Free, Light	8 oz	120	21	0	0	0	<5	110	0	7	1 skim milk, 1/2 carb

MILK, YOGURT, SOY DRINKS

	Serving	Calories	Carb. (g)	Fat (g)	% Cal. Fat	Sat. Fat (g)	Chol. (mg)	Sod. (mg)	Fib. (g)	Prot. (g)	Servings/ Exchanges
Dannon											
Yogurt, Creamy Fruit Blends, Strawberry	6 oz	170	31	2	12	2	10	115	0	6	1 skim milk, 1 carb
Yogurt, DanActive, Original	3.3 oz	90	16	2	17	1	10	50	0	3	1/2 skim milk, 1 carb
Yogurt, DanActive, Strawberry	3.3 oz	100	18	2	15	1	5	50	0	3	1/2 skim milk, 1 carb
Yogurt, Danimals Drinkable, Strawberry Explosion	3.1 oz	90	16	2	17	1	5	55	0	4	1/2 skim milk, 1 carb
Yogurt, Danimals XL Cherry Berry Blast	5.75 oz	170	29	3	15	2	15	105	0	7	1 skim milk, 1 carb
Yogurt, Fruit-on-the-Bottom, Strawberry	6 oz	160	30	2	9	1	10	130	0	6	1 skim milk, 1 carb
Yogurt, Fusion, Banana Berry Blend	10 oz	270	52	4	11	2	15	130	0	8	1 low-fat milk, 2 1/2 carb

Food	Serving										Exchange
Yogurt, Light 'n Fit Carb Control Smoothie, Strawberry 'n Cream	7 oz	70	4	3	36	2	10	35	0	6	1/2 low-fat milk
Yogurt, Light 'n Fit Creamy Strawberry	6 oz	100	16	0	0	0	<5	125	0	8	1 skim milk
Yogurt, Light 'n Fit Nonfat Strawberry	6 oz	90	17	0	0	0	<5	120	0	6	1 skim milk
Yogurt, Light 'n Fit Nonfat Smoothie Strawberry	7 oz	80	14	0	0	0	0	85	0	5	1 skim milk
Yogurt, Light 'n Fit with Fiber, Strawberry	4 oz	70	13	0	0	0	<5	55	3	4	1 skim milk
Yogurt, Lowfat, Plain	6 oz	110	14	3	23	2	15	140	0	9	1 skim milk
Yogurt, Natural Flavors, Vanilla	6 oz	150	26	3	17	2	10	115	0	7	1 skim milk, 1 carb
Yogurt, Plain, Natural	8 oz	160	14	8	43	5	35	150	0	9	1 whole milk
Yogurt, Plain, Nonfat	6 oz	90	14	0	0	0	<5	140	0	9	1 skim milk

MILK, YOGURT, SOY DRINKS

	Serving	Calories	Carb. (g)	Fat (g)	% Cal. Fat	Sat. Fat (g)	Chol. (mg)	Sod. (mg)	Fib. (g)	Prot. (g)	Servings/ Exchanges
Yogurt, Sprinkl'ins Strawberry	4.1 oz	120	22	2	13	1	5	65	0	4	1 skim milk, 1/2 carb
Lactaid											
Milk, Lactaid, Fat-Free	1 cup	90	13	0	0	0	<5	130	0	9	1 skim milk
Milk, Lactaid, Lowfat	1 cup	110	13	3	18	2	15	125	0	8	1 skim milk
Milk, Lactaid, Reduced-Fat	1 cup	130	13	5	35	3	20	125	0	8	1 low-fat milk
Milk, Lactaid, Whole	1 cup	160	12	9	50	5	35	125	0	8	1 whole milk
Pet											
Milk, Regular Evaporated	2 Tbsp	40	3	2	45	2	10	30	0	2	1 fat
Milk, Skimmed Evaporated	2 Tbsp	25	4	0	0	0	0	40	0	2	free
Silk											
SoyMilk, Chocolate	1 cup	140	23	4	21	<1	0	100	0	5	1 lowfat milk, 1 carb
SoyMilk, Plain	1 cup	100	8	4	35	<1	0	120	0	7	1 low-fat milk
SoyMilk, Vanilla	1 cup	100	10	4	30	<1	0	95	0	6	1 low-fat milk

Yoplait

Yogurt, Carb Monitor, Strawberry Crème	6 oz	90	8	3	30	2	15	45	0	8	1 skim milk, 2 carb
Yogurt, Custard Style Thick & Creamy Strawberry	6 oz	190	32	4	16	2	15	100	0	7	1 lowfat milk, 1 carb
Yogurt, GoGurt	2.25 oz tube	80	13	2	19	1	5	40	0	2	1 carb
Yogurt, GoGurt Smoothie Strawberry Splash	5 oz	120	23	<1	0	0	5	100	0	4	1/2 skim milk, 1 carb
Yogurt, Healthy Heart Strawberry	6 oz	180	35	2	8	<1	10	95	0	5	1 skim milk, 1 1/2 carb
Yogurt, Light Fat-Free Strawberry	6 oz	100	19	0	0	0	<5	85	0	5	1 skim milk, 1/2 carb
Yogurt, Nouriche Breakfast Smoothie, Strawberry	11 oz	290	60	0	0	0	5	290	6	10	1 skim milk, 3 carb

MILK, YOGURT, SOY DRINKS

	Serving	Calories	Carb. (g)	Fat (g)	% Cal. Fat	Sat. Fat (g)	Chol. (mg)	Sod. (mg)	Fib. (g)	Prot. (g)	Servings/ Exchanges
Yogurt, Nouriche Light Breakfast Smoothie, Strawberry	11 oz	170	33	0	0	0	10	250	5	10	1 skim milk, 1 1/2 carb
Yogurt, Scooby-Doo GoGurt	2.25 oz tube	80	13	2	19	1	5	40	0	2	1 carb
Yogurt, Whips! Strawberry Mist	6 oz	140	25	3	14	2	10	75	0	5	1 skim milk, 1 carb
Yogurt, Yumsters	4 oz	120	21	2	17	2	10	60	0	5	1 skim milk, 1/2 carb

NUTS, SEEDS, NUT/SEED PRODUCTS

	Serving	Calories	Carb. (g)	Fat (g)	% Cal. Fat	Sat. Fat (g)	Chol. (mg)	Sod. (mg)	Fib. (g)	Prot. (g)	Servings/ Exchanges
Almond Butter, Plain	1 Tbsp	101	3	10	89	<1	0	2	<1	2	2 fat
Almond Butter, Salted	1 Tbsp	98	3	9	83	<1	0	70	<1	2	2 fat
Almonds, Dried, Whole	1 oz	165	6	15	82	1	0	3	4	5	1 med-fat meat, 2 fat
Almonds, Dry-Roasted	1 oz	166	7	15	81	1	0	221	4	5	1 med-fat meat, 2 fat
Almonds, Dry-Roasted, Whole, Unsalted	1 oz	166	7	15	81	1	0	3	4	5	1 med-fat meat, 2 fat
Almonds, Oil-Roasted	1 oz	175	5	16	82	2	0	221	3	6	1 med-fat meat, 2 fat
Almonds, Toasted	1 oz	167	7	14	75	1	0	3	3	6	1 med-fat meat, 2 fat
Beechnuts, Dried	1 oz	164	10	14	77	2	0	11	<1	2	1/2 strch, 3 fat
Brazilnuts, Dried	1 oz	186	4	19	92	5	0	<1	2	4	1 med-fat meat, 3 fat
Cashew Butter, Unsalted	1 Tbsp	94	4	8	77	2	0	2	<1	3	2 fat
Cashews, Dry-Roasted	1 oz	161	9	13	73	3	0	179	<1	5	1/2 strch, 3 fat
Cashews, Oil-Roasted	1 oz	163	8	14	77	3	0	178	1	5	1/2 strch, 3 fat

NUTS, SEEDS, NUT/SEED PRODUCTS

	Serving	Calories	Carb. (g)	Fat (g)	% Cal. Fat	Sat. Fat (g)	Chol. (mg)	Sod. (mg)	Fib. (g)	Prot. (g)	Servings/ Exchanges
Chinese Chestnuts, Dried	1 oz	103	23	<1	0	<1	0	1	<1	2	1 1/2 strch
Chinese Chestnuts, Roasted	1 oz	68	15	<1	0	<1	0	1	<1	1	1 strch
Coconut, Dried, Shredded, Sweetened	1/4 cup	117	11	8	62	7	0	61	1	<1	1 strch, 2 fat
Coconut, Fresh	2.5 × 2-inch piece	159	7	15	85	13	0	9	4	2	1/2 strch, 3 fat
Coconut, Toasted	1 oz	168	13	13	70	12	0	11	2	2	1 strch, 3 fat
Coconut Milk, Raw	1 cup	552	13	57	92	51	0	36	5	6	1 strch, 11 fat
English Walnut Halves, Dried	1 oz	182	5	18	89	2	0	3	1	4	1 med-fat meat, 3 fat
European Chestnuts, Roasted	1 oz	69	15	<1	0	<1	0	<1	2	<1	1 strch
Filberts/Hazelnuts, Dried, Whole	1 oz	177	4	18	92	1	0	<1	2	4	1 med-fat meat, 3 fat

Food	Serving										Exchanges
Filberts/Hazelnuts, Dry Roasted, Salted	1 oz	188	5	18	86	1	0	221	2	3	3 fat
Filberts/Hazelnuts, Oil Roasted, Salted	1 oz	187	6	18	87	1	0	223	2	4	1/2 strch, 3 fat
Hickory Nuts, Dried	1 oz	186	5	18	87	2	0	<1	2	4	4 fat
Japanese Chestnuts, Dried	1 oz	101	23	<1	0	<1	0	10	<1	2	1 1/2 strch
Japanese Chestnuts, Roasted	1 oz	57	13	<1	0	<1	0	5	<1	<1	1 strch
Macadamia Nuts	1 oz	199	4	21	95	3	0	1	3	2	4 fat
Macadamia Nuts, Oil Roasted	1 oz	204	4	22	97	3	0	74	3	2	4 fat
Mixed Nuts, Dry Roasted	1 oz	168	7	15	80	2	0	190	3	5	1/2 strch, 3 fat
Mixed Nuts, Oil Roasted	1 oz	175	6	16	82	4	0	185	3	5	1/2 strch, 3 fat
Mixed Nuts, Oil Roasted, No Peanuts	1 oz	172	6	16	84	3	0	196	2	4	1/2 strch, 3 fat

NUTS, SEEDS, NUT/SEED PRODUCTS

	Serving	Calories	Carb. (g)	Fat (g)	% Cal. Fat	Sat. Fat (g)	Chol. (mg)	Sod. (mg)	Fib. (g)	Prot. (g)	Servings/ Exchanges
Mixed Nuts, Oil Roasted, Unsalted	1 oz	173	6	16	84	2	0	3	2	4	1 med-fat meat, 2 fat
Peanut Butter, Chunky	1 Tbsp	94	4	8	77	2	0	78	1	4	1 med-fat meat, 1 fat
Peanut Butter, Natural, Salted	1 Tbsp	94	3	8	77	1	0	40	1	4	1 med-fat meat, 1 fat
Peanut Butter, Natural, Unsalted	1 Tbsp	94	3	8	77	1	0	<1	1	4	1 med-fat meat, 1 fat
Peanut Butter, Smooth	1 Tbsp	94	3	8	77	2	0	77	<1	4	1 med-fat meat, 1 fat
Peanut Butter, Smooth, Salted	2 Tbsp	190	6	16	76	4	0	149	2	8	1 high-fat meat, 1 fat
Peanuts, Dry-Roasted, Unsalted	1 oz	166	6	14	76	2	0	2	2	7	1 med-fat meat, 2 fat
Peanuts, Oil-Roasted	1 oz	165	5	14	76	2	0	123	3	8	1 med-fat meat, 2 fat
Peanuts, Spanish, Raw	1 oz	167	5	14	76	2	0	6	3	8	1 med-fat meat, 2 fat

Food	Serving										Exchanges
Pecans, Dried Halves	1 oz	189	5	19	90	2	0	<1	2	2	4 fat
Pecans, Dry-Roasted	1 oz	187	6	18	87	2	0	222	3	2	3 fat
Pecans, Oil-Roasted	1 oz	194	5	20	93	2	0	214	2	2	4 fat
Pine Nuts (Pignoli), Dried	1 oz	178	6	17	86	3	0	20	3	3	1 med-fat meat, 2 fat
Pistachio Nuts, Dry-Roasted	1 oz	170	8	15	79	2	0	218	3	4	1/2 strch, 3 fat
Pumpkin Kernels, Roasted	1 oz	148	4	12	73	2	0	163	1	9	1 med-fat meat, 1 fat
Pumpkin Seeds, Roasted	1 oz	126	15	6	43	1	0	163	2	5	1 strch, 1 fat
Sesame Seeds, Dried, Whole	1 Tbsp	52	2	5	87	1	0	1	1	2	1 fat
Sunflower Seeds, Dry	1 oz	162	5	14	77	2	0	<1	3	7	1 med-fat meat, 2 fat
Sunflower Seeds, Dry-Roasted	1 oz	163	7	14	77	2	0	<1	3	6	1 med-fat meat, 2 fat
Sunflower Seeds, Oil-Roasted	1 oz	174	4	16	83	2	0	171	2	6	1 med-fat meat, 2 fat
Tahini/Sesame Butter	1 Tbsp	91	3	9	89	1	0	<1	1	3	2 fat

NUTS, SEEDS, NUT/SEED PRODUCTS

	Serving	Calories	Carb. (g)	Fat (g)	% Cal. Fat	Sat. Fat (g)	Chol. (mg)	Sod. (mg)	Fib. (g)	Prot. (g)	Servings/ Exchanges
Brands											
Baker's											
Coconut, Angel Flake	2 Tbsp	70	6	5	64	5	0	40	1	<1	1/2 carb, 1 fat
Beer Nuts											
Cashew Halves	1 oz	170	8	13	69	3	0	65	NA	5	1 med-fat meat, 2 fat
Peanuts	1 oz	170	7	14	74	3	0	80	2	7	1 med-fat meat, 2 fat
Blue Diamond											
Almonds, Whole, Roasted	1 oz	170	5	16	85	1	0	85	3	6	1 med-fat meat, 2 fat
Smokehouse Almonds	1 oz	170	5	16	82	1	0	150	3	6	1 med-fat meat, 2 fat
CornNuts											
Barbeque	1 oz	130	20	5	35	<1	0	170	2	2	1 strch, 1 fat
Chili Picante	1 oz	130	19	5	35	<1	0	280	2	2	1 strch, 1 fat
Nacho Cheese	1 oz	130	20	4	28	1	0	190	2	2	1 strch, 1 fat
Original	1 oz	120	20	5	38	<1	0	180	2	3	1 strch, 1 fat

Ranch	1 oz	130	19	5	35	1	0	230	2	3	1 strch, 1 fat
Estee										
Peanut Butter, Creamy/Chunky	2 Tbsp	190	7	15	71	3	0	0	2	7	1 high-fat meat, 1 fat
Fisher										
Butter Toffee Peanuts	1 oz	130	17	6	46	1	0	150	1	3	1 carb, 1 fat
Honey Roasted Peanuts	1 oz	170	7	13	69	3	0	70	2	7	1/2 carb, 1 med-fat meat, 2 fat
Mixed Nuts	1 oz	180	5	16	80	3	0	110	2	6	1 med-fat meat, 2 fat
Jif										
Peanut Butter, Creamy	2 Tbsp	190	7	16	76	3	0	150	2	8	1 high-fat meat, 2 fat
Peanut Butter, Extra Crunchy	2 Tbsp	190	7	16	76	3	0	130	2	8	1 high-fat meat, 2 fat
Peanut Butter, Reduced-Fat, Creamy	2 Tbsp	190	15	12	57	3	0	250	2	8	1 carb, 1 high-fat meat, 1 fat
Peanut Butter, Reduced-Fat, Crunchy	2 Tbsp	190	15	12	58	3	0	220	2	8	1 carb, 1 high-fat meat, 1 fat

NUTS, SEEDS, NUT/SEED PRODUCTS

	Serving	Calories	Carb. (g)	Fat (g)	% Cal. Fat	Sat. Fat (g)	Chol. (mg)	Sod. (mg)	Fib. (g)	Prot. (g)	Servings/ Exchanges
Peanut Butter, Simply Jif, Creamy	2 Tbsp	190	6	16	68	3	0	65	2	8	1 high-fat meat, 2 fat
Peanut Butter & Honey	2 Tbsp	190	11	15	68	3	0	120	2	6	1 carb, 1 high-fat meat, 1 fat
Laura Scudder's											
Peanut Butter, Nutty	2 Tbsp	210	6	16	68	3	0	120	2	8	1 high-fat meat, 2 fat
Peanut Butter, Smooth	2 Tbsp	210	6	16	68	3	0	120	2	8	1 high-fat meat, 2 fat
Peanut Butter, Smooth, Unsalted	2 Tbsp	210	6	16	68	3	0	5	2	8	1/2 carb, 1 high-fat meat, 1 fat
Peter Pan											
Peanut Butter, Creamy	2 Tbsp	190	6	17	81	4	0	140	2	7	1 high-fat meat, 2 fat
Peanut Butter, Crunchy	2 Tbsp	190	3	16	74	3	0	110	2	8	1 high-fat meat, 2 fat
Peanut Butter Spread, Reduced-Fat	2 Tbsp	190	15	11	52	2	0	160	2	8	1 carb, 1 high-fat meat, 1 fat
Peter Paul Mounds											
Sweetened Coconut Flakes	2 Tbsp	70	6	5	64	4	0	35	1	<1	1/2 carb, 1 fat

Planters

Cocktail Peanuts, Lightly Salted	1 oz	170	5	15	76	2	0	55	2	7	1 high-fat meat, 1 fat
Mixed Nuts	1 oz	170	6	15	82	2	0	105	2	5	1/2 carb, 1 high-fat meat, 1 fat
Peanuts, Dry Roasted, Lightly Salted	1 oz	170	5	14	76	2	0	95	2	8	1 high-fat meat, 1 fat
Peanuts, Dry Roasted, Unsalted	1 oz	170	5	14	76	2	0	0	2	8	1 high-fat meat, 1 fat
Peanuts, Honey-Roasted	1 oz	150	8	12	72	2	0	95	2	7	1/2 carb, 1 high-fat meat, 1 fat
Redskin Spanish Peanuts	1 oz	180	5	14	67	2	0	100	2	8	1 high-fat meat, 1 fat
Sweet Roasts Honey Roasted Peanuts & Cashews	1 oz	160	10	12	68	2	0	120	2	5	1/2 carb, 1 high-fat meat, 1 fat

Reese's

Peanut Butter, Creamy	2 Tbsp	200	8	15	68	2	0	140	2	7	1/2 carb, 1 high-fat meat, 2 fat

NUTS, SEEDS, NUT/SEED PRODUCTS

	Serving	Calories	Carb. (g)	Fat (g)	% Cal. Fat	Sat. Fat (g)	Chol. (mg)	Sod. (mg)	Fib. (g)	Prot. (g)	Servings/ Exchanges
Peanut Butter, Extra Crunchy	2 Tbsp	200	6	16	72	3	0	80	2	7	1 high-fat meat, 2 fat
Skippy											
Carb Options Creamy Peanut Spread	2 Tbsp	190	5	17	81	4	0	150	2	7	1 high-fat meat, 2 fat
Peanut Butter, Creamy	2 Tbsp	190	7	17	81	4	3	150	2	7	1/2 carb, 1 high-fat meat, 2 fat
Peanut Butter, Reduced-Fat Creamy	2 Tbsp	190	15	12	57	3	0	190	2	7	1 carb, 1 high-fat meat, 1 fat
Peanut Butter, Reduced-Fat Super Chunk	2 Tbsp	190	14	12	57	3	0	170	2	7	1 carb, 1 high-fat meat, 1 fat
Peanut Butter, Super Chunk	2 Tbsp	190	7	17	81	3	0	140	2	7	1/2 carb, 1 high-fat meat, 2 fat
Squeez'It Creamy Peanut Butter	2 Tbsp	190	7	17	81	4	0	160	2	7	1/2 carb, 1 high-fat meat, 2 fat

SAUCES, GRAVIES, CONDIMENTS, RELISHES

	Serving	Calories	Carb. (g)	Fat (g)	% Cal. Fat	Sat. Fat (g)	Chol. (mg)	Sod. (mg)	Fib. (g)	Prot. (g)	Servings/ Exchanges
Apple Butter	2 Tbsp	65	17	<1	0	0	0	0	<1	<1	1 carb
Catsup/Ketchup	1 Tbsp	16	4	<1	0	<1	0	182	<1	<1	free
Catsup/Ketchup, Low-Sodium	1 Tbsp	16	4	<1	0	<1	0	3	<1	<1	free
Chutney	1 Tbsp	26	7	<1	0	<1	0	38	<1	<1	1/2 carb
Gravy, Au Jus, Canned	1/2 cup	19	3	<1	0	<1	0	60	0	1	free
Gravy, Beef, Canned	1/2 cup	62	6	3	43	1	4	652	<1	4	1/2 carb, 1 fat
Gravy, Beef, Homemade	1/2 cup	89	7	5	51	2	3	767	<1	4	1/2 carb, 1 fat
Gravy, Brown, Dry Mix with Water	1/2 cup	38	7	<1	0	<1	1	538	<1	1	1/2 carb
Gravy, Chicken, Canned	1/2 cup	94	7	7	67	2	2	687	<1	2	1/2 carb, 1 fat
Gravy, Chicken Giblet, Homemade	1/2 cup	97	6	5	46	1	55	683	<1	6	1/2 carb, 1 fat

SAUCES, GRAVIES, CONDIMENTS, RELISHES

	Serving	Calories	Carb. (g)	Fat (g)	% Cal. Fat	Sat. Fat (g)	Chol. (mg)	Sod. (mg)	Fib. (g)	Prot. (g)	Servings/ Exchanges
Gravy, Mushroom, Canned	1/2 cup	60	7	6	90	<1	0	678	<1	2	1/2 carb, 1 fat
Gravy, Sausage	1/2 cup	206	8	16	70	6	33	408	<1	8	1/2 carb, 3 fat
Gravy, Turkey, Canned	1/2 cup	61	6	3	44	<1	2	687	<1	3	1/2 strch, 1 fat
Guacamole with Tomatoes	1 Tbsp	17	1	2	100	<1	0	27	<1	<1	free
Honey	1 Tbsp	64	17	0	0	0	0	<1	<1	<1	1 carb
Horseradish, Prepared	1 Tbsp	7	2	<1	0	<1	0	47	<1	<1	free
Jam, Cherry/Strawberry	1 Tbsp	54	14	<1	0	0	0	2	<1	<1	1 carb
Jam, Not Cherry or Strawberry	1 Tbsp	54	14	<1	0	0	0	2	<1	<1	1 carb
Jam/Marmalade, Artificially Sweetened	1 Tbsp	2	11	<1	0	<1	0	0	<1	<1	free
Jam/Marmalade/Preserves, Reduced-Sugar	1 Tbsp	36	9	<1	0	<1	0	5	<1	<1	1/2 carb
Jam/Preserves	1 Tbsp	48	13	<1	0	<1	0	8	<1	<1	1 carb

Jelly	1 Tbsp	52	14	<1	0	0	0	7	<1	<1	1 carb
Jelly, Blackberry	1 Tbsp	50	13	0	0	0	0	10	0	0	1 carb
Jelly, Dietetic	1 Tbsp	6	11	0	0	0	0	<1	<1	<1	free
Jelly, Reduced-Sugar	1 Tbsp	34	9	<1	0	0	0	<1	<1	<1	1/2 carb
Marmalade, Orange	1 Tbsp	49	13	0	0	0	0	11	<1	<1	1 carb
Mustard, Dijon	1 Tbsp	19	2	1	47	<1	0	379	<1	<1	free
Mustard, Honey	1 Tbsp	50	7	3	54	<1	0	91	<1	<1	1/2 carb
Mustard, Prepared	1 Tbsp	12	1	<1	0	<1	0	196	<1	<1	free
Olives, Green, Pitted	10	45	<1	5	45	<1	0	936	<1	<1	1 fat
Olives, Green, Stuffed	10	41	<1	5	100	<1	0	827	<1	<1	1 fat
Olives, Small Ripe, Canned	10	37	2	3	73	<1	0	279	1	<1	1 fat
Peppers, Pickled Hot Jalapeño	2	8	2	<1	0	<1	0	121	<1	<1	free
Pickle, Dill	1	12	3	<1	0	<1	0	833	<1	<1	free
Pickle, Dill, Low-Sodium	1	12	3	<1	0	<1	0	12	<1	<1	free

SAUCES, GRAVIES, CONDIMENTS, RELISHES

	Serving	Calories	Carb. (g)	Fat (g)	% Cal. Fat	Sat. Fat (g)	Chol. (mg)	Sod. (mg)	Fib. (g)	Prot. (g)	Servings/ Exchanges
Pickle, Sour	1	4	<1	<1	0	<1	0	423	<1	<1	free
Pickle, Sweet	1 medium	41	11	<1	0	<1	0	329	<1	<1	1/2 carb
Pickle Slices, Dill	10	11	3	<1	0	<1	0	769	<1	<1	free
Pickle Slices, Dill, Low-Sodium	10	11	3	<1	0	<1	0	11	<1	<1	free
Pickle Slices, Fresh Pack	4	22	5	<1	0	0	0	202	<1	<1	free
Pickle Slices, Sour	10	8	2	<1	0	<1	0	846	<1	<1	free
Relish, Hot Dog	1 Tbsp	14	4	<1	0	<1	0	167	<1	<1	free
Relish, Sweet Pickle	1 Tbsp	20	5	<1	0	<1	0	124	<1	<1	free
Sauce, Bearnaise, Homemade	1/2 cup	321	1	34	95	20	237	444	<1	2	7 fat
Sauce, Black Bean	1/2 cup	129	14	6	42	1	0	1322	2	3	1 strch, 1 fat
Sauce, Cheese	1/2 cup	221	9	16	64	10	36	515	<1	10	1/2 carb, 1 med-fat meat, 2 fat
Sauce, Curry	1/2 cup	74	3	6	73	1	0	392	3	3	1 fat

Sauce, Hollandaise, Dry Mix & Water	1/2 cup	119	7	10	76	6	26	783	<1	2	1/2 carb, 2 fat
Sauce, Hot Chili/Red Pepper	2 Tbsp	7	1	<1	0	<1	0	8	<1	<1	free
Sauce, Hot Green Chili	1 Tbsp	6	2	<1	0	0	0	4	<1	<1	free
Sauce, Marinara Tomato	1/2 cup	85	13	4	42	<1	0	786	1	2	1 carb, 1 fat
Sauce, Salsa/Mexican, Homemade	1/2 cup	23	5	<1	0	<1	0	468	1	<1	1 vegetable
Sauce, Soy	1 Tbsp	10	2	<1	0	<1	0	1028	0	<1	free
Sauce, Spanish-Style Tomato	1/2 cup	40	9	<1	0	<1	0	576	2	2	1/2 carb
Sauce, Tartar	1 Tbsp	74	<1	8	97	2	7	99	<1	<1	2 fat
Sauce, Teriyaki	1 Tbsp	15	3	0	0	0	0	690	<1	1	free
Sauce, White, Homemade	1/2 cup	178	10	14	71	4	14	185	<1	4	1/2 strch, 3 fat
Sauce, Worcestershire	1 Tbsp	11	3	0	0	0	0	167	0	0	free
Spaghetti Sauce, Meat, Canned	1/2 cup	150	19	7	42	1	8	590	4	4	1 carb, 2 fat

SAUCES, GRAVIES, CONDIMENTS, RELISHES

	Serving	Calories	Carb. (g)	Fat (g)	% Cal. Fat	Sat. Fat (g)	Chol. (mg)	Sod. (mg)	Fib. (g)	Prot. (g)	Servings/ Exchanges
Spaghetti Sauce, Meat, Homemade	1/2 cup	145	11	8	50	2	23	565	2	8	2 carb, 1 med-fat meat, 1 fat
Spaghetti Sauce, Canned	1/2 cup	136	20	6	40	<1	0	618	4	2	1 carb, 1 fat
Syrup, Maple	1 Tbsp	52	13	<1	0	0	0	2	0	0	1 carb
Syrup, Pancake	1 Tbsp	57	15	0	0	0	0	17	0	0	1 carb
Brands											
A.1. Steakhouse											
Marinade, Chicago Steakhouse	1 Tbsp	20	3	1	45	0	0	270	0	0	free
Marinade, Classic	1 Tbsp	15	4	0	0	0	0	290	0	0	free
Marinade, Jamaican Jerk	1 Tbsp	25	5	<1	0	0	0	190	0	0	free
Marinade, Mesquite	1 Tbsp	15	4	0	0	0	0	400	0	0	free
Marinade, New Orleans Cajun	1 Tbsp	25	5	0	0	0	0	180	0	0	free

Food	Amount	Cal					Sod			Exch
Marinade, Steakhouse Teriyaki	1 Tbsp	25	5	0	0	0	490	0		free
Steak Sauce	1 Tbsp	15	3	0	0	0	280	0		free
Aunt Jemima										
Butter Lite Syrup	1/4 cup	100	26	0	0	0	180	0		2 carb
Butter Rich Syrup	1/4 cup	210	52	0	0	0	170	0		3 1/2 carb
Country Rich Regular Syrup	1/4 cup	210	53	0	0	0	120	0		3 1/2 carb
Lite Syrup	1/4 cup	100	26	0	0	0	180	0		2 carb
Original Syrup	1/4 cup	210	52	0	0	0	120	0		3 1/2 carb
Betty Crocker										
Bac-Os, Salad Topping Bits or Chips	1 1/2 Tbsp	30	2	2	60	0	120	0	3	1 fat
Bigelow										
Black Currant Honey Spread	1 Tbsp	70	17	0	0	0	0	0		1 carb

SAUCES, GRAVIES, CONDIMENTS, RELISHES

	Serving	Calories	Carb. (g)	Fat (g)	% Cal. Fat	Sat. Fat (g)	Chol. (mg)	Sod. (mg)	Fib. (g)	Prot. (g)	Servings/ Exchanges
Cinnamon Honey Spread	1 Tbsp	70	17	0	0	0	0	0	0	0	1 carb
Orange Honey Spread	1 Tbsp	70	17	0	0	0	0	0	0	0	1 carb
Braswell's											
Mango Butter	1 Tbsp	40	11	0	0	0	0	0	0	0	1 carb
Pear Preserves	1 Tbsp	50	14	0	0	0	0	0	0	0	1 carb
Campbell's											
Gravy, Beef	1/4 cup	25	3	1	40	<1	<5	270	0	1	free
Gravy, Chicken	1/4 cup	40	3	3	75	1	5	260	0	0	1 fat
Gravy, Country Style Cream Gravy	1/4 cup	50	3	4	60	1	5	190	0	1	1 fat
Gravy, Cream Style Sausage Gravy	1/4 cup	70	3	6	71	2	10	270	0	2	1 fat
Gravy, Turkey	1/4 cup	25	3	1	40	<1	0	270	0	1	free
Spaghetti Sauce, Italian-Style	1/2 cup	50	12	0	0	0	0	360	2	2	1 carb

Spaghetti Sauce, Marinara, Homestyle	1/2 cup	40	0	0	0	0	360	2	2	1/2 carb
Spaghetti Sauce, Mushroom	1/2 cup	50	11	1	20	0	330	2	2	1 1/2 carb
Spaghetti Sauce, Mushroom Garlic	1/2 cup	50	11	1	20	0	330	2	2	1 carb
Spaghetti Sauce, Traditional	1/2 cup	50	12	0	0	0	360	2	2	1 1/2 carb
Cary's										
Syrup, Maple	1/4 cup	210	53	0	0	0	5	0	0	3 1/2 carb
Syrup, Sugar-Free	1/4 cup	30	12	0	0	0	115	0	0	1 carb
Claussen										
Pickle Relish, Sweet	1 Tbsp	14	3	<1	0	0	90	NA	<1	free
Pickles, Bread 'n Butter Chips	1	7	2	0	0	0	61	NA	<1	free
Pickles, Hamburger Dill Chips	10	<1	<1	<1	0	0	42	<1	<1	free

SAUCES, GRAVIES, CONDIMENTS, RELISHES

	Serving	Calories	Carb. (g)	Fat (g)	% Cal. Fat	Sat. Fat (g)	Chol. (mg)	Sod. (mg)	Fib. (g)	Prot. (g)	Servings/ Exchanges
Pickles, Kosher Dill Halves	1	9	1	<1	0	<1	0	769	NA	<1	free
Pickles, Kosher Dill Slices	1	1	<1	<1	0	<1	0	107	NA	0	free
Pickles, Kosher Dill Spears	1	4	<1	<1	0	<1	0	312	<1	<1	free
Pickles, Kosher Mini Dills	1	4	<1	<1	0	<1	0	300	<1	<1	free
Contadina											
Pizza Sauce, Flavored with Pepperoni	1/4 cup	35	5	1	26	0	0	390	<1	1	1/2 carb
Pizza Sauce, Four Cheese	1/4 cup	30	6	<1	0	0	0	390	<1	<1	1/2 carb
Pizza Sauce, Original	1/4 cup	30	6	0	0	0	0	340	1	1	1/2 carb
Pizza Squeeze Sauce	1/4 cup	30	6	0	0	0	0	340	1	1	1/2 carb
Del Monte											
Sloppy Joe Sauce	1/4 cup	70	16	0	0	0	0	680	0	1	1 carb
Spaghetti Sauce, Traditional	1/3 cup	70	11	2	26	NA	NA	430	NA	1	1 carb

Spaghetti Sauce with Garlic & Onion	1/2 cup	70	10	2	26	0	NA	430	NA	1	1 carb
Spaghetti Sauce with Meat	1/2 cup	70	9	2	26	NA	NA	440	NA	2	1 carb
Spaghetti Sauce with Mushrooms	1/2 cup	70	11	2	26	NA	NA	440	NA	1	1 carb

Di Giorno

Sauce, Alfredo	1/4 cup	180	3	18	90	7	25	600	0	3	4 fat
Sauce, Alfredo, Light	1/4 cup	140	9	10	64	6	30	600	0	5	1/2 carb, 1 med-fat meat, 1 fat
Sauce, Basil Pesto	1/4 cup	320	2	31	87	6	15	530	<1	7	1 med-fat meat, 5 fat
Sauce, Four-Cheese	1/4 cup	160	3	15	84	7	30	410	0	5	1 med-fat meat, 2 fat
Sauce, Garlic Pesto	1/4 cup	340	3	33	87	7	15	540	<1	7	1 med-fat meat, 6 fat
Sauce, Marinara	1/2 cup	70	15	0	0	0	0	220	2	2	1 carb
Sauce, Plum Tomato & Mushroom	1/2 cup	50	3	0	0	0	0	260	2	2	1 carb

Dynasty

Chinese Duck Sauce	2 Tbsp	80	19	0	0	0	0	95	0	0	1 carb

SAUCES, GRAVIES, CONDIMENTS, RELISHES

	Serving	Calories	Carb. (g)	Fat (g)	% Cal. Fat	Sat. Fat (g)	Chol. (mg)	Sod. (mg)	Fib. (g)	Prot. (g)	Servings/ Exchanges
Chinese Stir-Fry Sauce	2 Tbsp	40	3	3	25	0	0	500	0	1	1 fat
Hoisin Sauce	2 Tbsp	50	9	1	20	0	0	410	0	0	1/2 carb
Hot Chili Oil	1 tsp	40	0	4	100	<1	0	0	0	0	1 fat
Plum Sauce	2 Tbsp	60	15	0	0	0	0	180	0	1	1 carb
Sweet & Sour Sauce	2 Tbsp	60	14	<1	0	0	0	90	0	0	1 carb
Szechwan Chili Sauce	1 tsp	10	1	<1	0	0	0	70	0	0	free
Fifty50											
Low Calorie, No-Sugar-Added Spread, All Varieties	1 Tbsp	10	4	0	0	0	0	10	0	0	free
Reduced-Calorie Blueberry Syrup	1/4 cup	70	18	0	0	0	0	80	0	0	1 carb
Reduced-Calorie Maple Syrup	1/4 cup	70	18	0	0	0	0	75	0	0	1 carb

Franco-American

Food	Serving									
Gravy, Brown, Slow Roast Turkey Gravy	1/4 cup	20	4	0	0	<5	320	0	1	free
Gravy, Slow Roast Beef Gravy	1/4 cup	20	3	0	0	<5	360	0	1	free
Gravy, Slow Roast Chicken Gravy	1/4 cup	15	3	0	0	<5	240	0	<1	free

Golden Valley Applicious

Food	Serving									
Applicious Peach & Orange Spread	1 Tbsp	33	8	0	0	0	3	0	0	1/2 carb
Applicious Raspberry Spread	1 Tbsp	33	8	0	0	0	2	0	0	1/2 carb
Applicious Strawberry Spread	1 Tbsp	33	8	0	0	0	2	0	0	1/2 carb
Sauce, Sloppy Joe Sandwich	1/4 cup	50	11	<1	<1	0	423	2	2	1 carb

SAUCES, GRAVIES, CONDIMENTS, RELISHES

	Serving	Calories	Carb. (g)	Fat (g)	% Cal. Fat	Sat. Fat (g)	Chol. (mg)	Sod. (mg)	Fib. (g)	Prot. (g)	Servings/ Exchanges
Grey Poupon											
Country Dijon Mustard	1 tsp	5	0	0	0	0	0	120	0	0	free
Healthy Choice											
Pasta Sauce, Garlic & Herbs	1/2 cup	60	13	0	0	0	0	320	3	2	1 carb
Pasta Sauce, Super Chunky Tomato, Mushroom & Garlic	1/2 cup	45	10	0	0	0	0	340	7	2	1/2 carb
Pasta Sauce, Super Chunky Vegetable	1/2 cup	60	13	0	0	0	0	390	3	2	1 carb
Pasta Sauce, Traditional	1/2 cup	60	13	0	0	0	0	370	3	3	1 carb
Heinz											
57 Sauce	1 Tbsp	20	4	0	0	0	0	190	0	0	free
Chili Sauce	1 Tbsp	20	5	0	0	0	0	230	0	0	free

	Serving Size	Calories	Fat (g)	% Calories from Fat	Saturated Fat (g)	Cholesterol (mg)	Sodium (mg)	Carbohydrate (g)	Fiber (g)	Protein (g)	Exchanges/Choices
Cocktail Sauce	1/4 cup	60	0	0	0	0	690	15	0	1	1 carb
Gravy, Classic Chicken	1/4 cup	25	1	40	0	0	310	4	0	0	free
Gravy, Homestyle Savory Beef	1/4 cup	25	<1	0	0	0	210	4	0	1	free
Gravy, Rich Mushroom Gravy	1/4 cup	20	<1	0	0	0	320	3	0	<1	free
Gravy, Roasted Turkey	1/4 cup	20	<1	0	0	0	270	3	0	0	free
Worcestershire Sauce	1 tsp	0	0	0	0	0	60	0	0	0	free
Hormel											
Real Bacon Bits, 50% Less Fat	1 Tbsp	30	2	50	1	5	250	0	0	3	1 fat
Real Bacon Pieces, 50% Less Fat	1 Tbsp	25	2	60	<1	10	180	0	0	3	1 fat
Hunt's											
BBQ Sauce, Hickory & Brown Sugar	2 Tbsp	70	0	0	0	0	340	16	0	0	1 carb

SAUCES, GRAVIES, CONDIMENTS, RELISHES

	Serving	Calories	Carb. (g)	Fat (g)	% Cal. Fat	Sat. Fat (g)	Chol. (mg)	Sod. (mg)	Fib. (g)	Prot. (g)	Servings/ Exchanges
BBQ Sauce, Mesquite	2 Tbsp	40	10	0	0	0	0	380	0	0	1/2 carb
BBQ Sauce, Original	2 Tbsp	60	15	0	0	0	0	240	0	0	1 carb
Spaghetti Sauce, Chunky Vegetable	1/2 cup	50	12	1	18	<1	0	470	2	1	1 carb
Spaghetti Sauce, Home Style	1/2 cup	60	10	1	15	0	0	560	3	2	1/2 carb, 1 fat
Spaghetti Sauce, Flavored with Meat	1/2 cup	70	12	2	26	<1	2	570	2	2	1 carb
Spaghetti Sauce, Four Cheese	1/2 cup	50	10	1	20	0	0	600	3	3	1/2 carb
Spaghetti Sauce, Italian Sausage	1/2 cup	60	10	2	30	0	0	590	3	2	1/2 carb
Spaghetti Sauce, Original Traditional	1/2 cup	70	12	2	26	<1	0	530	2	2	1 carb

Spaghetti Sauce with Mushrooms, Original	1/2 cup	50	10	1	18	0	0	600	3	2	1/2 carb
Spaghetti Sauce with Tomato & Basil, Classic Italian	1/2 cup	50	8	2	36	<1	0	550	NA	1	1/2 carb
Jack Daniel's											
Barbeque Sauce, Honey Smokehouse	2 Tbsp	50	12	0	0	0	0	290	0	0	1 carb
Grilling Sauce, Tennessee Hickory	2 Tbsp	50	3	0	0	0	0	300	0	0	free
Steak Sauce, Original	1 Tbsp	20	4	0	0	0	0	210	0	0	free
Steak Sauce, Smokey	1 Tbsp	20	0	0	0	0	0	200	0	0	free
Karo											
Dark Corn Syrup	2 Tbsp	120	31	0	0	0	0	45	0	0	2 carb
Light Corn Syrup	2 Tbsp	120	31	0	0	0	0	35	0	0	2 carb
Pancake Syrup	4 Tbsp	240	63	0	0	0	0	85	0	0	4 carb

SAUCES, GRAVIES, CONDIMENTS, RELISHES

	Serving	Calories	Carb. (g)	Fat (g)	% Cal. Fat	Sat. Fat (g)	Chol. (mg)	Sod. (mg)	Fib. (g)	Prot. (g)	Servings/ Exchanges
KC Masterpiece											
BBQ Sauce, Hickory Brown Sugar	2 Tbsp	60	15	0	0	0	0	300	0	0	1 carb
BBQ Sauce, Mesquite	2 Tbsp	60	13	0	0	0	0	210	0	0	1 carb
BBQ Sauce, Original	2 Tbsp	60	15	0	0	0	0	240	0	0	1 carb
Marinade, Ginger & Garlic	1 Tbsp	30	7	0	0	0	0	270	0	<1	1/2 carb
Marinade, Golden Honey Dijon	1 Tbsp	40	9	0	0	0	0	400	0	0	1/2 carb
Marinade, Honey Teriyaki	1 Tbsp	40	8	0	0	0	0	320	0	<1	1/2 carb
Marinade, Spiced Caribbean Jerk	1 Tbsp	25	6	0	0	0	0	320	0	0	1/2 carb
Marinade, Zesty Lemon Pepper	1 Tbsp	25	1	0	0	0	0	310	0	0	free

Kitchen Bouquet

Browning & Seasoning Sauce	1 tsp	15	3	0	0	0	10	0	free

Knott's Berry Farm

100% Spreadable Fruit, All Varieties	1 Tbsp	40	10	0	0	0	0–5	0	1/2 carb
Apple Cinnamon Jelly	1 Tbsp	50	13	0	0	0	10	0	1 carb
Apricot & Pineapple Light Preserves	1 Tbsp	20	5	0	0	0	0	0	free
Apricot Syrup	1/4 cup	210	52	0	0	0	30	0	3 1/2 carb
Bing Cherry Preserves	1 Tbsp	50	13	0	0	0	10	0	1 carb
Blackberry Syrup	1/4 cup	210	52	0	0	0	50	0	3 1/2 carb
Blueberry Syrup	1/4 cup	210	52	0	0	0	50	0	3 1/2 carb
Boysenberry Light Preserves	1 Tbsp	20	5	0	0	0	0	0	1 carb
Boysenberry Preserves	1 Tbsp	50	13	0	0	0	10	0	1 carb

SAUCES, GRAVIES, CONDIMENTS, RELISHES

	Serving	Calories	Carb. (g)	Fat (g)	% Cal. Fat	Sat. Fat (g)	Chol. (mg)	Sod. (mg)	Fib. (g)	Prot. (g)	Servings/ Exchanges
California Plum Jelly	1 Tbsp	50	13	0	0	0	0	10	0	0	1 carb
Crabapple Jelly	1 Tbsp	50	13	0	0	0	0	10	0	0	1 carb
Light Boysenberry Syrup	1/4 cup	100	25	0	0	0	0	20	0	0	1 1/2 carb
Mint Flavored Jelly	1 Tbsp	50	13	0	0	0	0	10	0	0	1 carb
Red Currant Jelly	1 Tbsp	50	13	0	0	0	0	10	0	0	1 carb
Red Raspberry Light Preserves	1 Tbsp	20	5	0	0	0	0	0	0	0	free
Red Raspberry Syrup	1/4 cup	210	52	0	0	0	0	50	0	0	3 1/2 carb
Seedless Red Raspberry Jam	1 Tbsp	50	13	0	0	0	0	10	0	0	1 carb
Strawberry Preserves	1 Tbsp	50	13	0	0	0	0	10	0	0	1 carb
Strawberry Syrup	1/4 cup	210	52	0	0	0	0	50	0	0	3 1/2 carb
Tomato Preserves	1 Tbsp	50	13	0	0	0	0	10	0	0	1 carb

Kozlowski Farms

100% Fruit Blueberry Spread	1 Tbsp	30	8	0	0	0	0	0	1/2 carb
100% Fruit Boysenberry Spread	1 Tbsp	45	11	0	0	0	0	0	1 carb
100% Fruit Cherry Spread	1 Tbsp	30	7	0	0	0	0	0	1/2 carb
100% Fruit Sweetened Apple Butter	1 Tbsp	25	6	0	0	0	20	0	1/2 carb
100% Fruit Sweetened Plum Butter	1 Tbsp	35	8	0	0	0	0	0	1/2 carb

Kraft

BBQ Sauce, Carb Well Original	2 Tbsp	15	3	0	0	0	390	0	free
BBQ Sauce, Hickory Smoke	2 Tbsp	40	9	0	0	0	420	0	1/2 carb
BBQ Sauce, Honey Hickory Smoke	2 Tbsp	60	14	0	0	0	360	0	1 carb

SAUCES, GRAVIES, CONDIMENTS, RELISHES

	Serving	Calories	Carb. (g)	Fat (g)	% Cal. Fat	Sat. Fat (g)	Chol. (mg)	Sod. (mg)	Fib. (g)	Prot. (g)	Servings/ Exchanges
BBQ Sauce, Honey	2 Tbsp	50	13	0	0	0	0	360	0	0	1 carb
BBQ Sauce, Honey Roasted Garlic	2 Tbsp	50	12	0	0	0	0	350	0	0	1 carb
BBQ Sauce, Mesquite Smoke	2 Tbsp	40	9	0	0	0	0	420	0	0	1/2 carb
BBQ Sauce, Original	2 Tbsp	40	11	0	0	0	0	420	0	0	1 carb
Sauce, Cocktail	1/4 cup	60	13	<1	0	0	0	800	1	1	1 carb
Sauce, Horseradish	1 tsp	20	<1	2	90	0	<5	35	0	0	free
Sauce, Horseradish, Cream-Style	1 tsp	0	0	0	0	0	0	50	0	0	free
Sauce, Horseradish, Mustard	1 tsp	0	0	0	0	0	0	55	0	0	free
Sauce, Lemon Herb Tartar	2 Tbsp	150	<1	16	96	3	15	170	0	0	3 fat
Sauce, Prepared Horseradish	1 tsp	0	0	0	0	0	0	50	0	0	free

Food	Serving											Exchanges
Sauce, Sauceworks Sweet & Sour	2 Tbsp	60	14	0	0	0	125	0	0			1 carb
Sauce, Tartar	2 Tbsp	90	90	4	40	9	2	10	170	0	0	
Sauce, Tartar, Fat-Free	2 Tbsp	25	5	0	0	0	200	0	0			free
La Choy												
Sauce, Brown Gravy	1 Tbsp	90	24	6	60	0	0	90	1	6		1 1/2 carb, 1 fat
Sauce, Plum	1 oz	45	11	<1	0	0	17	NA	<1			1 carb
Sauce, Soy	1 Tbsp	11	1	<1	0	0	1315	0	1			free
Sauce, Soy, Lite	1 Tbsp	15	2	<1	0	0	505	0	1			free
Sauce, Stir-Fry Mandarin Soy	1/2 cup	71	16	<1	0	0	851	1	2			1 carb
Sauce, Stir-Fry Szechwan	1/2 cup	73	16	<1	0	0	612	2	3			1 carb
Sauce, Stir-Fry Teriyaki	1/2 cup	90	21	<1	0	0	997	1	2			1 1/2 carb
Sauce, Sweet & Sour	1 Tbsp	26	7	<1	0	0	59	0	<1			1/2 carb
Sauce, Teriyaki	1 Tbsp	17	3	<1	0	0	917	0	1			free
Sauce, Teriyaki, Light	1 Tbsp	18	4	<1	0	0	439	0	1			free

SAUCES, GRAVIES, CONDIMENTS, RELISHES

	Serving	Calories	Carb. (g)	Fat (g)	% Cal. Fat	Sat. Fat (g)	Chol. (mg)	Sod. (mg)	Fib. (g)	Prot. (g)	Servings/ Exchanges
La Victoria											
Enchilada Sauce, Green Chili	1/4 cup	15	3	0	0	0	0	310	0	0	free
Enchilada Sauce, Hot Picante	1/4 cup	25	2	2	40	0	0	330	0	0	free
Green Taco Sauce	1 Tbsp	0	<1	0	0	0	0	70	0	0	free
Red Taco Sauce	1 Tbsp	5	1	0	0	0	0	90	0	0	free
Lawry's											
Carb Options, Asian Teriyaki	1 Tbsp	5	<1	<1	0	0	0	500	0	0	free
Carb Options, Steak Sauce	1 Tbsp	5	1	0	0	0	0	200	0	0	free
Marinade, Baja Chipotle	1 Tbsp	15	4	0	0	0	0	390	0	0	free
Marinade, Herb & Garlic	1 Tbsp	10	2	0	0	0	0	420	0	0	free
Marinade, Lemon Pepper	1 Tbsp	10	2	0	0	0	0	390	0	0	free
Marinade, Mesquite	1 Tbsp	5	1	0	0	0	0	350	0	0	free

Marinade, Sesame Ginger	1 Tbsp	30	7	0	0	0	0	580	0	0	1/2 carb
Marinade, Steak & Chop	1 Tbsp	5	<1	0	0	0	0	400	0	0	free
Marinade, Tequila Lime	1 Tbsp	15	4	0	0	0	0	490	0	0	free
Marinade, Teriyaki	1 Tbsp	20	5	0	0	0	0	560	0	0	free
Steak Sauce	1 Tbsp	10	3	0	0	0	0	250	0	0	free
Las Palmas											
Enchilada Sauce	1/4 cup	15	2	<1	0	0	0	310	1	0	free
Green Chili Enchilada Sauce	1/4 cup	25	3	1	60	0	0	260	0	0	free
Red Chili Sauce	1/4 cup	15	2	0	0	0	0	310	1	0	free
Libby's											
Gravy, Country Chicken	1/4 cup	60	3	4	60	<1	5	330	0	1	1 fat
Gravy, Country Sausage	1/4 cup	90	3	7	70	2	5	280	0	1	2 fat
Sauce, Sloppy Joe	1/3	45	10	0	0	0	0	430	1	1	1/2 carb
Sauce, Tomato	1/4 cup	20	4	0	0	0	0	280	<1	0	free
Log Cabin											
Country Kitchen Butter Syrup	1/4 cup	200	50	0	0	0	0	140	0	0	3 carb

SAUCES, GRAVIES, CONDIMENTS, RELISHES

	Serving	Calories	Carb. (g)	Fat (g)	% Cal. Fat	Sat. Fat (g)	Chol. (mg)	Sod. (mg)	Fib. (g)	Prot. (g)	Servings/ Exchanges
Country Kitchen Lite Syrup	1/4 cup	100	26	0	0	0	0	160	0	0	2 carb
Country Kitchen Original Syrup	1/4 cup	200	50	0	0	0	0	55	0	0	3 carb
Original Syrup	1/4 cup	210	53	0	0	0	0	100	0	0	3 1/2 carb
Sugar-Free Low Calorie Syrup	1/4 cup	35	12	0	0	0	0	100	0	0	1 carb
Maple Grove Farms Cozy Cottage											
Maple Syrup	1/4 cup	200	53	0	0	0	0	5	0	0	3 1/2 carb
Sugar-Free Low Calorie Syrup	1/4 cup	10	4	0	0	0	0	120	0	0	free
McCormick											
Bac 'n Pieces, Bits	1 1/2 Tbsp	30	2	2	50	0	0	220	0	3	1 fat
Salad Toppings	1 1/2 Tbsp	35	2	2	43	0	0	90	0	1	1 fat

Mezzetta

Cantina Antipasto	4 pieces	25	1	2	72	0	0	300	<1	0	1 fat
Cocktail Onions	12 pieces	5	1	0	0	0	0	300	0	0	free
Dilled Brussels Sprouts	1 1/2 sprouts	10	2	0	0	0	0	90	1	1	free
Garlic Olives	3	25	0	3	100	<1	0	260	<1	0	1 fat
Gourmet Baby Corn	4 pieces	4	1	0	0	0	0	120	0	0	free
Grape Leaves	1 leaf	5	1	0	0	0	0	100	0	0	free
Hors D'oeuvre Gourmet Okra	3 pieces	10	2	0	0	0	0	260	1	0	free
Hors D'oeuvre Onions	5 pieces	5	1	0	0	0	0	300	0	0	free
Hot Banana Wax Peppers	1/4 cup	10	2	0	0	0	0	310	0	0	free
Hot Pepper Relish	· Tbsp	25	6	0	0	0	0	60	0	0	1/2 carb
Italian Wax Peppers	8–10 pieces	10	1	0	0	0	0	320	0	0	free
Jalapeño Stuffed Olives	1 1/2 olives	15	1	1	100	0	0	170	0	0	free
Marinated Artichoke Hearts	2 pieces	20	2	2	90	0	0	80	1	0	free
Roasted Bell Peppers	1 1/2 Tbsp	10	1	0	0	0	0	110	0	0	free

SAUCES, GRAVIES, CONDIMENTS, RELISHES

	Serving	Calories	Carb. (g)	Fat (g)	% Cal. Fat	Sat. Fat (g)	Chol. (mg)	Sod. (mg)	Fib. (g)	Prot. (g)	Servings/ Exchanges
Sliced Jalapeño Peppers	1/4 cup	5	1	0	0	0	0	380	0	0	free
Spanish Queen Olives	3	15	0	2	100	0	0	160	1	0	free
Sweet Bell Pepper Relish	1 Tbsp	25	6	0	0	0	0	55	0	0	1/2 carb
Mrs. Butterworth's											
Original Syrup	1/4 cup	220	55	0	0	0	0	130	0	0	4 carb
Reduced Calorie Lite	1/4 cup	100	25	0	0	0	0	130	0	0	1 1/2 carb
Mrs. Dash											
10 Minute Marinade, Lemon Herb Peppercorn	1 Tbsp	25	2	2	60	0	0	0	0	0	free
10 Minute Marinade, Mesquite Grille	1 Tbsp	25	2	2	15	0	0	0	0	0	free
10 Minute Marinade, Southwestern Chipotle	1 Tbsp	20	2	2	75	0	0	0	0	0	free
10 Minute Marinade, Zesty Garlic Herb	1 Tbsp	25	3	2	15	0	0	0	0	0	free

Musselman's

	Serving									Exchanges
Apple Butter	1 Tbsp	30	8	0	0	0	0	0	0	1/2 carb

Ocean Spray

	Serving									Exchanges
Jellied Cranberry Sauce	1/4 cup	110	27	0	0	0	35	1	0	2 carb
Whole Berry Cranberry Sauce	1/4 cup	110	28	0	0	0	35	1	0	2 carb

Old El Paso

	Serving									Exchanges
Enchilada Sauce, Green Chili	1/4 cup	25	3	1	60	0	260	0	0	free
Enchilada Sauce, Mild	1/4 cup	25	3	1	36	0	270	0	1	free
Grilling Sauce, Chili Pepper & Spice	2 Tbsp	60	14	0	0	0	380	0	<1	1 carb
Grilling Sauce, Sweet 'N Smoky	2 Tbsp	60	14	0	0	0	380	0	<1	1 carb
Relish, Jalapeño	1 Tbsp	5	1	0	0	0	110	0	0	free
Taco Sauce, Hot	1 Tbsp	5	1	0	0	0	90	0	0	free

SAUCES, GRAVIES, CONDIMENTS, RELISHES

	Serving	Calories	Carb. (g)	Fat (g)	% Cal. Fat	Sat. Fat (g)	Chol. (mg)	Sod. (mg)	Fib. (g)	Prot. (g)	Servings/ Exchanges
Taco Sauce, Medium	1 Tbsp	5	1	0	0	0	0	70	0	0	free
Taco Sauce, Mild	1 Tbsp	5	1	0	0	0	0	85	0	0	free
Tomatoes & Green Chilis	1/4 cup	10	2	0	0	0	0	300	0	0	free
Open Pit											
BBQ Sauce, Hickory Flavor	2 Tbsp	50	11	0	0	0	0	380	0	0	1 carb
BBQ Sauce, Hot	2 Tbsp	50	11	0	0	0	0	380	0	0	1 carb
BBQ Sauce, Mesquite	2 Tbsp	50	11	<1	0	0	0	440	0	0	1 carb
BBQ Sauce, Onion Flavor	2 Tbsp	50	11	0	0	0	0	480	0	0	1 carb
BBQ Sauce, Original Flavor	2 Tbsp	50	11	0	0	0	0	450	0	0	1 carb
BBQ Sauce, Sweet Flavor	2 Tbsp	50	12	0	0	0	0	300	0	0	1 carb
BBQ Sauce, Sweet & Sour	2 Tbsp	45	10	0	0	0	0	420	0	0	1/2 carb
BBQ Sauce, Thick Tangy Onion	2 Tbsp	50	12	0	0	0	0	380	0	0	1 carb

BBQ Sauce, Thick Tangy Hickory	2 Tbsp	50	12	0	0	0	390	0	1 carb
BBQ Sauce, Thick Tangy Honey Spice	2 Tbsp	45	11	0	0	0	340	0	1 carb
Ortega									
Enchilada Sauce	1 oz	12	3	0	0	0	280	0	free
Green Chilis, Strips	2	10	3	0	0	0	25	<1	<1 free
Sauce/Puree, Green Chili	1/4 cup	15	3	0	0	0	0	1	free
Sauce/Puree, Jalapeño	1/4 cup	15	3	0	0	0	0	1	free
Sauce/Puree, Red Chili	1/4 cup	15	3	0	0	0	0	1	free
Sauce/Puree, Red Jalapeño	1/4 cup	15	3	0	0	0	0	1	free
Taco Sauce, Mexican Style	1 Tbsp	10	3	0	0	0	170	0	free
Taco Sauce, Original	1 Tbsp	10	0	0	0	0	120	0	free
Taco Sauce, Red Chili	1 Tbsp	10	3	0	0	0	130	0	free
Taco Sauce, Smokey Chipotle	1 Tbsp	10	3	0	0	0	170	0	free

SAUCES, GRAVIES, CONDIMENTS, RELISHES

	Serving	Calories	Carb. (g)	Fat (g)	% Cal. Fat	Sat. Fat (g)	Chol. (mg)	Sod. (mg)	Fib. (g)	Prot. (g)	Servings/ Exchanges
Oscar Mayer											
Bacon Bits	1 Tbsp	20	1	1	45	<1	5	180	0	3	free
Pace											
Enchilada Sauce	1/4 cup	25	5	0	0	0	0	520	1	1	free
Prego											
Chunky Garden Pasta Sauce, Garden Combination	1/2 cup	90	17	2	20	<1	0	470	3	2	1 carb
Chunky Garden Pasta Sauce, Mushrooms & Green Pepper	1/2 cup	110	17	4	33	1	0	470	4	2	1 carb, 1 fat
Chunky Garden Pasta Sauce, Mushroom Supreme	1/2 cup	120	20	4	30	1	0	470	4	2	1 carb, 1 fat
Hearty Meat Sauce, Authentic Sausage	1/2 cup	150	16	7	42	3	15	600	2	6	1 carb, 1 fat

Hearty Meat Sauce, Classic Meat Sauce with Fresh Mushroom	1/2 cup	130	14	6	28	3	10	660	2	6	1 carb, 1 fat
Hearty Meat Sauce, Meatball Parmesan	1/2 cup	160	16	8	45	3	10	690	2	7	1 carb, 1 med-fat meat, 1 fat
Hearty Meat Sauce, Three Meat Supreme	1/2 cup	170	12	10	53	4	15	600	3	7	1 carb, 1 med-fat meat, 1 fat
Pasta Bake Sauce, Three Cheese Marinara	1/2 cup	100	11	5	45	1	5	650	2	3	1 carb, 1 fat
Pasta Bake Sauce, Tomato, Garlic & Basil	1/2 cup	80	11	4	45	<1	0	530	2	1	1 carb, 1 fat
Pasta Sauce, Flavored with Meat	1/2 cup	130	19	5	35	1	5	570	3	2	1 carb, 1 fat
Pasta Sauce, Fresh Mushroom	1/2 cup	110	18	4	32	1	0	550	3	2	1 carb, 1 fat

SAUCES, GRAVIES, CONDIMENTS, RELISHES

	Serving	Calories	Carb. (g)	Fat (g)	% Cal. Fat	Sat. Fat (g)	Chol. (mg)	Sod. (mg)	Fib. (g)	Prot. (g)	Servings/ Exchanges
Pasta Sauce, Garlic Supreme	1/2 cup	120	17	5	38	2	0	470	3	2	1 carb, 1 fat
Pasta Sauce, Marinara	1/2 cup	100	11	5	45	1	0	550	4	2	1 carb, 1 fat
Pasta Sauce, Marinara with Cheese	1/2 cup	100	11	5	45	1	5	550	4	3	1 carb, 1 fat
Pasta Sauce, Mini Meatball	1/2 cup	150	20	6	36	2	10	650	3	4	1 carb, 1 fat
Pasta Sauce, Mushroom Parmesan	1/2 cup	130	22	4	28	2	5	480	3	3	1 1/2 carb, 1 fat
Pasta Sauce, Ricotta Parmesan	1/2 cup	120	20	4	30	2	5	500	3	3	1 carb, 1 fat
Pasta Sauce, Roasted Red Pepper & Garlic	1/2 cup	120	19	4	30	<1	0	530	3	2	1 carb, 1 fat
Pasta Sauce, Three Cheese	1/2 cup	90	17	2	20	1	5	430	3	2	1 carb

Food	Serving										Exchanges
Pasta Sauce, Tomato, Basil & Cheese	1/2 cup	90	17	2	20	1	0	420	3	2	1 carb
Pasta Sauce, Traditional	1/2 cup	120	19	4	30	1	0	580	3	2	1 carb, 1 fat
Progresso											
Artichoke Hearts	2 pieces	30	6	0	0	0	0	240	1	2	1/2 carb
Pasta Sauce, Meat-Flavored	1/2 cup	100	12	5	45	1	5	610	3	4	1 carb, 1 fat
Pizza Sauce	1/4 cup	20	4	0	0	0	0	170	1	<1	free
Sauce, Authentic Alfredo	1/2 cup	200	7	15	68	10	50	850	1	8	1/2 carb, 1 med-fat meat, 3 fat
Sauce, Authentic White Clam	1/2 cup	150	5	10	60	2	20	710	0	9	1 med-fat meat, 1 fat
Sauce, Creamy Clam	1/2 cup	110	8	6	49	2	10	440	0	5	1/2 carb, 1 fat
Sauce, Lobster	1/2 cup	100	6	7	63	1	2	430	2	3	1/2 carb, 1 fat
Sauce, Marinara	1/2 cup	100	12	4	36	1	<5	590	3	4	1 carb, 1 fat
Sauce, Red Clam	1/2 cup	60	8	1	15	0	10	350	1	4	1/2 carb, 1 very lean meat
Spaghetti Sauce	1/2 cup	100	12	5	45	1	<5	620	2	3	1 carb, 1 fat

SAUCES, GRAVIES, CONDIMENTS, RELISHES

	Serving	Calories	Carb. (g)	Fat (g)	% Cal. Fat	Sat. Fat (g)	Chol. (mg)	Sod. (mg)	Fib. (g)	Prot. (g)	Servings/ Exchanges
Ragú											
Carb Options, Alfredo Sauce	1/4 cup	110	2	10	82	4	30	390	0	1	2 fat
Carb Options, Double Cheddar	1/4 cup	90	2	8	78	3	25	480	0	0	2 fat
Carb Options, Garden Style Sauce	1/4 cup	80	7	5	50	<1	0	540	2	2	1/2 carb, 1 fat
Cheese Creations, Classic Alfredo	1/4 cup	110	3	10	82	4	30	400	0	1	2 fat
Cheese Creations, Parmesan Mozzarella	1/4 cup	60	3	5	67	3	25	460	0	2	1 fat
Cheese Creations, Roasted Garlic Parmesan	1/4 cup	110	3	10	82	3	20	400	0	2	2 fat

Meat Sauce, Rich & Meaty Classic Italian	1/2 cup	130	10	8	54	3	15	550	2	5	1/2 carb, 2 fat
Pasta Sauce, Chunky Garden Style Tomatoes, Garlic & Onion	1/2 cup	110	21	3	23	0	0	510	2	2	1 1/2 carb, 1 fat
Pasta Sauce, Flavored with Meat	1/2 cup	70	7	3	36	<1	0	750	2	2	1/2 carb, 1 fat
Pasta Sauce, Old World Style Traditional	1/2 cup	70	10	3	36	0	0	770	2	2	1/2 carb, 1 fat
Pasta Sauce, Traditional	1/2 cup	70	8	3	36	0	0	770	2	2	1/2 carb, 1 fat
Pizza Quick Snack Sauce, Traditional	1/4 cup	40	4	2	50	0	0	380	1	1	1/2 carb
Robusto, Pasta Sauce, Six Cheese	1/2 cup	90	12	4	33	1	<5	580	2	3	1 carb, 1 fat
Regina										
Cooking Wine, Burgundy	1/4 cup	20	1	1	45	0	0	365	0	1	free

SAUCES, GRAVIES, CONDIMENTS, RELISHES

	Serving	Calories	Carb. (g)	Fat (g)	% Cal. Fat	Sat. Fat (g)	Chol. (mg)	Sod. (mg)	Fib. (g)	Prot. (g)	Servings/ Exchanges
Cooking Wine, Sherry	1/4 cup	20	5	0	0	0	0	70	0	1	1/2 carb
Vinegar, Red Wine, 50 Grain	1 oz	4	0	0	0	0	0	0	0	0	free
Vinegar, White Wine	1 oz	4	1	0	0	0	0	0	0	0	free
Roland											
Cornichons Gherkins	6 pieces	5	1	0	0	0	0	360	1	0	free
Green Peppercorns in Wine Vinegar	2 Tbsp	15	3	0	0	0	0	430	1	0	free
Heart of Palm	1/2 cup	25	4	<1	0	0	0	450	2	2	free
Smucker's											
Apricot-Pineapple Preserves	1 Tbsp	50	13	0	0	0	0	0	0	0	1 carb
Apricot Preserves	1 Tbsp	50	13	0	0	0	0	0	0	0	1 carb
Blueberry Syrup	1/4 cup	210	52	0	0	0	0	0	0	0	3 1/2 carb
Boysenberry Preserves	1 Tbsp	50	13	0	0	0	0	0	0	0	1 carb

Food	Serving									
Boysenberry Syrup	1/4 cup	210	52	0	0	0	0	0	0	3 1/2 carb
Cider Apple Butter	1 Tbsp	45	11	0	0	0	0	10	0	1 carb
Concord Grape Jam	1 Tbsp	50	13	0	0	0	0	0	0	1 carb
Currant Jelly	1 Tbsp	50	13	0	0	0	0	0	0	1 carb
Light Sugar-Free Apricot Preserves	1 Tbsp	10	5	0	0	0	0	0	0	free
Light Sugar-Free Blackberry Jam	1 Tbsp	10	5	0	0	0	0	0	0	free
Light Sugar-Free Strawberry Preserves	1 Tbsp	10	5	0	0	0	0	0	0	free
Low Sugar Apricot Preserves	1 Tbsp	25	6	0	0	0	0	0	0	1/2 carb
Low Sugar Concord Grape Jelly	1 Tbsp	25	6	0	0	0	0	0	0	1/2 carb
Low Sugar Strawberry Preserves	1 Tbsp	25	6	0	0	0	0	0	0	1/2 carb

SAUCES, GRAVIES, CONDIMENTS, RELISHES

	Serving	Calories	Carb. (g)	Fat (g)	% Cal. Fat	Sat. Fat (g)	Chol. (mg)	Sod. (mg)	Fib. (g)	Prot. (g)	Servings/ Exchanges
Low Sugar Sweet Orange Marmalade	1 Tbsp	25	6	0	0	0	0	0	0	0	1/2 carb
Peach Butter	1 Tbsp	45	11	0	0	0	0	10	0	0	1 carb
Red Raspberry Preserves	1 Tbsp	50	13	0	0	0	0	0	0	0	1 carb
Simply 100% Fruit Spreadable Fruit, All Varieties	1 Tbsp	40–45	10–11	0	0	0	0	0–10	0	0	1/2 carb
Squeeze Grape Jelly	1 Tbsp	50	13	0	0	0	0	0	0	0	1 carb
Squeeze Strawberry Fruit Spread	1 Tbsp	50	13	0	0	0	0	0	0	0	1 carb
Strawberry Jam	1 Tbsp	50	13	0	0	0	0	0	0	0	1 carb
Strawberry Preserves	1 Tbsp	50	13	0	0	0	0	0	0	0	1 carb
Sweet Orange Marmalade	1 Tbsp	50	13	0	0	0	0	0	0	0	1 carb

Sorrell Ridge

100% Spreadable Fruit, All Varieties	1 Tbsp	36	9	0	0	0	0	0	0	1/2 carb

Tabasco

Sauce, Pepper	1 tsp	0	0	0	0	0	0	30	0	free
Sauce, Green Pepper	1 tsp	0	0	0	0	0	0	140	0	free

Trappy's Red Devil

Cayenne Pepper Sauce	1 tsp	0	0	0	0	0	0	150	0	free

Vermont

Sugar-Free Low Calorie Syrup	1/4 cup	10	4	0	0	0	0	120	0	free

Vlasic

Mild Pepperoncini Peppers	2 peppers	5	1	0	0	0	0	440	0	free
Stackers Mild Pepper Rings	12	5	1	0	0	0	0	480	0	free

SAUCES, GRAVIES, CONDIMENTS, RELISHES

	Serving	Calories	Carb. (g)	Fat (g)	% Cal. Fat	Sat. Fat (g)	Chol. (mg)	Sod. (mg)	Fib. (g)	Prot. (g)	Servings/ Exchanges
Sweet Gherkins	3	35	9	0	0	0	0	170	0	0	1/2 carb
Zesty Cherry Peppers	2	10	1	0	0	0	0	480	0	0	free
Zesty Jalapeño Peppers	2	5	1	0	0	0	0	470	0	0	free
Welch's											
Concord Grape Jam	1 Tbsp	50	13	0	0	0	0	15	0	0	1 carb
Concord Grape Jelly	1 Tbsp	50	13	0	0	0	0	15	0	0	1 carb
Squeezable Concord Grape Jelly	1 Tbsp	50	13	0	0	0	0	15	0	0	1 carb
Squeezable Strawberry Spread	1 Tbsp	50	13	0	0	0	0	10	0	0	1 carb
Strawberry Spread	1 Tbsp	50	13	0	0	0	0	10	0	0	1 carb

SNACKS, CRACKERS, CHIPS, POPCORN, SNACK BARS

	Serving	Calories	Carb. (g)	Fat (g)	% Cal. Fat	Sat. Fat (g)	Chol. (mg)	Sod. (mg)	Fib. (g)	Prot. (g)	Servings/ Exchanges
Chips, Bagel	5	298	52	7	21	1	0	419	6	6	3 1/2 strch, 1 fat
Chips, Yogurt	1 oz	148	16	8	49	2	1	13	<1	3	1 strch, 2 fat
Cracker Crumbs, Graham	1/2 cup	254	46	6	21	1	0	363	2	4	3 strch, 1 fat
Crackers, Animal	8	45	7	1	20	<1	0	39	<1	<1	1/2 strch
Crackers, Graham	8	89	16	2	20	<1	0	127	<1	1	1 strch
Crackers, Matzoh, Plain	1 oz	112	24	<1	0	<1	0	<1	<1	3	1 1/2 strch
Crackers, Matzoh, Whole-Wheat	1	100	22	<1	0	<1	0	<1	3	4	1 1/2 strch
Crackers, Norwegian Flatbread	5	106	24	<1	0		0	77	5	2	1 1/2 strch
Crackers, Rye Crispbread	2	59	13	<1	0	<1	0	150	2	2	1 strch
Crispbread, Rye	1	37	8	<1	0	<1	0	26	2	<1	1/2 strch
Melba Toast	2	39	8	<1	0	<1	0	83	<1	1	1/2 strch

SNACKS, CRACKERS, CHIPS, POPCORN, SNACK BARS

	Serving	Calories	Carb. (g)	Fat (g)	% Cal. Fat	Sat. Fat (g)	Chol. (mg)	Sod. (mg)	Fib. (g)	Prot. (g)	Servings/ Exchanges
Oriental Snack Mix	1 oz	155	9	12	70	5	0	235	4	5	1/2 strch, 2 fat
Popcorn, Air-Popped	1 cup	31	6	<1	0	<1	0	<1	1	<1	1/2 strch
Popcorn, Caramel	1 cup	152	28	5	30	1	2	73	2	1	1 strch, 1 fat
Popcorn, Cheese	1 cup	58	6	4	62	<1	1	98	1	1	1/2 strch, 1 fat
Popcorn, Oil-Popped, Salted	1 cup	55	6	3	49	<1	0	97	1	4	1/2 strch, 1 fat
Popcorn Cakes	2	76	16	<1	0	<1	0	58	<1	2	1 strch
Pretzel Twists, Hard, Unsalted	1 oz	108	23	<1	0	<1	0	486	<1	3	1 1/2 strch
Pretzels, Whole-Wheat	1 oz	103	23	<1	0	<1	0	58	2	3	1 1/2 strch
Pretzels, Yogurt-Covered	5	96	14	4	38	3	<1	13	<1	2	1 strch, 1 fat
Rice Cakes, Brown, Plain	2	70	15	<1	0	<1	0	59	<1	2	1 strch
Rice Cakes, Brown, Sesame Seed	2	71	15	<1	0	<1	0	41	<1	1	1 strch

Trail Mix	1/4 cup	173	17	11	57	2	0	86	2	5	1 strch, 2 fat
Brands											
Act II											
Microwave Popcorn, 94% Fat-Free Butter	1 cup	15	4	0	0	0	0	30	<1	<1	free
Microwave Popcorn, Butter Lover's	1 cup	40	4	3	68	<1	0	80	<1	<1	1 fat
Microwave Popcorn, Kettle Corn	1 cup	15	4	0	0	0	0	25	<1	<1	free
Microwave Popcorn, Light Butter	1 cup	25	5	1	40	0	0	60	<1	<1	1/2 carb
Austin											
Cracker Sandwiches, Cheese & Peanut Butter	1 pkg	190	22	10	47	2	0	310	1	4	1 1/2 strch, 2 fat
Cracker Sandwiches, Toast & Peanut Butter	1 pkg	200	23	10	45	2	0	380	1	4	1 1/2 strch, 2 fat

SNACKS, CRACKERS, CHIPS, POPCORN, SNACK BARS

	Serving	Calories	Carb. (g)	Fat (g)	% Cal. Fat	Sat. Fat (g)	Chol. (mg)	Sod. (mg)	Fib. (g)	Prot. (g)	Servings/ Exchanges
Cracker Sandwiches, Wheat & Cheddar	1 pkg	200	24	10	45	2	0	370	<1	3	1 1/2 strch, 2 fat
Barbara's Bakery											
Nature's Choice Multigrain Cereal Bars, All Varieties	1 bar	120	25	1	13	0	0	65	2	1	1 1/2 carb
Puffins Cereal & Milk Bars, French Toast	1 bar	130	25	1	7	1	0	100	3	5	1 1/2 carb
Puffins Cereal & Milk Bars, Strawberry Yogurt	1 bar	130	24	2	12	1	0	90	3	5	1 1/2 carb
Betty Crocker											
Fruit By The Foot	1 roll	80	17	2	23	1	0	50	0	0	1 carb
Fruit Gushers	1 pouch	90	20	1	11	0	0	55	0	0	1 carb
Fruit Roll-Ups, Strawberry Kiwi	1	50	12	1	10	0	0	55	0	0	1 carb

Fruit Smoothie Blitz Fruit Snacks	1 pouch	140	32	1	7	0	0	70	0	0	2 carb
Pop-Secret Popcorn, Butter	1 cup	40	4	3	68	<1	0	50	<1	<1	1 fat
Pop-Secret Popcorn, Movie Theater Butter	1 cup	40	3	3	68	<1	0	55	<1	<1	1 fat
Pop-Secret Popcorn, Natural	1 cup	35	4	3	77	<1	0	65	<1	<1	1 fat
Cracker Jack											
Butter Toffee Clusters	3/4 cup	140	22	4	26	2	0	100	1	2	1 1/2 carb, 1 fat
Original	1/2 cup	120	23	2	15	0	0	70	1	2	1 1/2 carb
Entenmann's											
Multi-Grain Chewy Cereal Bars, Chocolate Chip with Raisins	1 bar	140	28	3	18	1	0	100	2	2	2 carb, 1 fat
Multi-Grain Chewy Cereal Bars, Oatmeal Apple Raisin	1 bar	140	27	3	18	0	0	110	2	2	2 carb, 1 fat

SNACKS, CRACKERS, CHIPS, POPCORN, SNACK BARS

	Serving	Calories	Carb. (g)	Fat (g)	% Cal. Fat	Sat. Fat (g)	Chol. (mg)	Sod. (mg)	Fib. (g)	Prot. (g)	Servings/ Exchanges
Multi-Grain Fruit-Filled Cereal Bar, Strawberry	1 bar	140	26	2	18	0	0	110	0	1	2 carb, 1 fat
Franklin											
Crunch 'N Munch	2/3 cup	150	23	6	36	2	10	100	<1	2	1 1/2 carb, 1 fat
Crunch 'N Munch, Buttery Toffee	2/3 cup	150	22	6	36	2	5	170	<1	2	1 1/2 carb, 1 fat
Frito-Lay											
Baken-ets Fried Pork Rind, Hot 'N Spicy Cracklins	8	80	<1	5	56	2	20	330	<1	7	1 med-fat meat
Baken-ets Fried Pork Rind, Regular	8	90	<1	6	56	2	15	550	<1	7	1 med-fat meat
Cheetos, Baked	1 oz	130	19	5	35	1	0	240	0	2	1 strch, 1 fat
Cheetos, Crunchy	1 oz	160	15	10	56	3	0	290	<1	2	1 strch, 2 fat

Cheetos, Flamin' Hot	1 oz	170	11	11	65	2	0	250	<1	2	1 strch, 2 fat
Cheetos, Golden Toast Crackers	1 pkg	240	25	14	53	4	5	440	1	4	1 1/2 strch, 3 fat
Cheetos, Puffs	1 oz	160	13	10	56	2	0	350	<1	2	1 strch, 2 fat
Chester's Butter Popcorn	3 cups	170	16	12	64	2	0	330	3	2	1 strch, 2 fat
Chester's Cheddar Cheese Popcorn	3 cups	200	17	13	59	3	0	340	2	3	1 strch, 3 fat
Crackers, Cheese Sandwich Crackers	1 pkg	210	23	10	43	3	0	350	1	5	1 1/2 strch, 2 fat
Crackers, Peanut Butter Sandwich Crackers	1 pkg	210	23	10	43	3	0	350	<1	5	1 1/2 strch, 2 fat
Doritos, Baked, Cooler Ranch	1 oz	120	21	5	25	<1	0	200	2	2	1 1/2 strch, 1 fat
Doritos, Cooler Ranch	1 oz	140	18	7	43	2	0	170	1	2	1 strch, 1 fat
Doritos, Four Cheese	1 oz	140	17	8	50	1	0	240	1	2	1 strch, 2 fat
Doritos, Guacamole	1 oz	150	16	8	48	2	0	230	1	4	1 strch, 2 fat

SNACKS, CRACKERS, CHIPS, POPCORN, SNACK BARS

	Serving	Calories	Carb. (g)	Fat (g)	% Cal. Fat	Sat. Fat (g)	Chol. (mg)	Sod. (mg)	Fib. (g)	Prot. (g)	Servings/ Exchanges
Doritos, Light Nacho Cheesier	1 oz	90	18	1	9	0	0	240	1	2	1 strch
Doritos, Nacho Cheesier	1 oz	140	17	7	50	1	0	200	1	2	1 strch, 1 fat
Doritos, Rollitos, Cooler Ranch	1 oz	140	17	8	50	2	0	250	1	2	1 strch, 2 fat
Doritos, Salsa	1 oz	140	17	7	45	1	0	170	1	3	1strch, 1 fat
Doritos, Spicier Nacho	1 oz	140	18	7	45	2	0	210	1	2	1 strch, 1 fat
Doritos, Toasted Corn	1 oz	140	18	7	45	1	0	120	1	2	1 strch, 1 fat
Fritos, BBQ	1 oz	150	16	10	60	2	0	280	1	2	1 strch, 2 fat
Fritos, Chili Cheese	1 oz	160	15	10	56	2	0	260	1	2	1 strch, 2 fat
Fritos, Flamin' Hot	1 oz	160	15	10	56	2	0	160	1	2	1 strch, 2 fat
Fritos, Flavor Twists, Cheddar Ranch	1 oz	150	17	9	53	2	0	230	1	2	1 strch, 2 fat
Fritos, Original	1 oz	160	15	10	56	2	0	170	1	2	1 strch, 2 fat

Food	Serving										
Fritos, Sabrositas Lime 'N Chili	1 oz	150	17	9	54	2	0	240	1	2	1 strch, 2 fat
Fritos, Scoops	1 oz	160	16	10	45	2	0	110	1	2	1 strch, 2 fat
Funyuns	1 oz	140	18	7	45	2	0	270	<1	2	1 strch, 1 fat
Lay's, Baked KC Masterpiece BBQ Potato Chips	1 oz	120	22	3	23	0	0	210	2	2	1 1/2 strch, 1 fat
Lay's, Baked Original Potato Chips	1 oz	110	23	2	16	0	0	150	2	2	1 1/2 strch
Lay's, Baked Sour Cream & Onion Potato Chips	1 oz	120	21	3	23	0	0	210	2	2	1 1/2 strch, 1 fat
Lay's, Classic Potato Chips	1 oz	150	15	10	60	3	0	180	1	2	1 strch, 2 fat
Lay's, Deli Style Original Potato Chips	1 oz	150	16	10	60	3	0	180	1	1	1 strch, 2 fat
Lay's, Flamin' Hot Potato Chips	1 oz	160	15	10	56	3	0	330	1	2	1 strch, 2 fat

SNACKS, CRACKERS, CHIPS, POPCORN, SNACK BARS

	Serving	Calories	Carb. (g)	Fat (g)	% Cal. Fat	Sat. Fat (g)	Chol. (mg)	Sod. (mg)	Fib. (g)	Prot. (g)	Servings/ Exchanges
Lay's, KC Masterpiece BBQ Potato Chips	1 oz	150	15	10	60	3	0	200	1	2	1 strch, 2 fat
Lay's, Kettle Cooked, Original	1 oz	150	16	8	53	3	0	190	1	2	1 strch, 2 fat
Lay's, Light Original Fat-Free	1 oz	75	18	0	0	0	0	200	1	2	1 strch
Lay's, Natural Sea Salted, Kettle Cooked	1 oz	150	15	9	53	1	0	180	1	2	1 strch, 2 fat
Lay's, Salt & Vinegar Potato Chips	1 oz	150	15	10	60	3	0	380	1	2	1 strch, 2 fat
Lay's, Stax, Original	1 oz	160	15	10	56	3	0	160	1	1	1 strch, 2 fat
Lay's, Wavy Original Potato Chips	1 oz	150	15	10	60	3	0	180	1	2	1 strch, 2 fat
Lay's, Wavy Au Gratin Potato Chips	1 oz	150	14	10	60	3	<5	200	1	2	1 strch, 2 fat

Lay's, Wavy Hidden Valley Ranch Potato Chips	1 oz	150	16	10	60	3	200	1	2	1 strch, 2 fat
Munchos	1 oz	160	16	10	56	2	230	1	1	1 strch, 2 fat
Munchies, Flamin Hot	3/4 cup	140	17	6	39	1	190	1	2	1 strch, 1 fat
Rold Gold, Cheddar Tiny Twists Pretzels	1 oz	110	22	1	8	0	370	1	3	1 1/2 strch
Rold Gold, Honey Mustard Tiny Twists Pretzels	1 oz	110	23	1	8	0	430	1	3	1 1/2 strch
Rold Gold, Sour Dough Pretzels	1 oz	110	23	<1	0	0	470	1	3	1 1/2 strch
Rold Gold, Stick Pretzels	1 oz	100	23	0	0	0	460	1	2	1 1/2 strch
Rold Gold, Tiny Twists Pretzels	1 oz	110	23	1	8	0	580	1	2	1 1/2 strch
Ruffles, Baked, Cheddar & Sour Cream	1 oz	120	22	3	25	<1	220	2	2	1 1/2 strch, 1 fat
Ruffles, Baked, Original	1 oz	120	21	3	25	0	200	2	2	1 1/2 strch, 1 fat

SNACKS, CRACKERS, CHIPS, POPCORN, SNACK BARS

	Serving	Calories	Carb. (g)	Fat (g)	% Cal. Fat	Sat. Fat (g)	Chol. (mg)	Sod. (mg)	Fib. (g)	Prot. (g)	Servings/ Exchanges
Ruffles, Cheddar & Sour Cream Potato Chips	1 oz	160	14	10	56	3	0	230	1	2	1 strch, 2 fat
Ruffles, KC Masterpiece Mesquite BBQ Potato Chips	1 oz	150	16	10	60	3	0	190	1	2	1 strch, 2 fat
Ruffles, Light Fat-Free Regular Potato Chips	1 oz	70	17	0	0	0	0	190	1	2	1 strch
Ruffles, Original Potato Chips	1 oz	160	14	10	56	3	0	160	1	2	1 strch, 2 fat
Ruffles, Sour Cream & Onion Potato Chips	1 oz	160	14	10	56	3	0	190	1	2	1 strch, 2 fat
Santitas White Corn Tortilla Chips	1 oz	130	19	6	42	1	0	110	1	2	1 strch, 1 fat

Santitas Yellow Corn Tortilla Strips	1 oz	130	19	6	42	1	0	110	1	2	1 strch, 1 fat
Smartfood White Cheddar Cheese Popcorn	1 pkg	160	14	10	56	2	5	290	2	3	1 strch, 2 fat
Smartfood White Cheddar Cheese Popcorn, Reduced-Fat	3 cups	140	19	6	39	2	<5	280	3	4	1 strch, 1 fat
Sunchips, French Onion	1 oz	140	18	6	39	1	0	160	2	2	1 strch, 1 fat
Sunchips, Harvest Cheddar	1 oz	140	19	6	39	1	0	170	2	2	1 strch, 1 fat
Sunchips, Original	1 oz	140	19	6	39	1	0	115	2	2	1 strch, 1 fat
Tostitos, Baked Bite Size	1 oz	110	24	1	8	0	0	200	2	3	1 1/2 strch
Tostitos, Bite Size	1 oz	140	17	8	50	1	0	110	1	2	1 strch, 2 fat
Tostitos, Crispy Rounds	1 oz	140	18	7	50	1	0	120	1	2	1 strch, 1 fat
Tostitos, Restaurant-Style	1 oz	130	19	6	42	1	0	80	1	2	1 strch, 1 fat
Tostitos, Restaurant-Style, Hint of Lime	1 oz	140	19	6	39	1	0	160	1	2	1 strch, 1 fat

SNACKS, CRACKERS, CHIPS, POPCORN, SNACK BARS

	Serving	Calories	Carb. (g)	Fat (g)	% Cal. Fat	Sat. Fat (g)	Chol. (mg)	Sod. (mg)	Fib. (g)	Prot. (g)	Servings/ Exchanges
Tostitos, Santa Fe Rounds	1 oz	140	19	6	39	1	0	80	1	2	1 strch, 1 fat
Gardetto's											
Snack Mix, Snak-ens, Original	1/2 cup	160	20	7	39	1	0	330	1	4	1 strch, 2 fat
General Mills											
Bugles, Baked, Original	1 1/3 cup	160	18	9	51	8	0	310	<1	1	1 strch, 2 fat
Chex Milk 'n Cereal Bars	1 bar	160	26	4	22	1	0	150	0	6	2 carb, 1 fat
Chex Mix, Bold Party Blend	1/2 cup	140	20	6	39	1	0	390	<1	3	1 strch, 1 fat
Chex Mix, Cheddar Cheese	2/3 cup	130	22	4	28	1	0	370	<1	2	1 1/2 strch, 1 fat
Chex Mix For Kids	2/3 cup	130	22	3	23	1	0	430	<1	2	1 1/2 strch, 1 fat
Chex Mix, Peanut Lovers	1/2 cup	140	19	6	36	1	0	340	1	3	1 strch, 1 fat
Chex Mix, Sweet 'n Salty Trail Mix	1/2 cup	140	22	5	29	2	0	230	1	2	1 1/2 strch, 1 fat
Chex Mix, Traditional	2/3 cup	130	1	4	27	<1	0	380	2	2	1 1/2 strch, 1 fat

Food	Serving										Exchanges/Choices
Cinnamon Toast Crunch Milk 'n Cereal Bar	1 bar	180	31	4	19	1	0	180	1	6	2 carb, 1 fat
Cocoa Puffs Milk 'n Cereal Bar	1 bar	160	26	4	22	1	0	130	1	6	2 carb, 1 fat
Honey Nut Cheerios Milk 'n Cereal Bar	1 bar	160	26	4	22	1	0	150	1	6	2 carb, 1 fat
Oatmeal Crisps Fruit 'n Cereal Bar, Strawberry	1 bar	140	30	2	11	0	0	115	1	2	2 carb, 1 fat
Health Valley											
Cereal Bars, Apple or Strawberry Cobbler	1 bar	130	27	2	15	0	0	50	1	2	2 carb
Fat-Free Apple Bakes	1 bar	70	19	0	0	0	0	30	3	2	1 carb
Fat-Free Raisin Bakes	1 bar	70	19	0	0	0	0	30	3	2	1 carb
Honey Corn Bread Crackers	4	60	11	2	25	0	0	140	1	1	1 strch
Low-Fat Sesame Crackers	5	60	10	2	25	0	0	140	1	2	1/2 strch

SNACKS, CRACKERS, CHIPS, POPCORN, SNACK BARS

	Serving	Calories	Carb. (g)	Fat (g)	% Cal. Fat	Sat. Fat (g)	Chol. (mg)	Sod. (mg)	Fib. (g)	Prot. (g)	Servings/ Exchanges
Low-Fat Stone Wheat Crackers	5	60	10	1	17	0	0	140	1	1	1/2 strch
Original Amaranth Graham Crackers	6	120	22	3	21	0	0	80	3	3	1 1/2 strch, 1 fat
Keebler											
Crackers, Club, Low-Salt	4	70	9	3	39	<1	0	80	0	1	1/2 strch, 1 fat
Crackers, Club, Original	4	70	9	3	39	1	0	140	0	1	1/2 strch, 1 fat
Crackers, Club, Reduced-Fat	5	70	12	2	26	0	0	200	0	1	1 strch
Crackers, Graham, Chocolate	8	140	23	4	25	1	0	105	1	2	1 1/2 strch, 1 fat
Crackers, Graham, Cinnamon Crisps	8	130	23	3	21	<1	0	140	1	2	1 1/2 strch
Crackers, Graham, Cinnamon Crisps, Low-Fat	8	110	23	2	16	0	0	135	1	2	1 1/2 strch

Crackers, Graham, Original	8	130	22	4	28	<1	0	150	1	2	1 1/2 strch, 1 fat
Crackers, Honey Graham	8	140	23	4	26	1	0	140	0	2	1 1/2 carb, 1 fat
Crackers, Honey Graham, Low-Fat	9	120	25	2	15	0	0	160	1	2	1 1/2 carb
Crackers, Toasteds, Buttercrisps	5	80	10	4	45	1	0	150	0	1	1/2 strch, 1 fat
Crackers, Toasteds, Onion	5	80	10	3	33	<1	0	150	0	1	1 strch, 1 fat
Crackers, Toasteds, Sesame	5	80	10	4	45	<1	0	135	<1	1	1 strch, 1 fat
Crackers, Toasteds, Wheat	5	80	10	4	45	<1	0	150	<1	1	1 strch, 1 fat
Crackers, Town House	5	80	9	5	56	1	0	150	<1	1	1/2 strch, 1 fat
Crackers, Town House, Low-Sodium	5	80	10	5	50	1	0	75	<1	1	1/2 strch, 1 fat
Crackers, Town House, Reduced-Fat	6	70	11	2	26	<1	0	180	<1	1	1 strch
Crackers, Zesta Saltines, Fat-Free	5	60	13	0	0	0	0	280	<1	1	1 strch

SNACKS, CRACKERS, CHIPS, POPCORN, SNACK BARS

	Serving	Calories	Carb. (g)	Fat (g)	% Cal. Fat	Sat. Fat (g)	Chol. (mg)	Sod. (mg)	Fib. (g)	Prot. (g)	Servings/ Exchanges
Crackers, Zesta Saltines, Original	5	60	11	2	30	<1	0	230	<1	1	1 strch
Crackers, Zesta Saltines, Reduced-Sodium	5	60	11	2	30	<1	0	115	<1	1	1 strch
Crackers, Zesta Saltines, Unsalted Tops	5	60	11	2	30	<1	0	100	1	1	1 strch
Crackers, Zesta Soup & Oyster	45	70	10	3	39	1	0	140	0	1	1/2 strch, 1 fat
Munch'ems, Seasoned	41	140	21	5	32	1	0	220	1	2	1 strch, 1 fat
Wheatables, Original Wheat	19	140	20	6	39	1	0	300	1	2	1 strch, 1 fat
Wheatables, Wheat Reduced-Fat	19	140	22	4	26	1	0	220	2	3	1 1/2 strch, 1 fat

Kellogg's

	Serving									
Froot Loops Cereal & Milk Bar	1 bar	110	16	3	25	2	0	75	0	2	1 carb, 1 fat
Frosted Flakes Cereal & Milk Bar	1 bar	110	19	3	25	2	0	90	0	2	1 carb, 1 fat
Fruit Streamers	1 pouch	80	17	1	13	0	0	80	0	1	1 carb
Fruit Twistables	1 pouch	70	17	<1	0	0	0	55	0	<1	1 carb
Nutri-Grain Cereal Bars, All Varieties	1 bar	140	27	3	18	0	0	110	1	2	2 carb, 1 fat
Nutri-Grain Minis Bite-Size Cereal Bar	1 pouch	160	32	3	16	0	0	115	1	2	2 carb, 1 fat
Nutri-Grain Minis Bite-Size Cereal Bars with Yogurt Icing, All Varieties	1 pouch	160	32	3	16	0	0	115	0	2	2 carb, 1 fat
Nutri-Grain Muffin Bar, Banana	1 bar	160	30	4	22	0	0	110	1	3	2 carb, 1 fat

SNACKS, CRACKERS, CHIPS, POPCORN, SNACK BARS

	Serving	Calories	Carb. (g)	Fat (g)	% Cal. Fat	Sat. Fat (g)	Chol. (mg)	Sod. (mg)	Fib. (g)	Prot. (g)	Servings/ Exchanges
Nutri-Grain Muffin Bar, Cinnamon Raisin	1 bar	170	32	4	21	0	0	100	1	2	2 carb, 1 fat
Nutri-Grain Twists Cereal Bars, Apple Cobbler	1 bar	140	27	3	18	0	0	105	1	1	2 carb, 1 fat
Nutri-Grain Twists Cereal Bars, Cappuccino & Crème	1 bar	140	26	3	18	0	0	90	1	1	1 carb, 1 fat
Nutri-Grain Yogurt Bars, All Varieties	1 bar	140	27	3	18	0	0	110	1	2	2 carb, 1 fat
Rice Krispies Treats, Original	1	90	18	2	20	<1	0	100	0	1	1 strch
Special K Bars	1 bar	90	18	1	10	1	0	100	0	2	1 carb, 1 fat
Kraft											
Handi-Snacks, Cheez 'n Breadsticks	1 pkg	110	14	5	41	1	5	340	0	3	1 strch, 1 fat

Product	Serving	Cal	Carb (g)	Fat (g)	% Cal Fat	Sat Fat (g)	Chol (mg)	Sodium (mg)	Fiber (g)	Prot (g)	Exchanges
Handi-Snacks, Cheez 'n Crackers	1 pkg	100	10	5	45	1	10	340	0	2	2 1/2 strch, 1 fat
Handi-Snacks, Cheez 'n Pretzels	1 pkg	90	12	4	40	1	5	380	0	3	1 strch, 1 fat
Nabisco											
Better Cheddars	22	150	18	7	42	2	<5	350	<1	3	1 strch, 2 fat
Better Cheddars, Reduced-Fat	23	140	20	5	32	2	<5	320	<1	3	1 strch, 1 fat
Cereal Bar, Snackwell's Apple Cinnamon	1	130	26	3		<1	0	70	1	1	1 1/2 carb, 1 fat
Cheese Nips	29	150	19	6	36	2	<5	340	<1	3	1 strch, 1 fat
Cheese Nips, Reduced-Fat	31	130	21	4	28	1	0	360	<1	3	1 1/2 strch, 1 fat
Chicken-In-A-Biskit	12	170	18	10	53	2	0	280	<1	2	1 strch, 2 fat
Chips, Ritz, Cheddar	14	140	20	6	36	1	0	320	<1	2	1 carb, 1 fat
Chips, Ritz, Original	15	140	23	5	29	1	0	350	<1	2	1 1/2 carb, 1 fat
Crackers, Barnum's Animal	10	120	22	4	30	<1	0	140	0	0	1 1/2 strch, 1 fat

SNACKS, CRACKERS, CHIPS, POPCORN, SNACK BARS

	Serving	Calories	Carb. (g)	Fat (g)	% Cal. Fat	Sat. Fat (g)	Chol. (mg)	Sod. (mg)	Fib. (g)	Prot. (g)	Servings/ Exchanges
Crackers, Honey Maid Chocolate Graham	8	130	22	3	21	<1	0	150	1	2	1 1/2 carb, 1 fat
Crackers, Honey Maid Graham, Low-Fat	8	120	25	2	15	0	0	190	<1	2	1 strch
Crackers, Honey Maid Honey Graham	8	140	22	3	19	<1	0	190	1	2	1 1/2 carb, 1 fat
Crackers, Honey Maid Low-Fat Cinnamon Graham	8	120	26	2	15	0	0	170	<1	2	2 strch
Crackers, Premium Saltine	5	70	11	2	26	0	0	220	0	1	1 strch
Crackers, Premium Saltine, Unsalted Tops	5	70	11	2	26	0	0	115	0	1	1 strch
Crackers, Ritz	5	80	10	4	45	1	10	135	0	1	1/2 strch, 2 fat
Crackers, Ritz Bits, Cheese	12	150	16	9	54	2	<5	260	0	2	1 strch, 2 fat

Food										
Crackers, Ritz Bits, Peanut Butter	12	140	16	8	51	2	0	240	1	3	1 strch, 2 fat
Crackers, Ritz, Reduced-Fat	5	70	11	2	26	0	0	150	0	1	1 strch
Crackers, Ritz Sticks	17	150	19	7	47	2	0	280	<1	2	1 carb, 1 fat
Crackers, Ritz, Whole-Wheat	5	70	11	3	29	0	0	125	<1	1	1 carb, 1 fat
Crackers, Swiss Cheese	15	140	18	7	45	2	0	360	<1	2	1 strch, 1 fat
Crackers, Triscuits	7	120	19	5	38	<1	0	180	3	3	1 strch, 1 fat
Crackers, Triscuits, Reduced-Fat	7	120	21	3	23	0	0	160	3	3	1 1/2 strch, 1 fat
Crackers, Triscuit Thin Crisps	15	130	21	5	35	1	0	180	3	3	1 1/2 strch, 1 fat
Crackers, Vegetable Thins	11	160	18	9	50	2	0	360	1	2	1 strch, 2 fat
Crackers, Wheat Thins, Original	16	150	21	6	36	1	0	270	1	3	1 strch, 1 fat
Crackers, Wheatsworth, Wheat Crackers	5	80	10	4	45	<1	0	170	1	2	1/2 strch, 1 fat

SNACKS, CRACKERS, CHIPS, POPCORN, SNACK BARS

	Serving	Calories	Carb. (g)	Fat (g)	% Cal. Fat	Sat. Fat (g)	Chol. (mg)	Sod. (mg)	Fib. (g)	Prot. (g)	Servings/ Exchanges
Crackers, Wheat Thins, Harvest Crisps, 5-Grain	13	140	23	4	26	<1	0	240	1	3	1 1/2 strch, 1 fat
Crackers, Wheat Thins, Reduced-Fat	16	130	21	4	28	<1	0	260	1	3	1 1/2 strch, 1 fat
Sociables	7	70	9	4	51	<1	0	140	0	1	1/2 strch, 1 fat
Twigs Snack Sticks	15	150	18	7	42	2	0	270	<1	3	1 strch, 1 fat
Pepperidge Farm											
Crackers, Butter Thins	4	70	10	3	39	1	10	95	0	1	1/2 strch, 1 fat
Crackers, Goldfish, Cheddar, 30% Less Sodium	60	140	18	5	32	1	10	170	<1	3	1 strch, 1 fat
Crackers, Goldfish, Flavor Blasted	51	140	18	6	39	2	0	250	1	3	1 strch, 1 fat
Crackers, Goldfish, Original	55	150	19	6	36	2	<5	250	<1	3	1 strch, 1 fat

Crackers, Goldfish, Parmesan	60	140	19	5	32	1	<5	300	1	4	1 strch, 1 fat
Crackers, Goldfish, Pizza Flavor	55	140	19	6	39	1	0	180	2	3	1 strch, 1 fat
Crackers, Goldfish, Pretze	43	110	22	1	8	1	0	430	<1	3	1 1/2 strch
Crackers, Goldfish, Sandwich Cheddar Snackers	11	140	18	6	43	2	0	280	<1	4	1 carb, 1 fat
Crackers, Hearty Wheat	3	80	10	4	45	0	0	100	1	2	1/2 strch, 1 fat
Cracker Trio	3	60	9	2	30	<1	<5	85	<1	1	1/2 strch
Snack Sticks, Sesame	9	130	19	5	35	1	0	290	2	3	1 strch, 1 fat
Planters											
Fiddle Faddle	3/4 cup	150	20	7	42	3	10	180	1	2	1 carb, 1 fat
Fiddle Faddle, Fat-Free	1 cup	110	28	0	0	0	0	210	0	2	2 carb
Trail Mix, Fruit & Nut Mix	2 Tbsp	120	14	7	50	2	0	10	2	3	1 strch, 1 fat
Trail Mix, Nut & Chocolate	3 Tbsp	170	16	11	53	3	0	15	2	4	1 strch, 2 fat

SNACKS, CRACKERS, CHIPS, POPCORN, SNACK BARS

	Serving	Calories	Carb. (g)	Fat (g)	% Cal. Fat	Sat. Fat (g)	Chol. (mg)	Sod. (mg)	Fib. (g)	Prot. (g)	Servings/ Exchanges
Trail Mix, Nuts, Seeds & Raisins	3 Tbsp	160	11	12	63	2	0	15	3	5	1 strch, 2 fat
Poore Brothers											
Chips, Original	1 oz	140	15	9	57	3	0	90	<1	2	1 carb, 2 fat
Chips, Salt & Vinegar	1 oz	140	15	9	57	3	0	300	1	2	1 carb, 2 fat
Power Bar											
Energy Bar, Chocolate	1	230	45	2	9	<1	0	95	3	10	3 carb
Energy Bar, Vanilla Crisp	1	230	45	3	11	<1	0	90	3	9	3 carb, 1 fat
Pringles											
Chips, Original	1 oz	160	15	11	56	3	0	170	1	1	1 strch, 2 fat
Chips, Original, Fat-Free	1 oz	70	15	0	0	0	0	160	2	2	1 carb
Chips, Original, Reduced-Fat	1 oz	140	19	7	43	2	0	135	1	2	1 carb, 1 fat

Chips, Sour Cream & Onion	1 oz	160	15	10	56	3	0	135	1	2	1 carb, 2 fat
Chips, Sour Cream & Onion, Reduced-Fat	1 oz	140	18	7	43	2	0	140	1	2	1 carb, 1 fat
Quaker											
Breakfast Squares, All Varieties	1 bar	220	43–44	4	16	1	15	220–240	2–3	4	3 carb, 1 fat
Fruit & Oatmeal Bites, Very Berry	1 bar	140	27	2	18	0	0	110	1	2	2 carb
Fruit & Oatmeal Cereal Bars, Apple Crisps	1 bar	130	26	3	21	0	0	90	1	1	2 carb, 1 fat
Mini Rice Cakes, Apple Cinnamon	8	60	15	0	0	0	0	50	0	1	1 carb
Mini Rice Cakes, Caramel Corn	7	60	13	0	0	0	0	150	0	1	1 carb
Oatmeal Crisps Fruit 'n Cereal Bar, Strawberry	1 bar	140	30	2	11	0	0	115	1	2	2 carb

SNACKS, CRACKERS, CHIPS, POPCORN, SNACK BARS

	Serving	Calories	Carb. (g)	Fat (g)	% Cal. Fat	Sat. Fat (g)	Chol. (mg)	Sod. (mg)	Fib. (g)	Prot. (g)	Servings/ Exchanges
Potato Stix, Sour Cream & Onion	1 oz	110	18	4	32	<1	0	280	1	1	1 strch, 1 fat
Rice Cakes, Apple Cinnamon	1	50	11	0	0	0	0	0	0	1	1/2 carb
Rice Cakes, Butter Popped Corn	1	35	7	0	0	0	0	45	0	1	1/2 carb
Rice Cakes, Caramel Corn	1	50	12	0	0	0	0	30	0	1	1 carb
Rice Cakes, Peanut Butter	1	60	12	1	15	0	0	65	0	1	1 carb
Rice Cakes, Salt Free	1	35	7	0	0	0	0	0	0	1	1 carb
Soy Crisps, White Cheddar	1 oz	120	14	5	33	5	0	270	2	7	1 strch, 1 fat
Wholesome Favorites Chewy Cereal Bars, Baked Apple	1 bar	110	22	2	18	0	0	70	1	1	1 1/2 carb
Ry Krisp											
Crackers, Seasoned Rye	2	60	10	2	30	0	0	90	3	1	1/2 strch

Crackers, Sesame Rye	2	60	11	2	30	0	0	80	3	2	1/2 strch

Slim Fast

Breakfast & Lunch Bars, Dutch Chocolate	1 bar	140	20	5	32	3	0	80	2	5	1 carb, 1 fat
Breakfast & Lunch Bars, Peanut Butter	1 bar	150	19	6	30	2	5	65	2	5	1 carb, 1 fat

Sunshine

Big Cheez-It	13	160	18	8	45	3	0	250	<1	4	1 strch, 2 fat
Cheez-It, Original	27	160	18	8	45	3	0	250	<1	4	1 strch, 2 fat
Cheez-It, Party Mix	1/2 cup	130	19	5	35	1	0	340	1	3	1 strch, 1 fat
Cheez-It, Reduced-Fat	29	130	20	5	35	2	0	360	<1	4	1 strch, 1 fat
Cheez-It, TwisterZ Cheddar & More Cheddar	17	140	19	6	36	3	0	270	<1	2	1 strch, 1 fat
Cheez-It, White Cheddar	26	150	18	7	42	2	<5	280	<1	3	1 strch, 1 fat
Krispy Saltines, Fat-Free	5	50	11	0	0	0	0	150	0	1	1 strch
Krispy Saltines, Original	5	60	10	2	30	0	0	180	<1	2	1/2 strch

SOUPS, STEW

READY-TO-SERVE CANNED SOUP

Brands

	Serving	Calories	Carb. (g)	Fat (g)	% Cal. Fat	Sat. Fat (g)	Chol. (mg)	Sod. (mg)	Fib. (g)	Prot. (g)	Servings/ Exchanges
Campbell's Carb Request											
Chicken Broccoli Cheese	1 cup	130	8	7	46	1.5	10	820	5	9	1/2 carb, 1 med-fat meat
Mediterranean Style Meatball	1 cup	90	5	4.5	44	2	20	890	2	8	1 med-fat meat
Savory Beef & Mushroom Medley	1 cup	70	7	2	29	1	10	870	1	7	1/2 carb, 1 lean meat
Spicy Sausage with Chicken & Bell Pepper Trio	1 cup	100	7	4	36	1.5	15	840	2	8	1/2 carb, 1 med-fat meat
Campbell's Chunky											
Baked Potato with Cheddar & Bacon Bits	1 cup	180	23	8	40	3	15	970	2	5	1 1/2 carb, 2 fat

Beef with Country Vegetables	1 cup	160	22	3	17	1.5	15	910	4	11	1 1/2 carb, 1 lean meat
Beef with White & Wild Rice	1 cup	150	24	2.5	15	1.5	10	960	2	9	1 1/2 carb, 1 lean meat
Cheese Tortellini with Chicken Vegetables	1 cup	110	18	2	16	1	10	890	2	5	1 carb
Chicken & Dumplings	1 cup	190	17	9	43	2	25	890	2	10	1 carb, 1 med-fat meat, 1 fat
Chicken Broccoli Cheese & Potato	1 cup	190	14	12	57	4	20	960	1	7	1 carb, 1 med-fat meat, 1 fat
Chicken Mushroom Chowder	1 cup	230	12	17	67	3	15	910	2	7	1 carb, 1 med-fat meat, 2 fat
Clam Chowder, Manhattan Style	1 cup	130	19	3.5	24	1	5	880	2	5	1 carb, 1 fat
Classic Chicken Noodle	1 cup	100	16	2.5	23	1	20	860	2	9	1 carb, 1 lean meat
Grilled Chicken & Sausage Gumbo	1 cup	140	21	2.5	16	1	15	890	3	9	1 1/2 carb, 1 lean meat

SOUPS, STEW

	Serving	Calories	Carb. (g)	Fat (g)	% Cal. Fat	Sat. Fat (g)	Chol. (mg)	Sod. (mg)	Fib. (g)	Prot. (g)	Servings/ Exchanges
Hearty Bean 'N Ham	1 cup	180	30	2	10	1	10	800	8	11	2 carb, 1 lean meat
Hearty Chicken & Vegetable	1 cup	100	14	1.5	14	0.5	15	790	2	7	1 carb, 1 lean meat
Hearty Chicken & Pasta	1 cup	130	23	2	14	0	<5	930	3	4	1 1/2 carb
New England Clam Chowder	1 cup	240	21	14	53	6	10	890	2	7	1 1/2 carb, 3 fat
Old Fashioned Vegetable Beef	1 cup	130	18	2.5	17	1.5	15	910	6	9	1 carb, 1 lean meat
Pepper Steak	1 cup	120	18	1.5	11	1	15	740	3	9	1 carb, 1 lean meat
Salisbury Steak Mushrooms & Onions	1 cup	150	18	4.5	27	2.5	20	890	2	9	1 carb, 1 med-fat meat
Sirloin Burger with Country Vegetables	1 cup	180	17	8	40	5	20	890	3	10	1 carb, 1 med-fat meat, 1 fat
Split Pea 'N Ham	1 cup	170	27	2.5	13	1	10	780	4	12	2 carb, 1 lean meat
Steak 'N Potato	1 cup	130	18	2	14	0.5	15	920	2	10	1 carb, 1 lean meat

Vegetable	1 cup	130	22	3.5	24	1	0	870	4	3	1 1/2 carb, 1 fat

Campbell's Kitchen Classics

Bean with Bacon	1 cup	180	28	4	20	1.5	5	820	8	9	2 carb, 1 fat
Chicken Noodle	1 cup	90	13	1	10	0.5	10	870	1	6	1 carb
Chicken with White & Wild Rice	1 cup	100	18	1	9	0.5	10	800	2	5	1 carb
Cream of Potato	1 cup	160	20	8	45	2	5	780	2	2	1 carb, 2 fat
Cream of Tomato	1 cup	140	24	3.5	23	1.5	10	730	2	3	1 1/2 carb, 1 fat
Lentil	1 cup	120	23	0.5	4	0.5	5	750	5	7	1 1/2 carb
Minestrone	1 cup	110	22	0.5	4	0.5	0	840	3	4	1 1/2 carb
New England Clam Chowder	1 cup	240	20	16	60	7	10	720	3	5	1 carb, 3 fat
Tomato	1 cup	100	22	0	0	0	0	820	3	3	1 1/2 carb
Vegetable	1 cup	100	22	0.5	5	0	0	820	3	3	1 1/2 carb

Campbell's Low Sodium

Chicken Broth	1 can	25	1	0.5	19	0.5	5	140	0	4	free
Chicken with Noodle	1 can	170	17	6	32	1.5	30	140	2	12	1 carb, 1 med-fat meat

SOUPS, STEW

	Serving	Calories	Carb. (g)	Fat (g)	% Cal. Fat	Sat. Fat (g)	Chol. (mg)	Sod. (mg)	Fib. (g)	Prot. (g)	Servings/ Exchanges
Chunky Vegetable Beef	1 can	160	17	4	23	1.5	40	90	6	14	1 carb, 2 lean meat
Cream of Mushroom	1 can	200	19	12	54	3.5	10	90	3	3	1 carb, 2 fat
Split Pea	1 can	240	38	4	15	1.5	5	50	6	12	2 1/2 carb, 1 med-fat meat
Tomato with Tomato Pieces	1 can	160	25	5	28	2	10	90	4	4	1 1/2 carb, 1 fat
Campbell's Select (Bean)											
Bean & Ham	1 cup	170	30	1	5	0.5	5	680	7	9	2 carb
Savory Lentil	1 cup	140	27	0.5	3	0.5	5	860	6	8	2 carb
Split Pea with Ham	1 cup	160	29	1	6	0.5	5	860	5	10	2 carb
Campbell's Select (Beef)											
Beef with Portabello Mushrooms & Rice	1 cup	110	15	1.5	12	1	10	860	1	8	1 carb, 1 lean meat
Beef with Roasted Barley	1 cup	150	24	1.5	9	1	10	860	3	9	1 1/2 carb
Italian Style Wedding	1 cup	120	16	2.5	19	2	10	850	2	8	1 carb, 1 lean meat

	Serving	Cal.						Sod.			Exchanges
Vegetable Beef	1 cup	110	16	2	16	1	15	910	3	8	1 carb, 1 lean meat
Campbell's Select (Chicken)											
Chicken & Pasta with Roasted Garlic	1 cup	110	16	1.5	12	0.5	10	840	2	7	1 carb, 1 lean meat
Chicken Rice	1 cup	100	17	1	9	0.5	5	990	2	6	1 carb
Chicken Vegetable	1 cup	100	18	0.5	5	0	10	830	3	7	1 carb, 1 lean meat
Chicken with Egg Noodles	1 cup	100	14	1.5	14	0.5	15	990	1	9	1 carb, 1 lean meat
Creamy Chicken Alfredo	1 cup	220	16	12	49	5	25	860	2	12	1 carb, 2 med-fat meat
Grilled Chicken with Sundried Tomatoes & Mushrooms	1 cup	110	17	1	8	0.5	15	780	2	8	1 carb, 1 lean meat
Herbed Chicken with Roasted Vegetables	1 cup	90	14	0.5	6	0.5	15	890	1	7	1 carb, 1 very lean meat
Honey Roasted Chicken with Golden Potatoes	1 cup	100	16	1	9	1	10	860	1	7	1 carb, 1 very lean meat

SOUPS, STEW

	Serving	Calories	Carb. (g)	Fat (g)	% Cal. Fat	Sat. Fat (g)	Chol. (mg)	Sod. (mg)	Fib. (g)	Prot. (g)	Servings/ Exchanges
Roasted Chicken with Long Grain & Wild Rice	1 cup	100	17	0.5	5	0	5	870	2	6	1 carb
Roasted Chicken with Rotini & Penne Pasta	1 cup	100	16	1	9	0.5	10	860	2	7	1 carb, 1 very lean meat
Rosemary Chicken with Roasted Potatoes	1 cup	100	18	0.5	5	0	10	880	2	7	1 carb, 1 very lean meat
Campbell's Select (Chowder)											
98% Fat-Free New England Clam Chowder	1 cup	110	19	1.5	12	0.5	10	860	2	6	1 carb, 1 very lean meat
New England Clam Chowder	1 cup	200	19	11	50	2.5	10	870	2	6	1 carb, 2 fat
Campbell's Select (Vegetable)											
Creamy Potato with Roasted Garlic	1 cup	170	20	9	48	2.5	10	770	2	3	1 carb, 2 fat
Fiesta Vegetable	1 cup	120	24	0.5	4	0	0	760	4	4	1 1/2 carb

	Serving	Cal	Carb				Sodium			Exchanges
Minestrone	1 cup	100	20	0	0	0	790	4	5	1 carb
Tomato Garden	1 cup	100	21	0.5	5	0.5	700	3	3	1 1/2 carb
Vegetable	1 cup	100	21	0.5	5	0	900	3	3	1 1/2 carb
Health Valley (Fat-Free)										
Chicken Noodle	1 cup	130	20	2	14	0	390	2	9	1 carb, 1 lean meat
Italian Minestrone	1 cup	90	21	0	0	0	210	8	8	1 1/2 carb
Tomato Vegetable	1 cup	80	17	0	0	0	240	5	6	1 carb
Vegetable Barley	1 cup	90	19	0	0	0	210	4	6	1 carb
Health Valley (No Salt Added, Organic)										
Organic Minestrone	1 cup	70	17	0	0	0	45	3	3	1 carb
Organic Split Pea	1 cup	110	23	0	0	0	115	8	10	1 1/2 carb, 1 very lean meat
Organic Tomato	1 cup	80	18	0	0	0	35	1	3	1 carb
Organic Vegetable	1 cup	80	18	0	0	0	40	4	3	1 carb
Health Valley (Organic)										
Black Bean	1 cup	130	25	1	7	0	380	5	7	1 1/2 carb
Lentil	1 cup	100	21	1	9	0	380	8	8	1 1/2 carb

SOUPS, STEW

	Serving	Calories	Carb. (g)	Fat (g)	% Cal. Fat	Sat. Fat (g)	Chol. (mg)	Sod. (mg)	Fib. (g)	Prot. (g)	Servings/ Exchanges
Minestrone	1 cup	110	17	0	0	0	0	380	3	3	1 carb
Split Pea	1 cup	110	23	0	0	0	0	160	8	10	1 1/2 carb, 1 very lean meat
Tomato	1 cup	80	18	0	0	0	0	380	1	3	1 carb
Vegetable	1 cup	80	18	0	0	0	0	380	4	3	1 carb
Healthy Choice											
Bean & Ham	1 cup	170	29	2.5	12	1	10	480	6	11	2 carb, 1 lean meat
Chicken & Dumpling	1 cup	140	19	3	18	1	35	480	4	11	1 carb, 1 lean meat
Chicken & Rice	1 cup	90	12	3	28	1	15	480	2	7	1 carb, 1 lean meat
Chunky Beef & Potato	1 cup	110	19	1	9	0	10	480	2	8	1 carb, 1 very lean meat
Country Vegetable	1 cup	100	22	0.5	5	0	0	480	4	4	1 1/2 carb
Creamy Tomato	1 cup	100	22	1.5	15	1	0	480	2	3	1 1/2 carb
Fiesta Chicken	1 cup	100	17	2	15	0.5	5	480	3	6	1 carb
Garden Vegetable	1 cup	120	25	1	8	0	0	480	4	6	1 1/2 carb
Hearty Chicken	1 cup	120	20	2	10	0.5	20	480	3	8	1 carb, 1 lean meat

	Serving	Cal	Carb	Fat				Sodium			Exchanges
New England Clam Chowder	1 cup	110	21	1.5	9	1	15	480	3	4	1 1/2 carb
Old Fashioned Chicken Noodle	1 cup	110	16	2	18	0.5	20	480	3	7	1 carb, 1 lean meat
Roasted Chicken with Garlic	1 cup	120	21	2	13	0	0.5	480	2	8	1 1/2 carb
Roasted Italian Chicken	1 cup	120	19	2.5	17	1	15	480	4	9	1 carb, 1 lean meat
Split Pea & Ham	1 cup	170	30	2.5	12	1	5	480	4	11	2 carb, 1 lean meat
Vegetable Beef	1 cup	130	24	1	8	0	10	480	4	9	1 1/2 carb, 1 lean meat
Zesty Gumbo	1 cup	100	16	2	20	1	20	480	3	6	1 carb
Progresso (99% Fat-Free)											
Beef Barley	1 cup	130	20	2	15	0.5	10	710	4	9	1 carb, 1 lean meat
Chicken Noodle	1 cup	90	13	1.5	17	0	20	950	<1	7	1 carb, 1 lean meat
Lentil	1 cup	130	20	1.5	16	0	0	440	6	8	1 carb, 1 lean meat
Minestrone	1 cup	110	19	1	9	0	0	630	4	5	1 carb
New England Clam Chowder	1 cup	110	18	1.5	14	0	5	610	2	5	1 carb

SOUPS, STEW

	Serving	Calories	Carb. (g)	Fat (g)	% Cal. Fat	Sat. Fat (g)	Chol. (mg)	Sod. (mg)	Fib. (g)	Prot. (g)	Servings/ Exchanges
Roasted Chicken with Wild Rice	1 cup	90	12	1.5	17	0	10	700	<1	6	1 carb
White Cheddar Potato	1 cup	100	20	1.5	15	0.5	<5	680	2	2	1 carb
Progresso (Chowder)											
Creamy Cheddar Chicken	1 cup	210	25	9	38	2	10	890	2	6	1 1/2 carb, 2 fat
Manhattan Clam Chowder	1 cup	110	17	2	18	0	10	880	2	6	1 carb
New England Clam Chowder	1 cup	230	23	13	52	5	25	790	1	6	1 1/2 carb, 3 fat
Potato with Broccoli & Cheese	1 cup	160	21	6	31	2	<5	960	1	5	1 1/2 carb, 1 fat
Roasted Potato Garlic	1 cup	180	23	9	44	3	10	900	2	2	1 1/2 carb, 2 fat
Southwestern Style Corn Chowder	1 cup	200	29	7	30	2	5	780	3	4	2 carb, 1 fat
Progresso (Classics)											
Black Bean	1 cup	170	30	1.5	9	0	<5	730	10	8	2 carb

Creamy Mushroom	1 cup	180	12	14	72	6	30	930	<1	2	1 carb, 3 fat
Escarole in Chicken Broth	1 cup	25	3	1	40	0	<5	930	1	1	free
Green Split Pea	1 cup	170	25	3	15	1	5	870	5	10	1 1/2 carb, 1 fat
Hearty Penne in Chicken Broth	1 cup	80	14	1	13	0	0	1020	<1	4	1 carb
Lentil	1 cup	140	22	2	14	0	0	750	7	9	1 1/2 carb
Macaroni & Bean	1 cup	160	23	4	22	1	<5	800	6	7	1 1/2 carb, 1 fat
Minestrone	1 cup	120	21	2	17	0	0	960	5	5	1 1/2 carb
Vegetable	1 cup	90	17	1	11	0	0	930	2	3	1 carb
Progresso (Distinctive Recipes)										
French Onion	1 cup	50	9	1.5	30	0.5	<5	900	1	<1	1/2 carb
Split Pea with Ham	1 cup	150	20	4	23	1.5	15	830	5	9	1 carb, 1 med-fat meat
Vegetarian Vegetable with Barley	1 cup	100	20	0.5	5	0	0	990	4	4	1 carb
Progresso (Italian Recipes)										
Cheese & Herb Tortellini	1 cup	140	23	3	18	0.5	<5	700	2	4	1 1/2 carb, 1 fat

SOUPS, STEW

	Serving	Calories	Carb. (g)	Fat (g)	% Cal. Fat	Sat. Fat (g)	Chol. (mg)	Sod. (mg)	Fib. (g)	Prot. (g)	Servings/ Exchanges
Chickarina	1 cup	130	12	5	35	2	20	1010	<1	8	1 carb, 1 fat
Herb & Rotini Vegetable	1 cup	100	19	1	10	0	0	1100	5	4	1 carb
Herb & Shell Minestrone	1 cup	120	22	1.5	13	0	0	1050	4	5	1 1/2 carb
Progresso (Steak)											
Beef & Baked Potato	1 cup	100	15	2	20	1	10	860	1	6	1 carb
Beef & Mushroom	1 cup	100	14	1.5	15	1	10	1030	1	7	1 carb
Beef & Vegetable	1 cup	130	16	2.5	19	1.5	20	850	2	10	1 carb, 1 fat
Progresso (Tomato)											
Creamy Tomato	1 cup	190	30	6	26	2.5	15	900	1	4	2 carb, 1 fat
Hearty Tomato	1 cup	110	23	1	9	0	0	1110	2	2	1 1/2 carb
Tomato Basil	1 cup	160	29	3	16	0	0	1060	2	3	2 carb, 2 fat
Tomato Rotini	1 cup	140	30	0.5	4	0	0	1000	2	4	2 carb
Progresso (White Meat)											
Chicken & Wild Rice	1 cup	100	15	1.5	15	0	15	850	1	7	1 carb

Chicken Noodle	1 cup	90	9	2	22	0	25	950	<1	9	1/2 carb, 1 lean meat
Chicken Vegetable	1 cup	90	13	1.5	17	0	15	820	2	7	1 carb
Hearty Chicken Rotini	1 cup	90	12	1.5	17	0	15	970	<1	8	1 carb, 1 lean meat
Turkey Noodle	1 cup	90	11	1.5	17	0	20	1060	<1	7	1 carb, 1 lean meat
Turkey Rice with Vegetable	1 cup	110	18	1	9	0	15	910	1	7	1 carb, 1 very lean meat

CONDENSED CANNED SOUP

Brands

Campbell's Condensed (98% Fat-Free)

Cream of Broccoli	1/2 cup	60	12	1	15	0.5	5	700	2	2	1 carb
Broccoli Cheese	1/2 cup	70	12	1.5	19	1	5	790	1	3	1 carb
Cream Celery	1/2 cup	60	8	3	45	1	<5	780	1	1	1/2 carb, 1 fat
Cream Chicken	1/2 cup	70	10	2	25	1	10	890	<1	3	1 carb
Cream Mushroom	1/2 cup	70	9	3	39	1	5	900	1	1	1/2 carb, 1 fat
New England Clam Chowder	1/2 cup	80	13	2	23	0.5	<5	940	1	3	1 carb

Campbell's Condensed

Bean & Bacon	1/2 cup	170	25	4	21	1.5	5	860	8	8	1 1/2 carb, 1 fat

SOUPS, STEW

	Serving	Calories	Carb. (g)	Fat (g)	% Cal. Fat	Sat. Fat (g)	Chol. (mg)	Sod. (mg)	Fib. (g)	Prot. (g)	Servings/ Exchanges
Beef Broth	1/2 cup	15	1	0	0	0	0	860	0	3	free
Beef Consomme	1/2 cup	20	1	0	0	0	0	810	0	4	free
Beef Noodle	1/2 cup	70	9	2.5	32	0.5	15	870	<1	4	1/2 carb, 1 fat
Beefy Mushroom	1/2 cup	50	6	2	36	1	10	890	0	3	1/2 carb
Black Bean	1/2 cup	110	19	2	16	0	0	900	5	5	1 carb
Broccoli Cheese	1/2 cup	100	12	4.5	41	2	5	820	0	2	1 carb, 1 fat
Chicken & Dumpling	1/2 cup	80	10	3	35	1	15	960	1	4	1/2 carb, 1 fat
Chicken & Stars	1/2 cup	80	12	2	23	0.5	10	940	1	3	1 carb
Chicken & Alphabet	1/2 cup	80	12	2	23	1	10	880	1	4	1 carb
Chicken Broth	1/2 cup	20	1	1	45	0	<5	770	0	1	free
Chicken Gumbo	1/2 cup	60	10	1	15	0.5	5	870	1	2	1/2 carb
Chicken Noodle	1/2 cup	60	8	1.5	23	0.5	15	890	<1	3	1/2 carb
Chicken with Rice	1/2 cup	80	14	1.5	16	0.5	5	820	1	2	1 carb
Chicken Won Ton	1/2 cup	45	6	1	20	0.5	10	870	0	3	1/2 carb

Cream Asparagus	1/2 cup	100	10	7	63	2	5	870	1	2	1/2 carb, 1 fat
Cream Broccoli	1/2 cup	90	12	3.5	35	1	5	750	1	2	1 carb, 1 fat
Cream Celery	1/2 cup	100	10	6	54	1.5	5	860	1	1	1/2 carb, 1 fat
Cream Chicken	1/2 cup	120	11	7	53	2	10	870	1	3	1 carb, 1 fat
Cream Mushroom	1/2 cup	100	9	7	63	1.5	5	870	1	1	1/2 carb, 1 fat
Fiesta Chili Beef	1/2 cup	170	25	5	26	2	10	770	8	7	1 1/2 carb, 1 fat
Fiesta Nacho Cheese	1/2 cup	120	10	8	60	4	10	800	1	3	1/2 carb, 2 fat
French Onion	1/2 cup	45	6	1.5	31	0.5	<5	900	1	2	1/2 carb
Golden Mushroom	1/2 cup	80	10	3.5	40	1	5	890	1	2	1/2 carb, 1 fat
Green Pea	1/2 cup	180	28	3	15	1	5	870	4	9	2 carb, 1 fat
Hearty Vegetable with Pasta	1/2 cup	90	19	0.5	6	0	0	890	2	3	1 carb
Manhattan Clam Chowder	1/2 cup	70	12	0.5	7	0.5	<5	880	2	2	1 carb
Minestrone	1/2 cup	90	17	1	10	0.5	<5	960	3	4	1 carb
New England Clam Chowder	1/2 cup	90	12	2.5	25	0.5	5	880	1	4	1 carb, 1 fat
Oyster Stew	1/2 cup	80	5	6	67	3.5	20	910	0	2	1/2 carb, 1 fat
Pepper Pot	1/2 cup	90	9	4	40	1.5	20	940	1	4	1/2 carb, 1 fat

SOUPS, STEW

	Serving	Calories	Carb. (g)	Fat (g)	% Cal. Fat	Sat. Fat (g)	Chol. (mg)	Sod. (mg)	Fib. (g)	Prot. (g)	Servings/ Exchanges
Split Pea with Ham & Bacon	1/2 cup	180	27	3.5	18	2	5	850	5	10	2 carb, 1 med-fat meat
Tomato	1/2 cup	90	20	0	0	0	0	710	1	2	1 carb
Turkey Noodle	1/2 cup	70	9	2	26	1	10	890	1	3	1 carb
Vegetable	1/2 cup	100	20	0.5	5	0.5	5	890	3	4	1 carb
Campbell's Healthy Request Condensed											
Chicken Noodle	1/2 cup	60	8	2	30	1	10	450	1	3	1/2 carb
Chicken Rice	1/2 cup	80	13	2	23	1	5	420	1	2	1 carb
Cream Celery	1/2 cup	70	11	2	26	1	<5	430	0	1	1 carb
Cream Chicken	1/2 cup	70	12	2.5	32	1	10	450	1	2	1 carb
Cream Mushroom	1/2 cup	70	10	2.5	32	1	<5	460	1	1	1/2 carb, 1 fat
Hearty Chicken with White & Wild Rice	1/2 cup	110	17	2	16	1	10	360	2	5	1 carb
Minestrone	1/2 cup	80	15	0.5	6	0	5	460	3	3	1 carb

Tomato	1/2 cup	90	18	1.5	15	0.5	0	450	1	2	1 carb
Vegetable	1/2 cup	100	20	1	9	0	<5	480	3	4	1 carb
Vegetable Beef	1/2 cup	90	15	1	10	0.5	5	480	3	5	1 carb

READY-TO-SERVE SINGLE SERVING CANNED SOUP

Brands

Campbell's Soup @ Hand

Blended Vegetable Medley	1 container	110	21	2	16	1.5	10	970	3	3	1 1/2 carb
Chicken & Stars	1 container	70	11	1.5	19	0.5	5	960	2	3	1 carb
Chicken with Mini Noodles	1 container	80	12	1.5	17	0.5	10	980	2	4	1 carb
Classic Tomato	1 container	120	27	0	0	0	0	970	2	3	2 carb
Cream Broccoli	1 container	160	16	8	45	2	5	910	3	4	1 carb, 2 fat
Creamy Chicken	1 container	150	15	8	48	2.5	10	970	2	4	1 carb, 2 fat
Creamy Mushroom	1 container	120	8	8	60	2.5	5	890	2	2	1/2 carb, 2 fat
Creamy Tomato	1 container	190	34	4	19	1.5	5	940	4	4	2 carb, 1 fat
Mexican Style Fiesta	1 container	130	22	3	21	1	15	930	3	7	1 1/2 carb, 1 fat
New England Clam Chowder	1 container	110	12	6	49	1	5	980	4	3	1 carb, 1 fat

SOUPS, STEW

	Serving	Calories	Carb. (g)	Fat (g)	% Cal. Fat	Sat. Fat (g)	Chol. (mg)	Sod. (mg)	Fib. (g)	Prot. (g)	Servings/ Exchanges
Pizza	1 container	130	27	0.5	4	0.5	5	850	2	5	2 carb
Vegetable Beef	1 container	60	10	1	15	0.5	5	830	2	3	1/2 carb
Velvety Potato	1 container	150	21	6	36	2	5	860	4	2	1 1/2 carb, 1 fat

MULTI-SERVE SOUP MIX

Brands

Bear Creek Country Kitchen

	Serving	Calories	Carb. (g)	Fat (g)	% Cal. Fat	Sat. Fat (g)	Chol. (mg)	Sod. (mg)	Fib. (g)	Prot. (g)	Servings/ Exchanges
Cheddar Broccoli	1 cup	170	26	7	35	2	5	1000	<1	3	2 carb, 1 fat
Cheddar Potato	1 cup	190	29	7	32	2.5	5	990	<1	3	2 carb, 1 fat
Chicken Noodle	1 cup	120	22	1.5	13	0	15	820	1	4	1 1/2 carb
Creamy Chicken	1 cup	140	28	2	13	0.5	0	990	1	2	2 carb
Creamy Potato	1 cup	160	28	4	22	1	0	500	1	3	2 carb, 1 fat
Hot & Sour	1 cup	90	17	1.5	11	0	10	1000	<1	2	1 carb
Minestrone	1 cup	110	22	0.5	5	0	0	870	2	4	1 1/2 carb
Navy Bean	1 cup	130	25	4.5	31	0	0	980	4	5	1 1/2 carb, 1 fat

Santa Fe Chipotle	1 cup	110	22	1	9	0	0	1030	1	4	1 1/2 carb
Tortilla	1 cup	110	22	1	9	0	0	840	3	4	1 1/2 carb
Vegetable Beef	1 cup	100	20	0	0	0	0	650	2	3	1 carb
Fantastic Simmer Soups											
Creamy Potato	1 cup	130	22	3	21	2	10	680	1	4	1 1/2 carb, 1 fat
Split Pea	1 cup	125	22	1	7	0	0	580	6	8	1 1/2 carb
Vegetable Barley	1 cup	120	26	0	0	0	0	690	3	4	2 carb
Vegetarian Chicken Noodle	1 cup	120	22	0.5	4	0	0	690	2	6	1 1/2 carb
Knorr Recipe Classics											
Cream Broccoli	1 cup	70	10	2.5	29	0.5	0	730	1	2	1/2 carb, 1 fat
Cream Spinach	1 cup	70	10	2.5	29	0.5	0	760	<1	2	1/2 carb, 1 fat
French Onion	1 cup	35	6	1	26	0.5	0	790	0	1	1/2 carb
Leek	1 cup	70	9	2.5	36	1	<5	810	0	2	1/2 carb, 1 fat
Spring Vegetable	1 cup	25	5	0	0	0	0	610	1	1	free

SOUPS, STEW

	Serving	Calories	Carb. (g)	Fat (g)	% Cal. Fat	Sat. Fat (g)	Chol. (mg)	Sod. (mg)	Fib. (g)	Prot. (g)	Servings/ Exchanges
Knorr Hearty Soups											
Chunky Potato with Roasted Onion	1 cup	100	20	1	10	0	0	850	1	2	1 carb
Homestyle Chicken Noodle	1 cup	80	13	1.5	19	0.5	15	860	1	3	1 carb
Roasted Vegetable with Long Grain Rice	1 cup	90	17	1	11	0.5	0	830	1	2	1 carb
Knorr Savory Soups											
Chicken Noodle	1 cup	70	11	1.5	21	1	10	650	1	3	1 carb
Cream Vegetable	1 cup	100	12	4.5	40	1.5	0	870	1	2	1 carb, 1 fat
Creamy Chicken with Rice	1 cup	90	14	2.5	27	1.5	<5	860	0	3	1 carb
Minestrone	1 cup	100	18	2	20	1	0	810	3	2	1 carb
Lipton Soup Secrets											
Extra Noodle	1 cup	80	15	1	11	1	10	680	<1	4	1 carb

Noodle	1 cup	60	9	1.5	23	0	5	720	<1	2	1/2 carb

SINGLE-SERVING SOUP MIX

Brands

Fantastic Big Soup Cups

Hot & Sour	1/2 pkg	130	22	2	15	0	0	710	1	4	1 1/2 carb
Miso with Tofu	1/2 pkg	100	19	1	9	0	0	580	<1	4	1 carb
Spring Vegetable	1/2 pkg	90	19	0	0	0	0	590	<1	4	1 carb
Vegetarian Beef Noodle	1/2 pkg	100	21	0	0	0	0	580	2	5	1 1/2 carb

Fantastic Carb Tastic Soup Cups

Asian Ginger Broccoli	1 pkg	80	11	1.5	19	0	0	680	9	7	1 carb
Broccoli Cheddar	1 pkg	110	13	3	23	1.5	5	560	7	7	1 carb, 1 fat
Sundried Tomato Basil	1 pkg	70	10	1	14	0	0	440	7	5	1 carb
Vegetarian Chicken Gumbo	1 pkg	90	9	1.5	17	0	0	470	4	9	1 carb

Fantastic Creamy Soup Cups

Corn & Potato Chowder	1/2 pkg	130	26	1	8	0	0	340	2	5	2 carb
Creamy Broccoli Cheddar	1/2 pkg	130	21	2.5	15	1.5	10	490	2	5	1 1/2 carb, 1 fat

SOUPS, STEW

	Serving	Calories	Carb. (g)	Fat (g)	% Cal. Fat	Sat. Fat (g)	Chol. (mg)	Sod. (mg)	Fib. (g)	Prot. (g)	Servings/ Exchanges
Fantastic Hearty Soup Cups											
Cha Cha Chili	1/2 pkg	220	37	2	7	0	0	440	11	14	2 carb
Country Lentil	1/2 pkg	180	32	1.5	8	0	0	440	9	12	2 carb
Five Bean	1/2 pkg	180	33	1.5	6	0	0	470	9	10	2 carb
Minestrone	1/2 pkg	140	27	1.5	11	0	0	470	4	7	2 carb
Health Valley (Fat-Free Soup Cups)											
Chicken Noodle with Vegetable	1/2 cup	110	24	0	0	0	0	270	3	5	1 1/2 carb
Cream Potato	1/3 cup	80	17	0	0	0	0	290	3	4	1 carb
Garden Split Pea with Carrots	1/3 cup	110	22	0	0	0	0	270	2	7	1 1/2 carb
Spicy Black Beans with Couscous	1/3 cup	130	29	0	0	0	0	290	5	6	2 carb
Lipton Carb Options											
Chicken Noodle	1 envelope	25	4	0	0	0	5	710	0	2	free

	Serving										
Cream Chicken	1 envelope	35	6	1	29	0	0	720	0	<1	1/2 carb
Lipton Cup-a-Soup											
Chicken Noodle	6 oz	50	3	1	20	0	10	560	0	2	1/2 carb
Maruchan Noodle Cups											
Assorted Flavors	1 container	290–310	37–38	12–15	38–45	6–7	0–10	1120–1220	2	6	2 1/2 carb, 2 fat
Maruchan Ramen Noodle Soup											
Assorted Flavors	1/2 pkg	190	25	8	37	4	0	780–930	1	4	1 1/2 carb, 2 fat
Nile Spice											
Minestrone	1 pkg	140	30	1	6	0	0	590	8	8	2 carb
Split Pea	1 pkg	200	35	1	5	1	0	600	8	13	2 carb
Sweet Corn Chowder	1 pkg	110	22	2	16	1	5	400	3	3	1 1/2 carb
Nissin Noodle Cups											
Assorted Flavors	1 container	280–300	37–38	13	40–43	6–7	0–5	1060–1480	1–9	6–7	2 1/2 carb, 3 fat
Nissin Top Ramen Noodle Soup											
Assorted Flavors	1/2 pkg	190	26–27	7	32	3.5	0	660–910	2–5	5	2 carb, 1 fat

SOUPS, STEW

	Serving	Calories	Carb. (g)	Fat (g)	% Cal. Fat	Sat. Fat (g)	Chol. (mg)	Sod. (mg)	Fib. (g)	Prot. (g)	Servings/ Exchanges
The Spice Hunter Soup Mixes											
Chicken Noodle	1 bowl	150	24	3	17	0	30	950	2	8	1 1/2 carb, 1 fat
Creamy Thai Noodle	1 bowl	180	29	4.5	22	3.5	0	790	2	6	2 carb, 1 fat
Navy Bean	1 cup	160	30	1	6	0	0	560	9	8	2 carb
Split Pea	1 bowl	240	43	1.5	4	0	0	720	10	16	3 carb
STEW											
Brands											
Dinty Moore											
Beef Stew	1 cup	180	17	8	39	4	30	970	2	10	1 carb, 1 med-fat meat, 1 fat
Chicken Dumplings	1 cup	230	28	8	30	3	35	860	1	12	2 carb, 1 med-fat meat, 1 fat

SWEET BREADS, MUFFINS, PASTRIES, DONUTS

	Serving	Calories	Carb. (g)	Fat (g)	% Cal. Fat	Sat. Fat (g)	Chol. (mg)	Sod. (mg)	Fib. (g)	Prot. (g)	Servings/ Exchanges
Baklava	2 × 2-inch piece	333	29	23	62	9	36	291	2	5	2 carb, 4 fat
Bread, Banana	1 slice	203	33	7	31	2	26	119	<1	3	2 carb, 1 fat
Bread, Date Nut	1 slice	217	30	10	41	2	28	140	<1	3	2 carb, 2 fat
Bread, Fruit, No Nuts	1 slice	150	23	6	36	2	22	109	<1	2	1 1/2 carb, 1 fat
Cream Puff with Custard Filling	1	335	30	20	54	5	174	375	<1	9	2 carb, 4 fat
Crepe/French Pancake	1	239	22	13	49	4	163	274	<1	9	1 1/2 carb, 3 fat
Croissant, Cheese	1	236	27	12	46	6	37	316	2	5	2 carb, 2 fat
Danish Pastry, Cinnamon	1	349	47	17	44	4	28	326	<1	5	3 carb, 3 fat
Danish Pastry, Fruit-Filled	1	335	45	16	42	3	19	333	NA	5	3 carb, 3 fat
Doughnut, Cake	1	198	23	11	50	2	18	257	<1	2	1 1/2 carb, 2 fat

SWEET BREADS, MUFFINS, PASTRIES, DONUTS

	Serving	Calories	Carb. (g)	Fat (g)	% Cal. Fat	Sat. Fat (g)	Chol. (mg)	Sod. (mg)	Fib. (g)	Prot. (g)	Servings/ Exchanges
Doughnut, Cake, Sugared/ Glazed	1	192	23	10	47	2	14	181	<1	2	1 1/2 carb, 2 fat
Doughnut, Cake, with Chocolate Icing	1	204	21	13	57	4	25	184	<1	2	1 1/2 carb, 3 fat
Doughnut, Custard-Filled with Icing	1	261	34	13	45	6	21	125	1	3	2 carb, 3 fat
Doughnut, Yeast, Creme-Filled	1	307	26	21	62	6	20	263	<1	5	2 carb, 4 fat
Doughnut, Yeast, Glazed	1	242	27	13	48	4	4	205	1	4	2 carb, 2 fat
Doughnut, Yeast, Jelly-Filled	1	289	33	16	50	4	22	190	<1	5	1 1/2 carb, 2 fat
Eclair, Chocolate with Custard Filling	1	262	24	16	55	4	127	337	<1	6	1 1/2 carb, 3 fat
Muffin	1	133	19	5	34	1	18	210	1	3	1 carb, 1 fat

Food	Serving										
Muffin, Cheese	1	184	23	8	39	3	30	274	<1	5	1 1/2 carb, 2 fat
Muffin, Chocolate Chip	1	190	27	9	43	3	25	186	1	4	2 carb, 2 fat
Muffin, Cranberry Nut	1	164	25	5	27	2	39	326	<1	4	1 1/2 carb, 1 fat
Muffin, Oat Bran	1	154	28	4	23	<1	0	224	3	4	2 carb 1 fat
Muffin, Pumpkin with Raisins & Nuts	1	181	34	4	20	<1	26	154	1	3	2 carb, 1 fat
Muffin, Wheat Bran	1	161	24	7	39	2	19	335	2	4	1 1/2 carb, 1 fat
Muffin, Whole-Wheat	1	142	20	6	38	2	21	283	3	4	1 carb, 1 fat
Muffin, Zucchini with Nuts	1	210	26	11	47	2	37	169	<1	3	2 carb, 2 fat
Pannetone or Italian Sweetbread	1 slice	86	15	2	21	1	19	96	<1	2	1 carb
Sweet Roll, Cheese	1	238	29	12	45	4	40	236	<1	5	2 carb, 2 fat
Sweet Roll, Cinnamon Raisin	1	145	20	7	43	2	40	149	1	4	1 carb, 1 fat
Sweet Roll, Cinnamon with Raisins & Nuts, Homemade	1	196	30	7	32	2	13	185	1	4	2 carb, 1 fat

SWEET BREADS, MUFFINS, PASTRIES, DONUTS

Brands	Serving	Calories	Carb. (g)	Fat (g)	% Cal. Fat	Sat. Fat (g)	Chol. (mg)	Sod. (mg)	Fib. (g)	Prot. (g)	Servings/ Exchanges
Aunt Fanny's											
Honey Bun, Applesauce	1	330	43	17	46	4	0	300	1	6	3 carb, 3 fat
Honey Bun, Banana Cream	1	350	32	18	46	4	0	290	2	5	2 carb, 3 fat
Honey Bun, Iced Honey	1	350	32	18	46	4	0	290	2	5	2 carb, 3 fat
Honey Bun, Raspberry-Filled	1	350	45	17	44	5	0	290	2	5	3 carb, 3 fat
Honey Bun, Regular	1	360	41	20	50	5	0	300	2	5	3 carb, 3 fat
Honey Bun, Vanilla Creme	1	350	32	18	46	4	0	290	2	5	2 carb, 3 fat
Betty Crocker											
Muffin Mix, Apple Cinnamon	1	170	24	7	37	2	NA	220	NA	3	1 1/2 carb, 1 fat
Muffin Mix, Banana Nut	1	170	22	7	37	1	NA	250	0	3	1 1/2 carb, 1 fat
Muffin Mix, Blueberry	1	160	25	6	34	1	NA	220	NA	3	1 1/2 carb, 1 fat

Muffin Mix, Lemon-Poppy Seed	1	180	24	8	40	1	NA	190	0	3	1 1/2 carb, 2 fat
Quick Bread Mix, Banana	1 slice	170	25	7	37	1	NA	200	NA	3	1 1/2 carb, 1 fat
Quick Bread Mix, Cinnamon Streusel	1 slice	180	28	7	35	1	NA	160	NA	2	2 carb, 1 fat
Quick Bread Mix, Lemon-Poppy Seed	1 slice	170	25	7	37	1	NA	200	NA	3	1 1/2 carb, 1 fat
Duncan Hines											
Muffin Mix, All-Bran Blueberry	1	140	25	4	26	1	NA	230	5	4	1 1/2 carb, 1 fat
Muffin Mix, Blueberry Streusel	1	190	32	6	28	1	NA	260	NA	2	2 carb, 1 fat
Muffin Mix, Cranberry Orange	1	150	26	5	30	1	NA	260	NA	2	2 carb, 1 fat
Entenmann's											
Cinnamon Rolls	1/2 roll	220	33	8	32	2	25	190	<1	3	2 carb, 2 fat

SWEET BREADS, MUFFINS, PASTRIES, DONUTS

	Serving	Calories	Carb. (g)	Fat (g)	% Cal. Fat	Sat. Fat (g)	Chol. (mg)	Sod. (mg)	Fib. (g)	Prot. (g)	Servings/ Exchanges
Coffee Cake, Cheese-Filled Crumb	1/9	210	26	10	43	3	35	200	<1	4	2 carb, 2 fat
Danish, Cheese Crumb	1/8	220	27	12	49	4	25	190	<1	3	2 carb, 2 fat
Danish Pastry Ring, Pecan	1/6	250	25	15	54	3	30	160	1	3	1 1/2 carb, 3 fat
Danish Pastry Twist, Blueberry	1/8	230	29	11	43	4	30	180	<1	3	2 carb, 2 fat
Donuts, Glazed Popems	3	240	31	12	45	3	15	230	1	2	2 carb, 2 fat
Donuts, Rich Frosted Popettes	3	280	26	18	58	5	15	220	1	3	2 carb, 4 fat
Donuts, Rich Frosted Variety	1	310	34	19	55	5	15	170	2	3	2 carb, 4 fat
Hot Pockets											
Fruit Pastries, Apple	1 piece	240	39	9	33	3	15	160	2	3	2 1/2 carb, 2 fat
Fruit Pastries, Cream Cheese & Strawberry	1 piece	240	34	10	38	4	20	200	2	3	2 carb, 2 fat

Jiffy

Muffin Mix, Apple Cinnamon	1/4 cup	170	28	5	26	2	NA	300	1	2	2 carb, 1 fat
Muffin Mix, Banana Nut	1/4 cup	160	25	5	28	2	NA	300	2	2	1 1/2 carb, 1 fat
Muffin Mix, Blueberry	1/4 cup	160	28	5	28	2	NA	270	1	2	2 carb, 1 fat

Kellogg's

Pop-Tarts Pastry, Blueberry	1	200	37	5	23	1	0	170	1	2	2 1/2 carb, 1 fat
Pop-Tarts Pastry, Brown Sugar Cinnamon	1	210	35	6	26	1	0	190	1	3	2 carb, 1 fat
Pop-Tarts Pastry, Cherry, Frosted	1	200	38	5	23	1	0	170	1	2	2 1/2 carb, 1 fat
Pop-Tarts Pastry, Chocolate Chip Cookie Dough	1	200	35	5	25	1	0	190	<1	2	2 carb, 1 fat
Pop-Tarts Pastry, Chocolate Fudge, Frosted	1	200	37	5	23	1	0	220	1	3	2 1/2 carb, 1 fat

SWEET BREADS, MUFFINS, PASTRIES, DONUTS

	Serving	Calories	Carb. (g)	Fat (g)	% Cal. Fat	Sat. Fat (g)	Chol. (mg)	Sod. (mg)	Fib. (g)	Prot. (g)	Servings/ Exchanges
Pop-Tarts Pastry, Raspberry, Frosted	1	210	37	5	21	1	0	170	1	2	2 1/2 carb, 1 fat
Pop-Tarts Pastry, S'mores, Frosted	1	200	36	6	27	1	0	200	1	3	2 1/2 carb, 1 fat
Pop-Tarts Pastry, Strawberry	1	200	37	5	23	1	0	190	1	2	2 1/2 carb, 1 fat
Pop-Tarts Pastry, Strawberry, Frosted	1	200	38	5	23	1	0	170	1	2	2 1/2 carb, 1 fat
Krusteaz											
Muffin Mix, Almond Poppyseed	1	180	30	4	20	1	NA	230	1	2	2 carb, 1 fat
Muffin Mix, Fat-Free Banana Nut	1	140	33	0	0	0	0	330	2	2	2 carb
Muffin Mix, Lemon-Poppy Seed	1	160	30	4	23	1	NA	280	<1	2	2 carb, 1 fat

Muffin Mix, Oat Bran	1	190	31	5	24	1	NA	310	2	4	2 carb, 1 fat
Pepperidge Farm											
Apple Turnover	1	290	36	15	47	4	0	230	2	4	2 1/2 carb, 3 fat
Cherry Turnover	1	280	34	15	48	4	0	250	1	4	2 carb, 3 fat
Raspberry Turnover	1	290	35	15	47	4	0	230	2	4	2 carb, 3 fat
Pillsbury											
Cinnamon Raisin Rolls with Icing	1	170	26	6	32	2	NA	320	1	2	2 carb, 1 fat
Cinnamon Reduced-Fat Rolls with Icing	1	140	24	4	25	1	NA	340	<1	2	1 1/2 carb, 1 fat
Cinnamon Rolls (Frozen) with Icing	1	340	55	11	29	3	NA	560	1	6	4 carb, 2 fat
Sweet Rolls, Caramel Sticky Bun	1	170	24	7	37	2	NA	330	<1	2	1 1/2 carb, 1 fat
Toaster Strudel Pastries, Blueberry	1	190	<1	9	43	2	5	190	2	3	2 carb, 1 fat

SWEET BREADS, MUFFINS, PASTRIES, DONUTS

	Serving	Calories	Carb. (g)	Fat (g)	% Cal. Fat	Sat. Fat (g)	Chol. (mg)	Sod. (mg)	Fib. (g)	Prot. (g)	Servings/ Exchanges
Toaster Strudel Pastries, Cinnamon	1	190	26	8	38	2	5	200	1	3	2 carb, 2 fat
Toaster Strudel Pastries, Raspberry	1	180	26	9	45	2	5	190	0	2	2 carb, 1 fat
Rhodes											
Any Time! Cinnamon Rolls (Frozen)	1	320	50	11	31	3	NA	510	1	4	3 carb, 2 fat
Any Time! Cinnamon Rolls with Cream Cheese Cheese Frosting (Frozen)	1	310	51	10	29	2	NA	500	1	4	3 carb, 2 fat

VEGETABLES, VEGETABLE JUICES

	Serving	Calories	Carb. (g)	Fat (g)	% Cal. Fat	Sat. Fat (g)	Chol. (mg)	Sod. (mg)	Fib. (g)	Prot. (g)	Servings/ Exchanges
Alfalfa Sprouts	1 cup	10	1	<1	0	0	0	2	<1	1	free
Artichoke Hearts, Canned, Drained	1/2 cup	36	7	<1	0	0	0	42	<1	3	1 vegetable
Artichokes, Cooked	1/2	30	7	<1	0	0	0	57	3	2	1 vegetable
Arugula, Raw	1 cup	5	<1	0	0	0	0	6	0	<1	free
Asparagus, Fresh, Cooked	4 spears	14	3	0	0	0	0	7	1	2	free
Asparagus, Frozen	1/2 cup	23	4	<1	0	<1	0	3	3	2	1 vegetable
Asparagus, Spears, Canned, Drained	1/2 cup	23	3	<1	0	<1	0	472	2	3	1 vegetable
Bamboo Shoots, Canned	1 cup	25	4	<1	0	<1	0	9	2	2	1 vegetable
Bamboo Shoots, Sliced, Cooked	1 cup	14	2	<1	0	<1	0	5	1	2	free

VEGETABLES, VEGETABLE JUICES

	Serving	Calories	Carb. (g)	Fat (g)	% Cal. Fat	Sat. Fat (g)	Chol. (mg)	Sod. (mg)	Fib. (g)	Prot. (g)	Servings/ Exchanges
Bamboo Shoots, Sliced, Raw	1 cup	41	8	<1	0	0	0	6	3	4	1 vegetable
Beans, Green or Wax, Canned	1/2 cup	14	3	<1	0	0	0	171	1	<1	1 vegetable
Beans, Green, Frozen	1/2 cup	18	4	<1	0	0	0	9	2	<1	1 vegetable
Bean Sprouts, Raw	1 cup	31	6	<1	0	0	0	6	2	3	1 vegetable
Beets, Canned	1/2 cup	26	6	<1	0	0	0	233	2	<1	1 vegetable
Beets, Fresh, Cooked	1/2 cup	26	6	0	0	0	0	65	1	1	1 vegetable
Beets, Harvard, Diced	1/2 cup	136	25	4	26	<1	0	287	2	<1	1 carb, 1 vegetable, 1 fat
Beets, Pickled	1/2 cup	74	19	<1	0	<1	0	301	1	<1	1 carb, 1 vegetable
Broccoli, Cooked with Cheese Sauce	1/2 cup	110	6	7	57	4	15	365	2	6	1 vegetable, 1 fat
Broccoli, Cooked with Cream Sauce	1/2 cup	93	8	6	58	2	6	346	2	4	1 vegetable, 1 fat

Food	Serving									Exchange
Broccoli, Raw, Chopped	1 cup	25	5	<1	0	0	24	3	3	1 vegetable
Broccoli, Spears, Frozen	1/2 cup	26	5	<1	0	0	22	3	3	1 vegetable
Brussels Sprouts, Frozen Cooked	1/2 cup	33	7	<1	0	0	18	3	3	1 vegetable
Cabbage, Bok Choy, Cooked	1 cup	20	3	<1	0	0	58	3	3	1 vegetable
Cabbage, Chinese, Raw	1 cup	12	3	<1	0	0	7	<1	<1	1 vegetable
Cabbage, Fresh, Cooked	1/2 cup	16	3	<1	0	0	6	2	<1	1 vegetable
Cabbage, Raw, Green	1 cup	18	4	<1	0	0	13	2	1	1 vegetable
Cabbage, Red, Cooked	1/2 cup	16	4	<1	0	0	6	2	<1	1 vegetable
Carrot Juice, Canned	1/2 cup	47	11	<1	0	0	34	<1	1	2 vegetable
Carrots, Canned	1/2 cup	17	4	<1	0	0	176	1	<1	1 vegetable
Carrots, Fresh, Cooked	1/2 cup	35	8	<1	0	0	52	3	<1	1 vegetable
Carrots, Raw	1 cup	47	11	<1	0	0	38	3	1	2 vegetable
Cassava, Raw	1/4 cup	83	20	0	0	0	7	1	1	1 strch
Cauliflower, Frozen, Cooked	1/2 cup	17	3	<1	0	0	16	2	1	1 vegetable
Cauliflower, Raw	1 cup	25	5	<1	0	0	30	3	2	1 vegetable

VEGETABLES, VEGETABLE JUICES

	Serving	Calories	Carb. (g)	Fat (g)	% Cal. Fat	Sat. Fat (g)	Chol. (mg)	Sod. (mg)	Fib. (g)	Prot. (g)	Servings/ Exchanges
Celery, Fresh, Cooked	1/2 cup	14	3	<1	0	0	0	68	1	<1	1 vegetable
Celery, Raw	1 cup	19	4	<1	0	0	0	104	2	<1	1 vegetable
Chard, Swiss, Fresh, Cooked	1/2 cup	17	4	0	0	0	0	158	2	2	1 vegetable
Coleslaw	1/2 cup	97	9	7	65	1	3	178	1	<1	1 vegetable, 1 fat
Collard Greens, Fresh, Cooked	1/2 cup	17	4	<1	0	0	0	10	1	<1	1 vegetable
Corn, Canned	1/2 cup	83	20	<1	0	<1	0	286	6	3	1 strch
Corn, Cream-Style, Canned	1/2 cup	92	23	<1	0	<1	0	365	2	2	1 1/2 strch
Corn, Frozen, Cooked	1/2 cup	66	17	<1	0	0	0	4	2	3	1 strch
Corn on the Cob, Cooked	1 medium	83	19	1	0	<1	0	13	2	3	1 strch
Corn on the Cob, Frozen	1–3 inch	70	14	<1	0	NA	0	5	1	2	1 strch
Cucumber, Raw	1 cup	14	3	<1	0	0	0	2	<1	<1	1 vegetable

Food	Serving									Exchanges
Cucumber Salad, Marinated in Vinegar	1 cup	48	13	<1	0	0	350	1	<1	1/2 carb, 1 vegetable
Eggplant, Fresh, Cooked	1/2 cup	13	3	<1	0	0	1	1	<1	1 vegetable
Endive/Escarole, Raw	1 cup	9	2	<1	0	0	11	2	<1	1 vegetable
French Fries, Frozen, Oven-Heated	10	167	20	9	49	3	307	2	2	1 strch, 2 fat
Green Onions (Scallions), Raw	1 cup	32	7	0	0	0	16	3	2	1 vegetable
Hominy, Yellow, Canned	1/2 cup	58	12	<1	0	0	168	2	1	1 strch
Jicama	1 cup	46	11	<1	0	0	5	6	1	2 vegetable
Kale, Fresh, Cooked	1/2 cup	21	4	<1	0	0	15	1	1	1 vegetable
Kohlrabi, Cooked	1/2 cup	24	6	<1	0	0	17	<1	2	1 vegetable
Leeks, Cooked	1/2 cup	16	4	<1	0	0	6	1	<1	1 vegetable
Lettuce, Butterhead, Raw	1 cup	7	1	0	0	0	3	0	0	1 vegetable
Lettuce, Iceberg, Raw	1 cup	7	1	<1	0	0	5	<1	<1	1 vegetable
Lettuce, Romaine, Chopped	1 cup	9	1	<1	<1	0	5	1	<1	free

VEGETABLES, VEGETABLE JUICES

	Serving	Calories	Carb. (g)	Fat (g)	% Cal. Fat	Sat. Fat (g)	Chol. (mg)	Sod. (mg)	Fib. (g)	Prot. (g)	Servings/ Exchanges
Lettuce, Romaine, Raw	1 cup	9	1	<1	0	0	0	5	1	<1	1 vegetable
Lima Beans, Frozen, Cooked	1/2 cup	95	18	<1	0	<1	0	26	7	7	1 strch
Mixed Vegetables, No Corn, Peas, or Pasta	1/2 cup	20	3	0	0	0	0	15	1	1	1 vegetable
Mixed Vegetables with Corn	1/2 cup	80	18	0	0	0	0	80	4	4	1 strch
Mixed Vegetables with Pasta	1 cup	80	15	0	0	0	0	85	5	3	1 strch
Mushrooms, Canned	1/2 cup	19	4	<1	0	0	0	331	2	2	1 vegetable
Mushrooms, Fresh, Cooked	1/2 cup	21	4	0	0	0	0	2	2	2	1 vegetable
Mushrooms, Raw	1 cup	18	3	<1	0	0	0	3	<1	2	1 vegetable
Mustard Greens, Fresh, Cooked	1/2 cup	10	2	<1	0	0	0	11	1	2	1 vegetable

Okra, Batter-Fried	1/2 cup	88	6	7	0	1	8	67	1	1	1 vegetable, 1 fat
Okra, Frozen, Cooked	1/2 cup	34	8	<1	0	<1	0	3	3	2	1 vegetable
Onions, Creamed	1/2 cup	100	11	6	54	2	5	334	1	3	2 vegetable, 1 fat
Onions, Fresh, Cooked	1/2 cup	46	11	<1	0	0	0	3	2	1	2 vegetable
Onions, Green, Raw	1 cup	32	7	<1	0	0	0	16	3	2	1 vegetable
Onions, Raw	1 cup	61	14	<1	0	0	0	5	3	2	2 vegetable
Palm Hearts, Cooked	1/2 cup	75	20	<1	0	<1	0	10	1	2	1 strch
Parsnips, Raw Slices	1/2 cup	50	12	<1	0	<1	0	7	3	<1	2 vegetable
Pea Pods, Fresh, Ccoked	1/2 cup	34	6	<1	0	0	0	3	2	3	1 vegetable
Pea Pods, Raw	1 cup	61	11	<1	0	<1	0	6	4	4	2 vegetable
Peas, Green, Canned	1/2 cup	59	11	<1	0	<1	0	186	4	4	1 strch
Peas, Green, Fresh, Cooked	1/2 cup	67	13	<1	0	0	0	2	4	4	1 strch
Peas, Green, Frozen, Cooked	1/2 cup	62	11	<1	0	0	0	70	4	4	1 strch
Peppers, Green, Fresh, Cooked	1/2 cup	19	5	<1	0	0	0	1	<1	<1	1 vegetable

VEGETABLES, VEGETABLE JUICES

	Serving	Calories	Carb. (g)	Fat (g)	% Cal. Fat	Sat. Fat (g)	Chol. (mg)	Sod. (mg)	Fib. (g)	Prot. (g)	Servings/ Exchanges
Peppers, Green, Raw	1 cup	27	6	<1	0	0	0	2	2	<1	1 vegetable
Peppers, Hot Green Chili, Raw	1 cup	60	14	<1	0	0	0	10	2	3	2 vegetable
Peppers, Jalapeño, Canned	1/2 cup	16	3	<1	0	<1	0	995	1	<1	1 vegetable
Peppers, Sweet, Red, Cooked	1/2 cup	19	5	<1	0	<1	0	1	<1	<1	1 vegetable
Plantains, Cooked	1/2 cup	89	24	<1	0	0	0	4	2	<1	1 strch
Potatoes Au Gratin, Homemade with Margarine	1 cup	323	28	19	53	10	37	1060	4	13	2 strch, 4 fat
Potatoes, Baked with Skin	3 oz	93	22	<1	0	0	0	7	2	2	1 1/2 strch
Potatoes, Cooked, Peeled	3 oz	73	17	<1	0	0	0	4	2	2	1 strch
Potatoes, Hash Brown, Frozen, Cooked	1/2 cup	170	22	9	47	4	0	27	2	3	1 1/2 strch, 2 fat

Food	Serving										Exchanges
Potatoes, Mashed, Flakes, Milk/Fat Added	1/2 cup	119	16	6	45	4	0	349	2	2	1 strch, 1 fat
Potatoes, Scalloped	1 cup	211	27	9	38	3	15	821	5	7	2 strch, 2 fat
Potatoes, Sweet, Canned	1/2 cup	92	22	<1	0	0	0	53	3	2	1 1/2 strch
Radicchio, Raw	1 cup	9	2	0	0	0	0	9	0	0	1 vegetable
Radishes	1 cup	20	4	<1	0	0	0	28	2	<1	1 vegetable
Rutabagas, Fresh, Cooked	1/2 cup	33	8	0	0	0	0	17	2	1	1 vegetable
Sauerkraut, Canned	1/2 cup	22	5	<1	0	0	0	780	3	1	1 vegetable
Spinach, Canned	1/2 cup	25	4	<1	0	<1	0	29	3	3	1 vegetable
Spinach, Frozen, Ccoked	1/2 cup	27	5	<1	0	0	0	82	3	3	1 vegetable
Spinach, Raw	1 cup	12	2	<1	0	0	0	44	3	2	1 vegetable
Spinach Salad, No Dressing	1 cup	89	10	4	40	<1	0	157	2	4	2 vegetable, 1 fat
Squash, Spaghetti, Cooked	1/2 cup	23	5	<1	0	<1	0	14	1	<1	1 vegetable
Squash, Summer, Fresh, Cooked	1/2 cup	18	4	<1	0	<1	0	1	1	<1	1 vegetable
Squash, Summer, Raw	1 cup	26	6	<1	0	<1	0	3	3	2	1 vegetable

VEGETABLES, VEGETABLE JUICES

	Serving	Calories	Carb. (g)	Fat (g)	% Cal. Fat	Sat. Fat (g)	Chol. (mg)	Sod. (mg)	Fib. (g)	Prot. (g)	Servings/ Exchanges
Squash, Winter	1 cup	83	22	<1	0	0	0	8	7	2	1 1/2 strch
Succotash, Canned	1/2 cup	81	18	<1	0	<1	0	282	3	3	1 strch
Succotash, Cooked	1/2 cup	111	24	<1	0	<1	0	16	4	5	1 1/2 strch
Tater Tots, Frozen, Oven-Heated	3 oz	146	21	8	49	2	0	345	2	2	1 1/2 strch, 2 fat
Tomatillo, Raw	1 cup	42	8	0	0	0	0	1	3	1	1 vegetable
Tomato Juice	1/2 cup	21	5	<1	0	0	0	440	<1	<1	1 vegetable
Tomato Paste, Canned	1/2 cup	110	25	1	8	<1	0	1034	6	5	1 strch, 1 vegetable
Tomato Sauce	1/2 cup	37	9	<1	0	0	0	738	2	2	1 vegetable
Tomatoes, Canned	1/2 cup	24	5	<1	0	0	0	196	1	1	1 vegetable
Tomatoes, Raw	1 cup	38	8	<1	0	<1	0	16	2	2	1 vegetable
Tossed Green Salad	3/4 cup	19	4	<1	0	<1	0	11	1	<1	1 vegetable
Turnip Greens, Fresh, Cooked	1/2 cup	14	3	<1	0	0	0	21	2	<1	1 vegetable

Food	Serving										
Turnips, Fresh, Cooked	1/2 cup	14	4	<1	0	0	0	39	2	<1	1 vegetable
Vegetable Juice	1/2 cup	23	6	<1	0	0	0	442	1	<1	1 vegetable
Vegetable Juice Cocktail	1/2 cup	23	6	<1	0	<1	0	442	1	<1	1 vegetable
Water Chestnuts	1/2 cup	35	9	0	0	0	0	6	2	<1	1 vegetable
Watercress, Raw	1 cup	4	<1	0	0	0	0	14	<1	<1	1 vegetable
Yam, Plain	1/2 cup	79	19	<1	0	0	0	6	2	1	1 strch
Zucchini Squash, Fresh, Cooked	1/2 cup	14	4	0	0	0	0	3	1	<1	1 vegetable
Zucchini, Raw	1 cup	18	4	<1	0	0	0	4	2	2	1 vegetable
Brands											
Betty Crocker											
Mashed Potatoes, Four Cheese	1/2 cup	160	20	7	39	2	2	550	2	3	1 strch, 1 fat
Mashed Potatoes, Roasted Garlic	1/2 cup	120	19	4	29	1	<5	530	1	2	1 strch, 1 fat

VEGETABLES, VEGETABLE JUICES

	Serving	Calories	Carb. (g)	Fat (g)	% Cal. Fat	Sat. Fat (g)	Chol. (mg)	Sod. (mg)	Fib. (g)	Prot. (g)	Servings/ Exchanges
Mashed Potatoes, Sour Cream & Chives	1/2 cup	150	21	7	42	2	5	450	1	3	1 1/2 strch, 1 fat
Potatoes, Au Gratin	1/2 cup	150	23	6	36	2	<5	660	1	3	1 1/2 strch, 1 fat
Potatoes, Cheddar & Bacon	2/3 cup	130	21	4	31	2	<5	690	1	3	1 1/2 strch, 1 fat
Potatoes, Cheesy Scalloped, Homestyle	1/2 cup	150	22	8	40	2	<5	620	2	4	1 1/2 strch, 1 fat
Potatoes, Creamy Roasted Garlic Scalloped	2/3 cup	160	25	6	31	2	5	720	1	4	1 strch, 1 fat
Potatoes, Creamy Scalloped	2/3 cup	140	23	5	29	2	5	740	1	3	1 1/2 strch, 1 fat
Potatoes, Hash Browns	1/2 cup	160	26	5	28	0	0	320	2	2	2 strch, 1 fat
Potatoes, Julienne	2/3 cup	110	20	4	18	1	<5	660	1	2	1 strch, 1 fat
Potatoes, Loaded Au Gratin	1/2 cup	140	23	5	29	2	5	610	1	4	1 1/2 strch, 1 fat
Potatoes, Roasted Garlic & Olive Oil	3/4 cup	160	27	6	31	0.5	0	650	2	3	2 strch, 1 fat

Potatoes, Scalloped	1/2 cup	130	22	4	28	1	0	630	1	3	1 1/2 strch, 1 fat
Potatoes, Sour Cream 'n Chive	2/3 cup	120	21	4	30	1	<5	690	1	2	1 1/2 strch, 1 fat
Potatoes, Three Cheese	2/3 cup	190	24	9	43	3	5	720	1	4	1 1/2 strch, 2 fat
Birds Eye											
Artichoke Hearts	3 pieces	40	7	1	23	0	0	55	5	2	1 vegetable
Asian Vegetable in Sesame Ginger Sauce	1 cup	60	12	1	15	0	0	630	2	2	2 vegetable
Broccoli & Cheese Sauce	1/2 cup	90	8	5	50	3	5	490	1	3	1 vegetable, 1 fat
California Blend & Cheddar Cheese Sauce	1/2 cup	30	8	4	45	2	5	390	1	2	1 vegetable, 1 fat
Cauliflower & Garlic Sauce	1 1/4 cup	50	6	4	60	1	0	460	2	2	1 vegetable, 1 fat
Creamed Spinach	1/2 cup	100	7	7	63	3	35	630	1	3	1 vegetable, 1 fat
Garden Bean Medley & Toasted Almonds	1 cup	100	10	5	45	2	5	360	5	3	2 vegetable, 1 fat

VEGETABLES, VEGETABLE JUICES

	Serving	Calories	Carb. (g)	Fat (g)	% Cal. Fat	Sat. Fat (g)	Chol. (mg)	Sod. (mg)	Fib. (g)	Prot. (g)	Servings/ Exchanges
Peas & Pearl Onions in Lightly Seasoned Sauce	2/3 cup	90	17	0	0	0	0	510	4	5	1 strch
Roasted Potatoes & Broccoli	2/3 cup	100	15	4	36	2	0	470	1	2	1 strch, 1 fat
Szechuan Vegetable in Sesame Sauce	1 cup	60	9	2	30	0	0	460	2	1	1 vegetable
Campbell's											
Tomato Juice	8 oz	50	10	0	0	0	0	750	2	2	2 vegetable
Tomato Juice, Low-Sodium	8 oz	50	10	0	0	0	0	140	2	2	2 vegetable
Tomato Juice, Single Serving	5.5 oz can	30	6	0	0	0	0	470	1	1	1 vegetable
V8 A-C-E Vegetable Juice	8 oz	50	11	0	0	0	0	460	2	2	2 vegetable
V8 Diet Splash Juice Beverage	8 oz	10	3	0	0	0	0	30	0	0	free

V8 Diet Splash Juice Beverage, Single Serving	8 oz can	10	3	0	0	0	30–40	0	0	free
V8 Low-Sodium Vegetable Juice	8 oz	50	11	0	0	0	140	2	1	2 vegetable
V8 Spicy Hot Vegetable Juice	5.5 oz	35	7	0	0	0	510	1	1	1 vegetable
V8 Splash Juice Beverage, Assorted Varieties	8 oz	70–110	18–27	0	0	0	40–50	0	0	1–2 carb
V8 Splash Juice Beverage, Assorted Varieties, Single Serving	8 oz	110	27	0	0	0	50	0	0	2 carb
V8 Splash Smoothies	8 oz	90–130	20–27	0	0	0	50–70	0	3	1 1/2 carb
V8 Vegetable Juice	8 oz	50	10	0	0	0	520–620	2	2	2 vegetable
V8 Vegetable Juice, Single Serving	5.5 oz can	35	7	0	0	0	430	0	0	1 vegetable
V8 Vegetable Juice, Single Serving	12 oz can	70	15	0	0	0	880	3	3	3 vegetable

VEGETABLES, VEGETABLE JUICES

	Serving	Calories	Carb. (g)	Fat (g)	% Cal. Fat	Sat. Fat (g)	Chol. (mg)	Sod. (mg)	Fib. (g)	Prot. (g)	Servings/ Exchanges
Contadina											
Tomato Paste	2 Tbsp	30	6	0	0	0	0	20	1	2	1 vegetable
Tomato Paste, Italian	2 Tbsp	35	7	<1	0	0	0	290	1	1	1 vegetable
Tomato Puree	1/4 cup	20	4	0	0	0	0	15	<1	<1	1 vegetable
Tomato Sauce	1/4 cup	15	3	0	0	0	0	280	<1	<1	1 vegetable
Tomato Sauce, Italian	1/4 cup	15	4	0	0	0	0	320	1	<1	1 vegetable
Tomato Sauce, Thick & Zesty	1/4 cup	20	3	0	0	0	0	340	1	1	1 vegetable
Tomatoes, Crushed	1/4 cup	20	4	0	0	0	0	150	1	1	1 vegetable
Tomatoes, Italian (Pear)	1/2 cup	25	4	0	0	0	0	220	1	1	1 vegetable
Tomatoes, Italian Stewed	1/2 cup	35	8	0	0	0	0	260	1	1	1 vegetable
Tomatoes, Recipe-Ready	1/2 cup	25	5	<1	0	<1	0	570	1	1	1 vegetable
Tomatoes, Stewed	1/2 cup	35	9	0	0	0	0	220	1	1	2 vegetable
Tomatoes, Whole Peeled	1/2 cup	25	4	0	0	0	0	218	1	1	1 vegetable

Green Giant

Alfredo Vegetables	1/2 cup	60	9	2	25	1	0	390	2	3	1 vegetable
Au Gratin Potatoes	1/2 cup	140	19	5	32	2	10	620	1	5	1 strch, 1 fat
Baby Brussels Sprouts & Butter Sauce	1/2 cup	60	9	1	17	1	<5	300	3	3	2 vegetable
Broccoli & Zesty Cheese Sauce	3/4 cup	70	7	3	36	2	5	560	2	3	1 vegetable, 1 fat
Broccoli, Carrots, Cauliflower & Cheese Sauce	1/2 cup	50	7	2	30	1	<5	360	2	2	1 vegetable
Broccoli, Cauliflower, Carrots & Cheese Sauce	2/3 cup	60	8	3	42	1	<5	500	2	2	1 vegetable, 1 fat
Cauliflower & Cheese Sauce	1/2 cup	60	6	3	42	1	<5	460	1	2	1 vegetable, 1 fat
Creamed Spinach	1/2 cup	80	9	3	31	1	0	510	1	3	2 vegetable, 1 fat
Early June Peas & Butter Sauce	3/4 cup	90	14	2	17	1	<5	410	4	5	1 strch

VEGETABLES, VEGETABLE JUICES

	Serving	Calories	Carb. (g)	Fat (g)	% Cal. Fat	Sat. Fat (g)	Chol. (mg)	Sod. (mg)	Fib. (g)	Prot. (g)	Servings/ Exchanges
Garden Vegetable Medley	1/2 cup	70	14	1	7	0	0	270	2	3	1 strch
Niblets Corn & Butter Sauce	2/3 cup	110	22	2	14	1	<5	340	2	3	1 1/2 strch
Scalloped Potatoes	1/2 cup	120	19	4	25	2	5	590	1	4	1 strch, 1 fat
Shoepeg White Corn & Butter Sauce	3/4 cup	110	21	2	18	2	1	310	3	3	1 1/2 strch
Libby's											
Pumpkin, Solid Pack, Canned	1/2 cup	40	9	<1	0	0	0	5	5	2	2 vegetable
Sauerkraut	2 Tbsp	5	1	0	0	0	0	200	<1	0	free
Mrs. Paul's											
Onion Rings, Old-Fashioned	2.5 oz	200	24	10	45	NA	NA	367	NA	3	1 1/2 strch, 2 fat
Sweet Potatoes, Candied	1/2 cup	276	67	1	3	<1	0	109	2	<1	1 strch, 3 1/2 carb

Ore Ida

Cheddar Cheese Hash Browns	1 cup	130	14	7	46	2	5	460	1	4	1 strch, 1 fat
Country Style French Fries	3 oz	130	20	4	31	1	0	360	2	2	1 strch, 1 fat
Country Style Hash Browns	1 1/4 cup	70	16	0	0	0	0	20	1	2	1 strch
Country Style Steak Fries	3 oz	110	18	4	32	1	0	280	2	2	1 strch, 1 fat
Crispers	3 oz	210	23	12	52	3	0	430	2	2	1 1/2 strch, 2 fat
Crispy Crowns	11 pieces	170	21	9	47	2	0	460	2	1	1 1/2 strch, 2 fat
Extra Crispy Fast Food Fries	3 oz	180	21	7	33	7	0	390	1	2	1 1/2 strch, 1 fat
Extra Crispy Golden Crinkles	3 oz	160	20	6	38	1	0	490	1	2	1 strch, 1 fat
Extra Crispy Tater Tots	12 pieces	170	19	7	35	2	0	500	1	2	1 strch, 1 fat
Golden Crinkles	3 oz	130	17	12	27	4	0	340	2	2	1 strch, 2 fat
Golden Fries	3 oz	120	20	4	25	1	0	350	2	2	1 strch, 1 fat
Mini Tater Tots	19 pieces	190	19	10	47	2	0	470	2	2	1 strch, 2 fat
Onion Rings	3	190	24	9	42	2	0	530	1	3	1 1/2 strch, 2 fat

VEGETABLES, VEGETABLE JUICES

	Serving	Calories	Carb. (g)	Fat (g)	% Cal. Fat	Sat. Fat (g)	Chol. (mg)	Sod. (mg)	Fib. (g)	Prot. (g)	Servings/ Exchanges
Peppers & Onions Hash Browns	1 cup	90	12	4	44	1	0	360	2	1	1 strch, 1 fat
Potatoes O'Brien	3/4 cup	60	13	0	0	0	0	20	2	1	1 strch
Shoestrings	3 oz	150	19	6	30	1	0	370	2	2	1 strch, 1 fat
Shredded Potato Patties	1 pattie	70	16	0	0	0	0	40	2	2	1 strch
Southern Style Hash Browns	3/4 cup	80	18	0	0	0	0	55	2	2	1 strch
Steak Fries	3 oz	120	17	3	25	1	0	340	2	2	1 strch, 1 fat
Tater Tots	9 pieces	150	20	7	40	2	0	420	2	2	1 strch, 1 fat
Texas Crispers	3 oz	140	21	6	36	2	0	260	2	2	1 1/2 strch, 1 fat
Waffle Fries	3 oz	160	22	6	38	2	0	300	2	2	1 1/2 strch, 1 fat
Zesty Twirls	1 1/4 cup	150	22	6	40	2	0	370	2	2	1 1/2 strch, 1 fat

VEGETARIAN FOODS

	Serving	Calories	Carb. (g)	Fat (g)	% Cal. Fat	Sat. Fat (g)	Chol. (mg)	Sod. (mg)	Fib. (g)	Prot. (g)	Servings/ Exchanges
Miso	1/2 cup	284	39	8	25	1	0	5032	8	17	2 1/2 strch, 1 med-fat meat, 1 fat
Miso Sauce	1/2 cup	191	36	3	14	<1	0	2008	3	7	2 1/2 strch, 1 fat
Tempeh	1/2 cup	165	14	6	33	<1	0	5	5	16	1 strch, 2 lean meat
Tofu, Firm, Raw	1/2 cup	183	5	11	54	2	0	18	3	20	3 lean meat
Tofu, Regular	1/2 cup	94	2	6	57	<1	0	9	2	10	1 med-fat meat
Tofu Yogurt	1 cup	254	43	5	18	<1	0	92	<1	9	3 strch, 1 fat
Vegetarian Bacon Strips	3 strips	47	<1	4	77	<1	0	220	<1	2	1 fat
Vegetarian Breakfast Links	1 link	64	3	5	70	<1	0	222	<1	5	1 med-fat meat
Vegetarian Breakfast Patties	1	97	4	7	65	1	0	337	1	7	1 med-fat meat
Vegetarian Chicken Slices	2	132	4	8	55	1	0	474	3	10	1 med-fat meat, 1 fat
Vegetarian Chicken, Breaded, Fried	1 slice	97	3	7	65	1	0	228	3	6	1 med-fat meat
Vegetarian Chili	1 cup	282	30	4	13	<1	0	1052	8	38	2 strch, 4 very lean meat

VEGETARIAN FOODS

	Serving	Calories	Carb. (g)	Fat (g)	% Cal. Fat	Sat. Fat (g)	Chol. (mg)	Sod. (mg)	Fib. (g)	Prot. (g)	Servings/ Exchanges
Vegetarian Fillets	1	136	4	9	60	1	0	230	3	11	2 med-fat meat
Vegetarian Fish Sticks	2	165	5	10	55	2	0	279	4	13	2 med-fat meat
Vegetarian Frankfurter	1	102	4	5	44	<1	0	219	2	10	1 med-fat meat
Vegetarian Luncheon Meat	1 slice	188	6	11	53	2	0	576	3	17	1/2 strch, 2 med-fat meat
Vegetarian Meatballs	7	140	6	6	39	<1	0	385	3	15	1/2 strch, 2 lean meat
Vegetarian Meat Patties	1	142	6	6	38	1	0	391	3	15	1/2 strch, 2 lean meat
Vegetarian Pot Pie	1	524	41	34	58	10	20	538	5	15	3 strch, 1 med-fat meat, 6 fat
Vegetarian Sandwich Spread	3 Tbsp	72	4	4	50	<1	0	302	2	4	1 med-fat meat
Vegetarian Scallops, Breaded & Fried	1/2 cup	257	8	16	56	3	0	434	5	20	1/2 strch, 3 med-fat meat
Vegetarian Soyburger	1	142	6	6	38	1	0	391	3	15	1/2 strch, 2 lean meat
Brands											
Health Valley											
99% Fat-Free Vegetarian Spicy Black Bean Chili	1 cup	160	28	1	6	0	0	320	12	13	2 strch, 1 very lean meat

No-Added-Salt Spicy Vegetarian Chili	1 cup	160	30	1	6	0	0	65	11	14	2 strch, 1 very lean meat
Vegetarian Lentil Chili	1 cup	160	28	1	6	0	0	390	11	15	2 strch, 1 very lean meat

Lightlife Smart Deli (Meatless)

Country Ham Style	3 slices	60	3	0	0	0	0	300	0	11	2 very lean meat
Old World Bologna Style	3 slices	50	2	0	0	0	0	300	0	8	1 very lean meat
Roast Turkey Style	3 slices	40	1	0	0	0	0	290	0	9	1 very lean meat
Three Peppercorn Pastrami Style	3 slices	45	1	0	0	0	0	300	0	10	1 very lean meat

Loma Linda

Big Franks	1	110	2	5	41	1	0	240	2	10	1 med-fat meat
Big Franks, Low-Fat	1	80	3	3	33	<1	0	220	2	11	2 very lean meat
Dinner Cuts	2 sices	90	3	2	20	1	0	500	2	17	2 very lean meat
Fried Chik'n Gravy	1 piece	80	7	5	56	1	0	260	3	4	1 med-fat meat
Linketts	1	70	1	5	64	<1	0	160	1	7	1 med-fat meat
Little Links	2	70	1	5	64	<1	0	160	1	7	1 med-fat meat

VEGETARIAN FOODS

	Serving	Calories	Carb. (g)	Fat (g)	% Cal. Fat	Sat. Fat (g)	Chol. (mg)	Sod. (mg)	Fib. (g)	Prot. (g)	Servings/ Exchanges
Redi-Burger	1 slice	120	7	3	23	<1	0	450	4	18	1/2 strch, 2 very lean meat
Swiss Stake	1	140	4	9	51	2	0	440	4	9	1 high-fat meat
Tender Bits	6	110	7	5	41	<1	0	440	3	11	1/2 strch, 1 med-fat meat
Tender Rounds	8	120	5	5	38	1	0	330	3	14	2 lean meat
Vege-Burger	1/4 cup	70	2	2	26	<1	0	115	2	11	1 lean meat
Morningstar Farms											
American Original Veggie Dog	1	80	6	<1	0	0	0	580	1	11	1/2 strch, 1 very lean meat
Better 'n Burgers	1	100	6	2	18	0	0	310	3	13	1/2 strch, 1 very lean meat
Better 'n Eggs	1/4 cup	20	0	0	0	0	0	90	0	5	1 very lean meat
Breakfast Links	2	80	3	3	34	<1	0	320	2	9	1 med-fat meat
Breakfast Patties	1	80	3	3	34	<1	0	270	2	10	1 lean meat
Breakfast Sandwich with Scramblers/Pattie/Cheese	1	280	35	3	10	<1	10	1000	5	28	3 strch, 3 very lean meat

Food	Serving										Exchanges
Breakfast Strips	2	60	2	5	75	<1	0	220	<1	2	1 fat
Chik Nuggets	4	190	18	7	33	<1	0	490	2	12	1 strch, 1 med-fat meat
Chik Patties	1	150	16	6	36	1	0	540	2	9	1 strch, 1 med-fat meat, 1 fat
Fajita Burgers	1	130	7	7	54	2	5	290	3	8	1/2 strch, 1 med-fat meat
Garden Veggie Pattie	1	100	9	3	27	<1	0	350	4	10	1/2 strch, 1 lean meat
Grillers	1	170	5	9	48	1	0	390	2	15	2 med-fat meat
Grillers Recipe Crumbles	2/3 cup	80	4	3	34	0	0	210	2	10	1 very lean meat
Harvest Burger Original	1	140	8	4	26	2	0	390	5	18	1/2 strch, 2 lean meat
Italian Marinara Chix	1 piece	250	29	9	32	1	0	890	2	12	2 strch, 1 med-fat meat, 1 fat
Meatless Buffalo Wings	5	200	18	9	41	2	0	630	3	12	1 strch, 1 med-fat meat, 1 fat
Sausage Style Recipe Crumbles	2/3 cup	90	5	3	22	<1	0	440	1	11	1 med-fat meat
Scramblers	1/4 cup	35	2	0	0	0	0	95	0	6	1 very lean meat
Spicy Black Bean Burger	1	150	16	5	30	<1	0	470	5	11	1 strch, 1 med-fat meat
Tomato & Basil Pizza Burger	1	130	7	6	38	2	10	320	3	11	1/2 strch, 1 med-fat meat

VEGETARIAN FOODS

	Serving	Calories	Carb. (g)	Fat (g)	% Cal. Fat	Sat. Fat (g)	Chol. (mg)	Sod. (mg)	Fib. (g)	Prot. (g)	Servings/ Exchanges
Veggie Corn Dog	1	150	22	4	24	<1	0	500	3	7	1 1/2 strch, 1 med-fat meat
Veggie Mini Corn Dogs	4 pieces	170	21	5	24	<1	0	580	1	11	1 1/2 strch, 1 med-fat meat
Morningstar Farms with Natural Ingredients											
Lentil Rice Loaf	1 slice	160	16	7	44	1	0	350	4	8	1 strch, 1 med-fat meat
Nine Bean Loaf	1 slice	150	15	7	42	2	0	320	4	8	1 strch, 1 med-fat meat
Thai Burger	1	100	7	4	36	<1	0	380	3	10	1/2 strch, 1 med-fat meat
Veggie Corn Dog	1	170	22	1	29	1	0	530	3	8	1 1/2 strch, 1 very lean meat
Morningstar Farms with Organic Soy											
Breakfast Pattie	1	80	4	3	38	<1	0	250	1	8	1 med-fat meat
Classic Veggie Burger	1	150	10	7	40	1	0	340	3	14	1/2 strch, 2 lean meat
Okara Pattie	1	120	6	5	38	<1	0	300	3	12	1/2 strch, 2 lean meat
Roasted Herb Chik'n	1	110	9	3	18	<1	0	380	2	13	1/2 strch, 2 lean meat
Tex Mex Burger	1	120	17	2	13	0	0	330	2	9	1 strch, 1 lean meat
Vegan Burger	1	100	8	2	15	0	0	460	5	13	1/2 strch, 1 lean meat

Food	Serving										Exchanges
Veggie Medley Burger	1	120	11	4	33	<1	0	260	1	11	1 strch, 1 med-fat meat
Zesty Tomato Basil Burger	1	130	7	6	42	1	<5	290	4	12	1/2 strch, 2 lean meat
Worthington											
Low-Fat Vega Links	1	45	3	2	33	0	0	220	0	5	1 lean meat
Meatless Bolono	3 slices	80	2	3	38	1	0	720	0	10	1 lean meat
Meatless Salami	3 slices	130	2	8	54	1	0	800	0	12	2 med-fat meat
Meatless Smoked Turkey	3 slices	140	5	9	57	1	0	490	0	10	1 high-fat meat
Multi-Grain Cutlets	2 slices	100	5	1	10	<1	0	350	3	17	2 very lean meat
Prime Stakes	1 piece	120	7	6	42	1	0	440	1	9	1/2 strch, 1 med-fat meat
Saucettes	1 link	90	1	6	67	1	0	200	1	6	1 med-fat meat
Savory Sliced Meat Substitute	3 slices	140	7	8	50	1	0	420	2	12	1/2 strch, 2 med-fat meat
Sliced Chik'n	3 slices	80	3	<1	0	0	0	360	2	15	2 very lean meat
Sloppy Joe	1/2 cup	140	23	1	7	0	0	580	3	8	1 1/2 strch, 1 very lean meat
Super Links	1	110	2	8	64	1	0	350	1	7	1 high-fat meat
Turkee Slices	3 slices	180	5	12	61	2	0	530	0	14	2 med-fat meat

VEGETARIAN FOODS

	Serving	Calories	Carb. (g)	Fat (g)	% Cal. Fat	Sat. Fat (g)	Chol. (mg)	Sod. (mg)	Fib. (g)	Prot. (g)	Servings/ Exchanges
Vegetable Skallops	1/2 cup	90	4	1	11	0	0	390	3	17	2 very lean meat
Vegetarian Burger	1/4 cup	70	3	2	21	0	0	250	1	10	1 very lean meat
Vega-Links	1	50	1	3	50	<1	0	180	0	5	1 lean meat
Worthington/Loma Linda											
Big Franks	1 link	110	3	6	55	1	0	220	2	11	2 lean meat
Dinner Cuts	2 slices	90	4	1	11	0	0	500	2	18	2 very lean meat
Linketts	1 link	70	1	4	50	4	<1	160	1	7	1 med-fat meat
Little Links	2	90	3	5	50	<1	0	250	2	8	1 med-fat meat
Low-Fat Big Franks	1 link	80	3	3	25	<1	0	240	2	12	2 lean meat
Redi Burger	5/8-inch slice	120	7	3	21	<1	0	450	4	18	1/2 strch, 2 lean meat
Tender Bits	6 pieces	120	7	4	29	<1	0	440	3	13	1/2 strch, 2 lean meat
Tender Rounds	6 pieces	120	6	5	33	<1	0	340	1	13	1/2 strch, 2 lean meat
Vege Burger	1/4 cup	60	2	<1	0	0	0	130	2	12	2 very lean meat

Yves Veggie Cuisine

Veggie Bologna Deli Slices	2 oz	80	4	1	13	0	0	430	0	13	2 med-fat meat
Veggie Ham Deli Slices	2 oz	80	6	0	0	0	0	480	0	14	2 very lean meat
Veggie Turkey Deli Slices	2 oz	90	4	2	17	0	0	410	0	15	2 very lean meat

About the American Diabetes Association

The American Diabetes Association is the nation's leading voluntary health organization supporting diabetes research, information, and advocacy. Its mission is to prevent and cure diabetes and to improve the lives of all people affected by diabetes. The American Diabetes Association is the leading publisher of comprehensive diabetes information. Its huge library of practical and authoritative books for people with diabetes covers every aspect of self-care—cooking and nutrition, fitness, weight control, medications, complications, emotional issues, and general self-care.

To order American Diabetes Association books: Call 1-800-232-6733 or log on to http://store.diabetes.org

To join the American Diabetes Association: Call 1-800-806-7801 or log on to www.diabetes.org/membership

For more information about diabetes or ADA programs and services: Call 1-800-342-2383. E-mail: AskADA@diabetes.org or log on to www.diabetes.org

To locate an ADA/NCQA Recognized Provider of quality diabetes care in your area: www.ncqa.org/dprp

To find an ADA Recognized Education Program in your area: Call 1-800-342-2383. www.diabetes.org/for-health-professionals-and-scientists/recognition/edrecognition.jsp

To join the fight to increase funding for diabetes research, end discrimination, and improve insurance coverage: Call 1-800-342-2383. www.diabetes.org/advocacy-and-legalresources/advocacy.jsp

To find out how you can get involved with the programs in your community: Call 1-800-342-2383. See below for program Web addresses.

- *American Diabetes Month:* educational activities aimed at those diagnosed with diabetes—month of November. www.diabetes.org/communityprograms-and-localevents/americandiabetesmonth.jsp
- *American Diabetes Alert:* annual public awareness campaign to find the undiagnosed—held the fourth Tuesday in March. www.diabetes.org/communityprograms-and-localevents/americandiabetesalert.jsp
- *The Diabetes Assistance & Resources Program (DAR):* diabetes awareness program targeted to the Latino community. www.diabetes.org/communityprograms-and-localevents/latinos.jsp
- *African American Program:* diabetes awareness program targeted to the African American community. www.diabetes.org/communityprograms-and-localevents/africanamericans.jsp
- *Awakening the Spirit: Pathways to Diabetes Prevention & Control:* diabetes awareness program targeted to the Native American community. www.diabetes.org/communityprograms-and-localevents/nativeamericans.jsp

To find out about an important research project regarding type 2 diabetes: www.diabetes.org/diabetes-research/research-home.jsp

To obtain information on making a planned gift or charitable bequest: Call 1-888-700-7029. www.wpg.cc/stl/CDA/homepage/1,1006,509,00.html

To make a donation or memorial contribution: Call 1-800-342-2383. www.diabetes.org/support-the-cause/make-a-donation.jsp